www.harcourt-internatior

Bringing you products from all Harcourt Hea
companies including Baillière Tindall, Churcl
Mosby and W.B. Saunders

- ◉ **Browse** for latest information on new books, journals and electronic products

- ◉ **Search** for information on over 20 000 published titles with full product information including tables of contents and sample chapters

- ◉ **Keep up to date** with our extensive publishing programme in your field by registering with eAlert or requesting postal updates

- ◉ **Secure online ordering** with prompt delivery, as well as full contact details to order by phone, fax or post

- ◉ **News** of special features and promotions

If you are based in the following countries, please visit the country-specific site to receive full details of product availability and local ordering information

USA: www.harcourthealth.com

Canada: www.harcourtcanada.com

Australia: www.harcourt.com.au

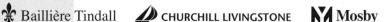 Baillière Tindall   CHURCHILL LIVINGSTONE   M Mosby   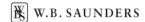 W.B. SAUNDERS

Integrating Complementary Therapies in Primary Care

For Churchill Livingstone:

Publishing Manager, Health Professions: Inta Ozols
Project Development Manager: Katrina Mather
Project Manager: Gail Murray
Designer: George Ajayi

Integrating Complementary Therapies in Primary Care

A Practical Guide for Health Professionals

David Peters MBChB DRCOG MFHom MLCOM

Clinical Director, School of Integrated Health, University of Westminster, London; Director, Complementary Therapies Unit and Osteopath, Marylebone Health Centre, London, UK

Leon Chaitow ND DO

Naturopath/Osteopath, Marylebone Health Centre, London; Senior Lecturer, School of Integrated Health, University of Westminster, London, UK

Gerry Harris BA LicAc BAcC

Associate Dean, Postgraduate General Practice Education, London; Senior Lecturer, School of Integrated Health, University of Westminster, London, UK

Sue Morrison MA FRCGP

Formerly Associate Dean Postgraduate General Practice, North Thames (West), London; Lead General Practitioner, Marylebone Health Centre, London; Director of Student Health Services and Visiting Lecturer, School of Integrated Health, University of Westminster, London, UK

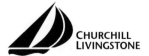

CHURCHILL
LIVINGSTONE

EDINBURGH LONDON NEW YORK PHILADELPHIA ST LOUIS SYDNEY TORONTO 2002

CHURCHILL LIVINGSTONE
An imprint of Harcourt Publishers Limited

© Harcourt Publishers Limited 2002

is a registered trademark of Harcourt Publishers Limited

The right of David Peters, Leon Chaitow, Gerry Harris and Sue Morrison to be identified as authors of this work has been asserted by them in accordance with the Copyright, Designs and Patents Act 1988

First published 2002

ISBN 0 443 06345 1

British Library Cataloguing in Publication Data
A catalogue record for this book is available from the British Library

Library of Congress Cataloging in Publication Data
A catalog record for this book is available from the Library of Congress

Note
Medical knowledge is constantly changing. As new information becomes available, changes in treatment, procedures, equipment and the use of drugs become necessary. The authors and the publishers have taken care to ensure that the information given in this text is accurate and up to date. However, readers are strongly advised to confirm that the information, especially with regard to drug usage, complies with the latest legislation and standards of practice.

The
publisher's
policy is to use
**paper manufactured
from sustainable forests**

Printed in China by RDC Group Limited

Contents

Preface

This is a book for clinicians. It is a snapshot of a prominent trend in health care: the increasing use of nonconventional treatments by the public and also by mainstream practitioners. The book also provides a moving picture of a reflective approach to using complementary therapies (CTs) in family practice. The story it tells is of work in a new area of health care and our attempts to map a route towards 'integration', a territory where two distinct cultures must somehow meet and strive to understand each other's ways. Consequently it will appeal to practitioners who feel they are in transit: collaborators, those working at the borders. It is for pioneers and would-be pioneers, looking across frontiers and wondering about new perspectives; having to explore different approaches and learn unfamiliar languages. But if you find these images – of refugees, explorers, bridge-builders – puzzling, even inappropriate, that does not mean this book will have nothing for you: it will still be a useful guidebook to CT clinical governance whether or not you are deeply curious about the place where the cultures merge.

Yet, unless you are intrigued by other systems of medicine and respect their integrity, then though you might incorporate some CT techniques into your work, you will not become a true integrator. On the other hand, this book will still interest you if you care to learn what it is like to pursue the clinical task in convoy with strangers who enrich your journey. If you have already embarked, you will recognize much of the scenery; should you be planning to, then we hope to point out some high points and hazards. But more than this, we are offering our communal map as a way of reaching out to fellow travellers who share our commitment to collaboration, interprofessional inquiry and the future of the healing team.

It is not entirely clear why practitioners with such disparate ways should want to work together. It is partly a matter of dissatisfaction: biomedicine may offer an illusion of concreteness and certainty, a sense that health can be reduced to biologically determinable elements, but day-to-day health care, far from having sure solutions to disease, is actually riven by uncertainties about causes and cures. People's shifting ideas about health and health problems and their changing relationship to medicine reflect this lively complexity. And it is in primary care, where they manage their own health problems, seek advice widely or confer with all kinds of professional—including family doctors—that complementary medicine has made most impression. Is that because the gulf between biomedical theory and people's experience has grown too great; or their perception of biomedical ineffectiveness; or a feeling that doctors are too busy, too tired, too distant? Whatever the explanation, it would be simplistic to take the rise of CT at face value; naive to believe that integration just means adding CTs to modern medicine. The effect is not additive and we are dealing here with a sociological event at least as much as a scientific one.

Why do general practitioners (GPs) seem so open to complementary therapies? The nature of family medicine is a clue: GPs deal mostly with acute disease, which would get better on its own, and with a great deal of chronic degenerative disease like arthritis and heart failure. True, they witness some (but not a great deal of) catastrophic disease like cancer and coronaries, but far more long-term relapsing disorders: asthma, digestive or skin problems; conditions where tissues are sound yet organs malfunction, often because of a 'stress-related' component. And a significant amount of GP time is taken up with patients' problems of daily living and their social crises, sometimes manifesting as bodily illness. Understandably we struggle with this array of suffering, knowing that health care is only partly a matter of science and that biomedicine has no 'cure' for ordinary unwellness and distress. Many patients still expect doctors to provide such a cure nonetheless, so it is disappointing that 30 years of pharmaceutical progress have delivered so few significant new treatments for common diseases.

Much discussion of integration of complementary and alternative and mainstream practice tends to focus on the needs, expectations and problems of medical professionals who are integrating CTs. But there are other issues relating particularly to the needs (and anxieties) of the complementary and alternative medicine (CAM) practitioner who intends to get involved in an integration project. Working collaboratively at close quarters with the medical profession can entail some loss of autonomy (for that is the nature of teamwork); and perhaps the acceptance of the doctor as the 'gatekeeper' would be high on the list of initial difficulties encountered.

Why then might complementary practitioners (CPs) want to work in the mainstream? Once again the issues are not just about effectiveness. Some experienced CPs having realized their own therapy is not a total 'alternative', want to reassess conventional medicine's strengths as well as its weaknesses; discover at first hand the worth and limitations of other CTs; treat a wider case mix and gain access to the state sector. This makes the idea of working in a group very interesting, compelling even. Although few have as yet been able to turn curiosity into the reality of teamwork, we predict that CPs and GPs will find ways to work together and that, for it to happen, all the members will have to be clear on why they are doing so and how best to go about it.

Successful integration entails a gradual acclimatization to what is in many ways a *foreign* environment, where the CAM practitioner will encounter language difficulties and perspectives quite different from those of the safe, self-directed world of independent private-sector CAM practice. What is more, working in an NHS setting usually involves a financial sacrifice. Why then might a CAM practitioner want to collaborate with a GP or work in a clinical setting with mainstream practitioners and therapists? The trade-off needs to make professional sense. One major reason why CAM practitioners choose to provide their particular skill or approach in a GP setting is for personal and professional development.

Yet, becoming enmeshed in teamwork is one of the first culture shocks involved; the tensions and challenges this involves, as well as the safety net it offers, mean abandoning the purely self-directed style of operation most CAM practitioners enjoy in private work. The integration exercise at Marylebone has involved the personal and professional growth of doctors as well as CAM therapists and practitioners. In fact, we suspect that the most critical factor for co-workers hoping to integrate their approaches is the availability of time for the sort of well organized group reflection where strongly held belief systems, and the therapeutic practices which flow from these, can be examined together.

Mainstream practice provides clinical challenges as well as opportunities to evaluate the relevance, practicability and effectiveness of one's own skills and approaches and those of others. CAM practitioners in private practice usually work solo, and if they interact with mainstream practitioners at all, it is only through occasional cross-referrals. However, when working in a team of GPs, counsellors and other CAM practitioners, detailed discussion of patients' individual needs and exploring therapeutic choices is possible. In this setting CAM practitioners will also be asked for evidence and explanations of what they do. Learning to discuss treatment approaches and clinical choices in a coherent way, using jargon-free language comprehensible to people from other disciplines, can be a profoundly educational experience. Multidisciplinary team-working requires co-workers to develop relationships with colleagues and build mutual confidence that patients will be safely cared for. Learning to understand the needs, methods and perspectives of other healthcare disciplines is an impetus for professional growth; for pre-existing prejudices slowly melt with the realization of our common aims.

The integration exercise calls for an ability to reflect honestly on the concepts and methods of one's own particular discipline while learning to appreciate the views and methods of others who see the world differently. Whether a team intends complementary therapies to be provided by conventional or by non-medically qualified practitioners, the need to plan and manage the project carefully will be paramount, because the decision to bring CTs into mainstream medical practice is a great challenge for any practice. We have therefore designed this book to help all practitioners discover their own best approach. It is based on our experience at Marylebone Health Centre (MHC) in central London, where we have been developing an integrated system since the mid-1980s. Our experience and the experience of other practices, have shaped this book, which has been 5 years in the writing.

David Peters
Leon Chaitow
Gerry Harris
London 2002   Sue Morrison

Why this book now?

The purpose of this book is to stimulate ideas and learning that will help you develop a framework to run a multidisciplinary primary care project.

WHAT IS CPD?

This approach brings together the key elements of education, service and research that combine in the workplace to produce effective and enjoyable practice-based learning. This can make a significant contribution to both Continuing Professional Development (CPD) and Clinical Governance agendas through the mechanism of lifelong learning and aims to ensure the delivery of high-quality health care.

HOW DO WE LEARN IN THE PRACTICE?

The purpose of CPD is to promote improvement in clinical practice. Learning as adults happens when we need to know something specific and is usually based on an experience (experiential learning). This book provides a format that will support a variety of practice-based learning activities such as individual self-directed learning, small group interaction, and learning in your organization as a whole. You will be able to consider and digest what has been learned by completing the reflective learning cycle audit at the end of each section.

Reflective Learning Cycle	
1. What did you need to know?	clarify learning objectives
2. What did you notice?	key points
3. What have you learned?	learning evaluation
4. How will you apply it to practice?	clinical relevance
5. What do I need to do next?	reflective educational audit

TRENDS IN CPD

There are worldwide trends in the professionalization of education, which is the process we have been considering. This means that professional learning can be seen only in its operational context (i.e. the practice) and any assessment of learning outcomes must evaluate self-directed learning and problem-solving rather than the factual recall of examinations. For example, a meaningful appraisal of the effectiveness of your CPD strategy in the use of this book as a learning tool may be to audit aspects of improved service delivery in some nominated areas.

RECERTIFICATION AND REACCREDITATION

This practice-based approach to CPD is inextricably linked with an accountability framework and paves the way for regulation of primary care services and the reaccreditation of its practitioners.

PRACTICE DEVELOPMENT PLANNING

It is clear that Personal Education Plans (PEPs) can be developed only in relation to the Practice Development Plan (PDP) and this in turn must be contextualized within the area Health Development agenda. In our own practices we need to develop our individual ability to link our professional development with an accountability framework, thereby strengthening the development and quality of the practice as a whole.

THE NEXT STEP

We will be motivated to learn as practitioners by our need for new competencies (e.g. in the area of complementary and alternative medicine), demonstrated by self-assessment (reflective learning cycle) and peer review (small group learning within the practice). This book will be a valuable item in the 'work-based learning toolkit'.

ADULT LEARNING: THEORY AND PRACTICE

Practice-based learning encourages us to develop relevant problem-solving skills and incorporate them into everyday work. Thinking about our actions and noticing that our professional behaviours change with experience is *reflection in action*, and allows us to become *reflective practitioners*. One of the most useful ways of reflecting on our practice is to record experiences in a 'portfolio'. This personal collection can help us demonstrate some of our skills, attitudes and achievements, and help us to understand our educational journey more fully.

This process of reflection and educational self-audit clarifies what you have learned and helps identify future learning needs. The reflective learning cycle audit at the end of Chapters 1–5 provides a framework for this process.

ABOUT THIS BOOK

You might be setting out to explore the relevance of complementary therapies (CTs) to your practice; wondering about referral, training or recruitment; working hard to keep your CT project on track; and finding ways to evaluate and develop your local Health Improvement Plan. When we did this at the Marylebone Health Centre (MHC), we asked about unmet needs, which medical conditions (and which patients) different CTs might be relevant for, and which of the approaches we had so far included at MHC were most appropriate. Next we looked at the available evidence base, the quality of the different research studies and the various research strategies that could be employed in evaluating complementary medicine.

With this information in mind, the next step was to design the most appropriate delivery system for integrating CTs into our medical service. We developed key materials at this stage, including referral guidelines for common conditions, forms to structure the service delivery process and assessment questionnaires, all of which are included in this book. The computer system developed to support the learning processes through data collection and monitoring is also described. We have included examples of the information sheets we produced for GPs and patients on CTs for common conditions, and a selection of patient self-help exercise and diet leaflets.

The development and management of a primary care CT service call for appropriate data collection and quality monitoring. Our experience of this aspect of the integration process, and that of others, is detailed, and in particular the issue of economic evaluation and cost-effectiveness is discussed.

Finally we consider the feedback we received from the participants in the project, including the patients themselves, look at some of the issues raised, and discuss some of the difficult and so far unresolved issues that integration can entail.

We are offering this book as work in progress because we hope colleagues will learn from our mistakes and our successes, and find some of our ideas, tools and insights useful. Although it is intended primarily for those conventional practitioners who consider no system of health care to have exclusive claim to completeness, it is also relevant to complementary practitioners who accept that aspects of conventional medicine definitely augment their traditional–natural approaches and who want to explore what non-conventional therapies can contribute to mainstream health care.

Acknowledgements

We would like to thank:

our patients, who endured the long haul as we developed CT clinical governance

the primary care team and its guardian angel hovering over our weekly meetings

long-suffering co-workers who waited patiently as we turned into data-freaks, trusting that one day we would become practitioners again

Hal Andrews, whose patience and skill produced the computer program those data-freaks so badly craved

those on the road towards integrative health care who use this book to create their own style of best practice

our fellow travellers, who we hope will treat our efforts compassionately. We hope they will send us occasional despatches from their part of the front line

Professor Patrick Pietroni, the visionary doctor and medical teacher who brought us together.

This book is the outcome of many years of teamwork. As well as the authors, it involved the participation of many others, whose contribution to developing the Marylebone model we want to acknowledge:

The Henry Smith's Charity for their generous funding of the three-year study which allowed us to develop the audit cycle and clinical guidelines for the use of complementary therapies in primary care

Current staff

Gabrielle Pinto	homeopath
Chrissie Melhuish	massage practitioner
Romain Jestry	counsellor
Alison Vaspe	counsellor
Richard Morrison	GP
Andy Godstone	GP
Bella Patel	GP
Lesley Ashdown Barr	nurse
Elizabeth Johnstone	nurse
Bunny Hoover	nurse
Jane Georgiadsis	nurse
Elizabeth Begley	health visitor
Geoff Wykurz	community development worker

Past team members

Mark Kane	osteopath
Brian Isbell	osteopath
Marilyn Miller Petroni	counsellor
Arnold Desser	acupuncturist
Francis Treuherz	homeopath
Dorothy Wallstein	homeopath
Vivien Weber	community outreach social worker and counsellor
Fran Robbe	practice nurse
Tania Eber	GP
Derek Chase	GP
Nadine Fox	massage practitioner
Sarah Martin	massage practitioner

Our reception staff

Martin Gerrish	centre manager
Gill Knight	
Fran Ward	
Janice Lancashire	
Leda Game	

The Patient Partnership Group

Members past and present, especially	
Peter Lucas	chair

We are also grateful to:

Dr Janet Richardson, Research Director, School of Integrated Health, University of Westminster, London, who supplied the example of how to develop a local CT service for GPs given in Chapter 4

Selina MacNair, acupuncture student, for material provided from her MYMOP project

The Glastonbury Health Centre for its contribution to Chapter 4

Joel Bonnet for the material we have used from his information pack on complementary therapies for Primary Care Groups, published by the Foundation for Integrated Medicine

Catherine Zollman and Andrew Vickers for material provided from their excellent and highly recommended book, ABC of Complementary Medicine, published by BMJ Books, London, 2000.

Background

1

Complementary medicine in practice

INTRODUCTION

Why integrate? Some issues to be considered when integration is on the agenda

Might there be advantages to providing complementary care alongside conventional medicine? In a resource-constrained system, any argument for diverting funds or seeking additional money would have to be made skilfully. For instance, within a framework of evidence-based medicine, NHS reorganizations and healthcare rationing, the further integration of complementary therapies (CTs) into conventional health care is bound to raise serious concerns. For those who intend to proceed the most important questions are:

- What reasons might doctors have for wishing to introduce CTs into their practice?
- Are there perceived unmet needs that might be met appropriately by integrating CTs?
- What concerns do doctors have about introducing CTs?
- Are unreasonable assumptions being made about CTs?
- What is the evidence base for their effectiveness?
- Which CTs might be particularly useful for particular conditions, and for particular patients?
- Are CTs safe?
- What are the clinical governance issues, including regulation, training and quality assurance?
- Can CTs be used cost effectively in mainstream health care?

Any developing project must face these issues. There are distinct challenges to integrating CTs into primary care practice. For example, groups need to achieve consensus on needs that are presently poorly met, and confirm these perceptions where possible with retrospective evaluation of service use—for example, external and internal referral rates and historical prescribing costs. Following this, there should be an assessment of which CTs are most likely be most relevant, and which could, practically speaking, be made available.

This chapter provides some necessary background for thinking about the prospects for integration. Chapter 2 will help you take account of the evidence base for some common conditions and widely available therapies. This is the beginning of a cyclical process of integration. Following this there are chapters on service design, delivery and evaluation. Finally clinical governance requires a process of feedback, discussion and reflection on the issues provoked by the implementation—most importantly intake and outcomes, but also problems and triumphs that have arisen and difficulties with interpersonal as well as organizational processes and management. Findings can then be fed back into the system to form the basis of improvements in professional development and service delivery.

Patient demand for complementary and alternative medicine (CAM) grew throughout the 1980s; by the end of the decade, more doctors were also becoming interested. In the early 1990s, ministers demonstrated the political will to make these approaches more available, and National Health Service (NHS) managers in some areas of the UK are now giving strong support to a variety of initiatives. Yet media reports, patients and their doctors generally show little insight into the differences between the various therapies; nor is it clear why general practitioners (GPs) have become so willing to collaborate with complementary practitioners (CPs).

Until recently, complementary and conventional medicine behaved like two separate cultures, kept apart by radically different languages and theories. Until the General Medical Council (GMC) reviewed its position in the 1970s, the traffic of patients between the two cultures was frankly illicit. Even today, despite an apparent convergence, each culture still tends to see the other as foreign. Nonetheless, it has been proposed that, by integrating certain aspects of CAM into the NHS, doctors' management of some common conditions could be improved.[1]

On the other hand, GPs whose patients visit CPs have described a number of difficulties. It is evident that there are a number of issues that need to be explored, including suitable conditions, and patients, for referral to CPs, the level of evidence for effectiveness of particular therapies, safety, possible interactions with prescription drugs, different methods for integration, and quality assurance. The continuity of care and clinical responsibility, as well as uncertainty about CPs' clinical competence and about doctors' own professional liability can also cause problems.[2]

Perhaps this will change as interdisciplinary academic units develop a dialogue between the cultures. The following important trends are at work:

- international peer-reviewed specialist journals in CTs are emerging, and studies of non-conventional practice already appear in established conventional publications
- in the UK, many GPs want to learn about and use CTs and the 1993 report of the British Medical Association's Board of Science was largely in their favour[3]
- the General Councils set up following the 1994 Osteopathic and Chiropractic Acts now ensure high standards of education, competence and ethics; practitioners' statutory recognition will bring the inclusion of these therapies in the NHS nearer
- several universities have developed degree programmes in complementary therapies, while the majority of medical schools have begun to include material dealing with these approaches in the undergraduate curriculum
- the Foundation for Integrated Medicine (FIM) has been established in the United Kingdom, as a result of an initiative by the Prince of Wales
- a similar body, the National Centers for Complementary and Alternative Medicine (NCCAM), has been established in the USA. It will receive $70 million a year to research these approaches
- there has been an increasing amount of research on the effectiveness of CTs in different conditions
- in November 2000 a subcommittee of the House of Lords Select Committee on Science and Technology reported to the government on Complementary Medicine. (A summary of the report and its recommendations appears in Appendix I, p. 317.)

Our changing visions of health and health care

In addition, if we are to understand fully the changes taking place in primary health care, and in particular the position of complementary medicine, we must appreciate that ways of thinking, both in the general population and in many scientific disciplines, are shifting in quite fundamental ways. Important cornerstones of this developing worldview have not been integrated into the biomedical frame, however, and this contributes in the eyes of many to a growing sense of the latter's inadequacy. Important amongst these new ideas are: the *ecological–evolutionary perspective*, which implies that organism and environment are not separate but have coevolved so that the organism itself is dynamically adapted to the world in a way that determines both its form and function; *homeostasis*, the organism's self-correcting capabilities, which can be stimulated and assisted to provide an internal stimulus for self-healing; and the mutual influence of *psychological and physical factors* on this self-regulation. All these are too little taken into account by clinical science, which tends still to focus largely on established end-stage disease in particular organs or systems, even though central nervous system effects are now known to penetrate via chemical receptors and neurotransmitter substances into every cell of the body. Psyche and physiology also have increasingly come to be understood as interdependent, with psychosocial pressures met by physiological and potentially pathophysiological responses. This emerging view can be generally termed the 'biopsychosocial model' of medicine. The need to incorporate such a framework into medical practice is at least unconsciously acknowledged by many doctors; hence in the 1990s 'whole person care' and 'holistic medicine' became a kind of professional shorthand for good practice.

For many people, the concept of health itself has become a metaphor for wholeness. The non-conventional approaches to treatment offered by practitioners of complementary medicine have come into their own within this holistic ethos, because their intent is to emphasize care in a wider context, mind–body–spirit interconnectedness, and the importance of catalysing homeostatic processes rather than simply confronting established disease. The ideas underlying systems such as traditional Chinese medicine (TCM), ayurveda and homeopathy appear to have some attributes of a more holistic approach. This might be why, despite a paucity of research, doctors as well as patients are attracted to them. Doctors' frustration at their inability to 'cure' many of the problems presenting, particularly those of the chronic variety, make them at least curious about whether complementary medicine could provide effective (and less potentially harmful) treatments, and a practical way of manipulating the self-regulation process. Finally, many people do report satisfaction with complementary therapies in a wide range of common illnesses and diseases even when conventional practitioners have failed to provide satisfactory treatment.[4] So, if there are features of complementary medicine that have a potential to improve management and quality of life for patients with such conditions, then investigating this role certainly ought to be worth while.

WHAT IS CAM?

A major problem in practice is the different usage of terms by different parties. In order to clarify the situation, we will therefore begin by offering definitions of some of the most common terms.

Definitions

Complementary and alternative medicine

Complementary medicine refers to 'a group of therapeutic and diagnostic disciplines that exist largely outside the institutions where conventional healthcare is taught and provided'.[5] It is an increasing feature of healthcare practice, but there is still considerable confusion about its exact nature. For instance, the catch-all term 'complementary and alternative medicine', or CAM, is persistently used to describe a complex field made confusing by ill-defined boundaries between apparently unrelated therapies.

The words *alternative* and *complementary* are, for instance, not synonymous, even though the less confrontational term is popular. In the 1970s and 1980s a number of disciplines were presented as *self-contained* and *alternative* medical systems, with their own distinct ideas about aetiology and diagnosis, as an alternative to conventional healthcare; hence they became known collectively as 'alternative medicine'. The name 'complementary medicine' developed as such systems were increasingly used alongside (to 'complement') mainstream medicine. Over the years, though, the term 'complementary' has changed from describing this relationship between unconventional healthcare disciplines and conventional care to a collective label for the disciplines themselves.

Furthermore, some authorities use the terms 'complementary medicine' and 'unconventional medicine' synonymously. 'Complementary medicine' is also used synonymously with the terms 'complementary therapies' and 'complementary and alternative medicine'. This changing and overlapping terminology may explain some of the confusion that surrounds the subject.

The following is the definition used by the Cochrane Collaboration.[5]

Complementary and alternative medicine (CAM) is a broad domain of healing resource that encompasses all health systems, modalities, and practices and their accompanying theories and beliefs, other than those intrinsic to the politically dominant health system of a particular society or culture in a given historical period. CAM includes all such practices and ideas self-defined by their users as preventing or treating illness or promoting health and well-being. Boundaries within CAM and between the CAM domain and that of the dominant system are not always sharp or fixed.

Treatment approaches commonly falling under the heading 'complementary medicine' include the following healthcare practices:

- acupressure
- acupuncture
- Alexander technique
- anthroposophical medicine
- applied kinesiology

- aromatherapy
- autogenic training
- ayurveda
- chiropractic
- cranial osteopathy
- environmental medicine
- healing
- herbal medicine
- homeopathy
- hypnosis
- massage
- meditation
- naturopathy
- nutritional therapy
- osteopathy
- qigong
- reflexology
- reiki
- relaxation and visualization techniques
- shiatsu
- tai chi
- therapeutic touch
- yoga.

This cannot be a final list, because new offshoots and newly named treatments continue to emerge. Nor is the frontier between complementary and conventional medicine always clear or constant. Osteopathy and chiropractic, for instance, have always been considered complementary therapies in the UK, even though these disciplines have, since the late 1990s, been regulated by statute and are now part of standard care guidelines (e.g. Royal College of General Practitioners).

Integrated medicine

The term 'integrated medicine' has become more common as a result of recent initiatives, such as those by the Foundation for Integrated Medicine (FIM),[6] aimed at integrating complementary therapies into the structure of mainstream medical care. It therefore is used to describe a system in which mainstream medical care and complementary therapies are integrated together within a practice, institution, etc., each complementing the other.

Holism

The word 'holistic' has several meanings, depending on the context in which it is used. In terms of healthcare, it implies that the therapy deals with illness as a dysfunction of the body and mind (and sometimes 'spirit') as an integrated whole, rather than focusing on ever more microscopic components.

THE PRESENT SITUATION

Trends in the use of CTs

UK

In the UK there is increasing public demand for complementary medicine, with an estimated 4–5 million people seeing a complementary therapist each year. The public popularity of complementary therapies grew throughout the 1980s.[7] At the end of that decade, a survey revealed that 74% of the population said they would use CTs if they were widely available in the NHS.[8] In a more recent study of lifetime use some 25% of the public said they had used one of the six main CTs (acupuncture, chiropractic, herbal medicine, homeopathy, hypnotherapy and osteopathy), and this proportion rises to one in three if reflexology and aromatherapy are also included.[9] A BBC poll of 1200 people in August 1999 estimated that 20% of the public are using CTs each year; this contrasts with a figure of 11% in a similar survey 6 years earlier.[4] Between 14% and 20% of those with chronic disease have consulted CPs of one of the six main therapies each year. Surveys of patients with chronic and difficult to manage diseases such as cancer, HIV infection, multiple sclerosis, psoriasis and rheumatological conditions show usage levels in such conditions to be possibly twice as high.

The number of CPs is growing rapidly: from 1981 to 1997 the number of registered practitioners in the UK trebled from about 13 500 to about 40 000.[4] Estimates based on the increased number of registered CPs suggest that at least 15 million complementary medicine consultations took place in 1997, which is about 5% of the number of general practice consultations. Most use of CT is confined to a few major disciplines. Osteopathy, chiropractic, homeopathy, acupuncture and herbalism are among the most popular in the UK, and spiritual healing and hypnotherapy are also often mentioned. In addition, approximately 25–35% of the public have used CT self-help (e.g. over the counter (OTC)) remedies or techniques (e.g. meditation).

CT is predominantly used in the private, paying sector; hence clients are often in higher socioeconomic groups and have higher levels of education than do users of conventional care. Yet, CT services are likely to be of particular benefit to socially deprived individuals with complex chronic problems.[11] There is also a big regional variation, with relatively more CT users living in the south of England, but this may reflect only differences in access and availability. There is a gender bias (55:45 female to male users) similar to that seen in conventional healthcare users; however, more men than women consult osteopaths and chiropractors. Finally, there are significant age differences: in contrast to conventional healthcare where users tend to be very old or very young, CT users are typically in their middle years (35–60), with relatively few children being seen (although some CTs such as homeopathy may see more). There has been little research into differences in CT use amongst various ethnic groups, though it can be anticipated that use of some therapies, such as TCM, ayurveda or massage/manipulative therapies, will reflect different cultural beliefs, traditions and taboos.

In surveys of users of CTs, about 80–90% were well or very well satisfied with their treatment.[4] Interestingly, this is not always dependent on an improvement in the presenting complaint—for example, cancer patients may include amongst the benefits of CT being emotionally stronger, less anxious and more hopeful about the future even if the cancer has remained unchanged.

In the UK and the Republic of Ireland common law has allowed the growth and development of CTs, as there is largely no direct regulation of professional non-medically qualified practitioners (PNMQPs) as such. However, as a result of moves to integrate CTs into the mainstream, a number of CT bodies have begun or completed the process of self-regulation (see Regulation and training, p. 18).[12]

International trends

This growth in CT use is reflected in other countries (Table 1.1).[4,13] For instance, in Australia in 1996 the total expenditure on CTs or remedies by private individuals was over a billion Australian dollars, where people spend approximately twice as much on such treatments as on orthodox medical drugs, whilst in the USA it doubled between 1990 and 1997 from 14 to 28 billion dollars.[14,15] In the United States, over 40% of the population uses CAM.[16]

The pattern of use of different therapies varies from country to country.[13,17] Although it is difficult to compare CAM use in different countries because of methodological differences between surveys, a recent review of Medline and CISCOM studies (638 in all) concluded that 'substantial proportions of the population in all the countries surveyed use complementary and alternative therapies'.[13] Overall a clearer picture emerges both of the growth in use of CAM and in the preferred treatments from country to country. For example, in Germany, France and Holland homeopathy is particularly popular (Fig. 1.1),[17] whereas in Australia acupuncture

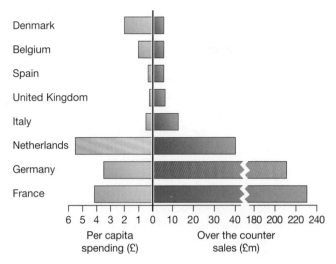

Figure 1.1 The market for complementary medicines in Europe 1991. (From Fisher P, Ward A 1994 Complementary medicine in Europe. British Medical Journal 309: 107–111, with permission of the British Medical Journal.)

is the treatment of choice.[15] This variation reflects differences both in medical culture and in the historical, political and legal position of CAM from country to country.

These cultural differences may be explained in part by historical and geographical factors such as distance from and links with country of origin of a therapy or system, or the location of training, particularly of early groups of practitioners; there are also important differences in legislation. For instance, within the European Union, the Belgian government has only recently legally recognized osteopathy, chiropractic, homeopathy and acupuncture and Belgian PNMQPs may treat patients only if referred by doctors and under the diagnostic supervision of a doctor, whilst homeopathy remains the sole preserve of doctors. State-registered UK osteopaths and chiropractors are even liable to arrest if they practise in France. European moves to 'harmonize' the provision of CTs may well curtail customary access to CAM.

Reasons for public interest

What is it about CAM that patients find worthwhile and what does this tell us about their expectations of healthcare services in general? A number of reasons have been cited. A report by FIM in 1997 suggested:

a degree of public dissatisfaction with what people see as the limitations of modern medicine and concern over the side effects of ever more potent drugs. Biotechnical approaches— pharmaceuticals and surgery—often have a limited amount to offer those with chronic, degenerative or stress-related diseases, mental disorders or addiction. In all developed countries there is a widespread recognition of the growing financial, social and personal cost involved, and of the need

Table 1.1 Use of complementary medicine worldwide (% of sample using complementary medicine employing any form of treatment)

Country	Past year (%)	Ever (%)
United Kingdom	10.5	33
Australia	20	46
United States	11	34
Belgium	24	66–75
France	No data	49
Netherlands	6–7	18
West Germany	5–12	20–30

Data from surveys during 1987–1996.

for a less fragmented, and more participative and humane, approach.[5]

In addition to this growing public scepticism, there are other possible reasons. The main one cited in the BBC poll of 1999 was that patients felt CTs had worked for them, sometimes when orthodox treatments had failed.[9] Some people said they found the treatments relaxing or felt they were safer, more 'natural' or helped in preventing further illness. The desire to take more responsibility for self-care may also be an important factor. There are, finally, an increasing number of reports in the media, largely expressing optimism and support for complementary therapies, which provide information for increasing numbers of people who wish to take more responsibility for health choices.

In March 2000 an international conference at the Wellcome Trust reached a number of conclusions about the increased use of CTs; these are listed in Box 1.1.

Increasing availability of and demand for complementary medicine is evidence of its popularity. The question this poses for public healthcare is: does this represent a passing fashion or a deeper need for change within the healthcare system?

Patterns of use of CAM

In private medicine

In the private sector, patients usually consult CPs with mild to moderate long-term, painful, functional and stress-related conditions[18]—disorders that occupy a great deal of the GP's time. Though conventional management for such disorders is often unsatisfactory, patients say that they are nonetheless satisfied with their non-conventional treatment. As doctors, we know that conventional approaches to undifferentiated illness, and chronic structural and relapsing functional disorders, are often unsatisfactory. There are good clinical trials suggesting that for certain conditions CTs might do better; for example, clinical trials of homeopathy have concluded that its effects are not a result of placebo.[19] There are well-designed studies on the effectiveness of other non-conventional approaches in a range of common problems, including anxiety, 'fibromyalgia', asthma, irritable bowel syndrome (IBS), eczema and migraine.

The following general points have emerged:

- people often choose complementary medicine to help with a chronic problem or to relieve stress
- complementary therapists deal with a high proportion of musculoskeletal problems (about 60%)
- the majority of clients already had conventional treatment for the same problems
- new consultations are mainly prompted by recommendation.

Box 1.1 Why are CTs so popular?

The Wellcome Trust 'Developing research capacity in complementary medicine' conference (10 March 2000) concluded that the increased use of CAM therapies could be attributed to:
- pressure on the health system
- lack of time spent with doctors
- the seeming success of CAM in fields of health care where orthodox medicine is failing
- the public concerns about the reductionist approach to illness
- the incidence of side-effects of conventional drugs.

In the public sector

Driven by concern for consumer choice, patient interest and client-centredness, doctors' attitudes to complementary medicine have become increasingly positive (e.g. the British Medical Association (BMA) now supports good practice[3] in cooperation, education and research). In the UK, the GMC has clarified that doctors may delegate treatment to non-medical CPs if satisfied of their competence and if they maintain overall clinical responsibility.

A growing number of GPs provide non-conventional therapies for their patients. A 1991 UK survey showed that 20–30% of UK GPs would like to provide main forms of complementary medicine through their practice[20]; a 1995 survey of typical UK GPs suggested 40% were offering some sort of access to CT, whereas other more recent surveys suggest as many as 60% either practise complementary therapies themselves, employ nurses who provide them or delegate treatment to complementary therapists working in the practice or elsewhere.[21]

Nearly 4000 conventional healthcare professionals also practise complementary medicine and are members of their own registers;[10] more than 1500 doctors are members of the Faculty of Homeopathy or the British Medical Acupuncture Society. Many more, especially GPs, have attended basic training courses and provide limited forms of complementary medicine. Although the reasons for this trend are still not fully understood, it is safe to assume these GPs believe CTs somehow augment conventional patient care. It might, for instance, be that rising healthcare costs and a widespread concern with the side-effects of drugs have encouraged them to use non-conventional therapies as a way of containing costs while maintaining patient satisfaction. There is some evidence that their implementation in the public sector can reduce resource use; for instance, a controlled study of acupuncture led to 25% fewer operations performed for osteoarthritis of the knee.[22] Perhaps, too, GPs' own clinical experience as well as the increasing amount of research published has raised their expectations.[5] Whatever the explanation, CTs have become a focus of public and professional aspirations for more acceptable or more effective forms of healthcare.

Exponents of CT systems such as classical homeopathy or TCM believe that their successful use demands the ability to diagnose from groupings of signs and syndromes that are mostly unrecognized by mainstream medicine. Only further research can prove or refute the validity of the ideas behind these methods. However, it is possible to separate certain non-conventional therapies from their system of origin and use them without a long training. Examples include elementary manipulation, simple homeopathic prescribing of the commonest remedies, needling of trigger points, nutritional interventions and basic hypnotherapy techniques. These are all widely practised by doctors elsewhere in Europe, where the law restricts their use by non-medics.

A case in point is musculoskeletal pain, which prompts about 20% of GP consultations and whose management is often problematic and costly. Recent guidelines on managing acute back pain recommend the early use of manipulative therapies.[23] Since few physiotherapists and even fewer doctors are trained to use them, this will stimulate collaboration with CPs. Establishment of the General Osteopathic Council (1993) and General Chiropractic Council (1994) has given professional status to UK manipulative therapists.

It is tempting to suppose that similar multidisciplinary approaches might help in managing other perplexing presentations. Perhaps this is why 20–30% of GPs say they want greater access to osteopathy, acupuncture, homeopathy and hypnotherapy.[24] Many CPs in turn want to develop working relationships with doctors and practise in mainstream healthcare, supporting NHS provision because it would improve equity of access, protect their right to practise and guarantee a caseload. Others, however, fear loss of their autonomy and domination by the medical profession.

PROVISION OF CAM IN MAINSTREAM MEDICAL CARE

Is there a place for CTs in the mainstream?

In the UK in 1991, the Department of Health (DoH) acknowledged consumer demand for NHS access to complementary medicine when it gave the go-ahead for family doctors to employ CPs as ancillary staff; many GPs were already funding complementary treatments through their health promotion clinics. Although no extra funding was then made available, this DoH policy change recognized a clinical pluralism that would have been incredible even 10 years previously. A clinically pluralistic NHS, where more doctors and nurses deliver non-conventional therapies, is no longer hard to imagine.

A 1993 report from the National Association of Health Authorities and Trusts indicated that, by that time, the Department of Health was spending over £1 million a year on non-conventional approaches.[25] Several health authorities and trusts have initiated small pilot projects to evaluate them, as detailed later in this book, but we are still a long way from understanding the cost–benefit implications for the NHS. Meanwhile, experience in some of these projects suggests that open-ended intake soon leads to overload with chronic problems and 'thick-notes patients'.[26]

Diversity versus equity

Fundholding and its variants have increased CT availability in the NHS, but how will the advent of primary care groups (PCGs) affect public sector access to these therapies? PCGs currently commission within the confines of their local health improvement programmes; as primary care trusts they will have to make their own rationing decisions in the light of assessments of local need including public priorities, costs and evidence for effectiveness.[27] Because commissioning will be shaped by local needs assessment we would expect the services to be appropriately diverse. The issue of whether to explore a role for CTs in the mainstream highlights some general difficulties with commissioning. Will PCGs find it hard to reconcile the drives for equity and diversity? And will the need to innovate cause a conflict with the pressure to provide similar services nationwide? Can people's perception that CTs have a part to play in their healthcare be reflected in evidence-based commissioning decisions?

Evidence-based medicine versus patient-centred medicine

Many important questions still need answering: for example, for which conditions are these diverse practices best indicated, how can treatment be quality assured and are they cost effective?[28] (These questions are discussed in more detail under Key issues later in the chapter.) In particular, it is the lack of cost-effectiveness studies that might discourage PCGs from supporting even the existing access to CTs. Indeed, early indications are that, in the current round of commissioning, CT access is being cut back. This is hardly surprising at a time when commissioning processes depend increasingly on evidence from RCTs. It has, however, been said that management of care through clinical guidelines based on RCTs can inadvertently suppress diversity, innovation or patient-centred care.[29] And if declining access to complementary therapies in the NHS illustrates this problem then this is a cause for concern, because important service developments have in the past been needs driven even when evidence for their effectiveness has been inconclusive.

Counselling services and hospice care are examples. Once considered marginal, both have—because they met previously unarticulated, unrecognized or poorly met needs—gradually been integrated into the NHS. Innovators within the NHS drew on pioneers' experience to develop provision in centres where research and education eventually legitimated these new areas of practice. In the UK a number of CT projects may currently be serving the same exemplary function,[30] although others have already succumbed in the face of funding changes.[31]

The question 'should CTs have a place in mainstream care?' must at least be asked, if only because over the last 20 years their public popularity has grown steadily: about 25% of the public have used them at some time. But there are other reasons to consider CTs: chronic illness, stress-related and painful conditions (all of which conventional practitioners tend to find problematic) appear to be complementary therapists' daily bread.[6] Their clients have usually received medical treatment already and surveys suggest high levels of satisfaction and useful outcomes. The growing acceptance of CTs coincides with an increased interest in lifestyle change, health promotion and low-technology treatments; approaches which, if they could be integrated into primary care, might provide inexpensive, safe ways to augment conventional healthcare. Such integrated delivery would be pluralist and centred on primary care, emphasizing prevention and based on modern medicine; it would also make other effective treatments available according to need and appropriateness.[5] Primary care groups may wonder whether the first round of health improvement programmes has adequately reflected the need for such integrated care. Yet, though these therapies apparently meet a need, it is not clear where access to CTs ranks in terms of the public's priorities.

Innovation versus resource management

Health professionals have a responsibility to meet patients' needs as well as a social responsibility to manage limited resources. However, the increasing emphasis on user-centredness and equity is difficult to reconcile with the imperative to limit healthcare costs. Continuing dispute over the appropriate limits to Viagra prescribing is a reminder both of how ambivalently doctors balance these responsibilities and of the difficulties of defining and implementing explicit rules.

Perhaps, in the past, uncritical acceptance of CTs has hindered their appropriate rigorous implementation as much as unyielding scepticism. In future, PCGs will have to ensure that the processes of clinical governance are extended to cover CTs and that clinical standards are well defined and can provide a basis for local audits. On this basis, could relevant aspects of complementary therapies

continue to be incorporated into the NHS? The possibility that they meet otherwise unmet needs, the expressions of professional support, as well as early indications of effectiveness and their popularity with patients, all imply that they will.

Although CM has taken root in the mainstream over the past few years, it is still a long way from thriving in the way counselling does. Those of us working towards an integrated holistic NHS hope that in time most NHS health centres will offer CTs just as, until recently, they did counselling. As the NHS 'modernizes' some parts of the UK are becoming less inclined to include either complementary therapists or counsellors—this might be a temporary glitch in the 10-year trend for more and more general practices to incorporate high-touch and listening therapies. Nevertheless the new PCGs are having to tighten their belts and set priorities. With limited budgets they are faced on the one hand by an ever-wider array of high-tech treatment options and on the other by an increasingly long-lived population with ever-higher expectations of healthcare. The new money in the NHS is earmarked for high-tech cancer services and more heart operations. Life-saving relief for catastrophic endstage disease calls for big money, yet this raises important questions about the kind of healthcare the public sector ought to provide. High-tech rescue is not enough; we have to find ways of building up national resources for prevention, health promotion and mind–body medicine too. With funds capped, how can the NHS ensure the high-tech meat in the sandwich is properly contained in a bread-and-butter package of skilled nursing, counselling and (feasibly) CTs? Apparently 60% of GPs have tried to do this in their own way, by including counselling and complementary therapies; by using their own CT skills, employing nurses who provide them or delegating treatment to complementary therapists.

Complementary therapies or integrated holistic healthcare?

We suspect the popularity of CTs is a coded message about aspirations for more acceptable or more effective healthcare. This is (ironically?) also what the NHS modernization project intends to achieve. Yet if 'modernization' allows the voices of poorly met needs to be heard, it will surely take more than high-tech medicine alone to satisfy them. Therefore if too few nurses, physios, health educators, counsellors (and osteopaths, homeopaths, herbalists, acupuncturists and massage practitioners) are working in the NHS then it may be a measure of how little holistic care is actually being delivered.

Current government health policy puts a high value on empowerment, diversity and equity: a levelling up of standards. It has also called for greater diversity—'a health service of all the talents'.[32] The job of the primary care organizations is to commission the local resources needed to make this happen. On these bodies GPs hold sway and British general practice at its best has pioneered a holistic approach since the 1950s: healthcare for people as minds and bodies, coping with their families and jobs and culture. Its great strength and a measure of its success have been a capacity for comprehensive, continuous, long-term care that reflects local need. Which is why, given the resources, GPs should be best placed to encourage more integrated holistic care, including access to CAM. But so far access has been haphazard and far from equitable, yet with an ageing population calls for evidence-based medicine get louder and what new funding should we expect—a levelling up or a levelling down of counselling and CT services as the NHS modernizes and equity takes centre stage? Research, and therefore the available evidence, still clusters round high-tech treatments rather than counselling and CT; that after all is where the research grants are. It seems ridiculous that the case for holism and humanity (whose lack is surely what the popularity of CT approaches signals)—both highly desirable aspects of a health service—should have to be made by randomized controlled trials (RCTs) and cost-effectiveness studies in order for them to survive!

Working together: some problems faced when integrating new approaches

Experience to date has shown that problems tend to arise when the skills of fully trained CPs are made available, partly because few doctors know how or when to refer to such practitioners. The BMA has emphasized the importance of doctors familiarizing themselves with complementary medicines. It is a sign of GPs' current confusion that, when some 300 were surveyed in 1994, most of them said they believed conventional medicine to be less effective than complementary medicine. Fantastic expectations actually impede the rational use of alternative approaches and, if experienced non-medical CPs are to work more closely with doctors in the NHS, then we will have to learn from one another. Glasgow's popular Certificate of Primary Care Homeopathy may be an important model, aiming as it does to give GPs the basic knowledge and skills, at the same time building up a referral network of experienced 'specialized' practitioners.

Complementary medicine is a relative newcomer to the NHS. Rather like counselling—another recent arrival that gradually became an essential part of primary care—it is most effective in the hands of practitioners with real knowledge and skill. And, like counselling, it works better for some problems (and for certain kinds of people) than it does for others. Consequently, making an inte-

grated health system work—emphasizing prevention and modern medicine in their place, while making a range of other treatments available according to need and appropriateness—is going to require discrimination and collaboration (see Figure 1.2).

One of the reasons that CTs will not go under in mainstream medicine is that too many doctors and nurses value job satisfaction and know it largely depends on having good enough relationships with patients. The truth is, when the gap between people's health beliefs

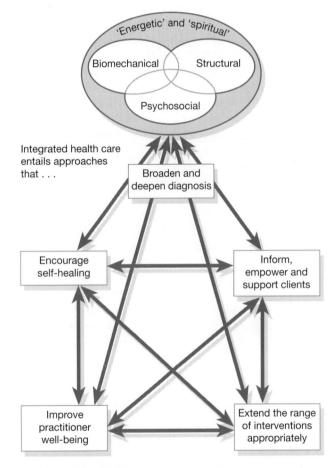

Figure 1.2 The integrated approach to health care.
The main elements in the integration process are interconnected. If the aim is to encourage better physiological and personal functioning then a broader approach to 'diagnosis' of what has disturbed the organism's normal state of self-organization will be needed. It may be that CAM approaches to diagnosis have something to add to conventional methods. If so then an extended range of interventions would have to follow and that could mean involving different kinds of practitioner in the care team. Because such reflective collaboration depends on interprofessional learning and careful organization, it requires considerable staff development. It is a challenge to work realistically and humanely in a team with a range of colleagues spanning the fields of medicine, CAM, nursing, social care and psychotherapy. Nor is the process of engaging with patients as co-workers and co-inquirers always easy or straightforward. 'Whole person' approaches to health care will call for practitioners who are prepared to become 'whole people', by cultivating their ability to collaborate, cope and care.

and perceived needs and health professionals' ideas, abilities and willingness to meet them gets too wide, then relationships strain and eventually fracture. That's why successful integration of CAM with mainstream approaches will only partly depend on the evidence base. It has as much to do with how doctors learn to share ideas with and hear what clients and colleagues can tell them about health and healthcare needs and wants. In our experience this kind of openness is what makes dialogue between experienced GPs and experienced CPs so creative and (ultimately) positive.

In the Centre for Community Care & Primary Health at the University of Westminster we are designing courses introducing GPs to the roles and realities of CAM (website: http//www.westminster.ac). Programmes like this are obviously important and not just because they are a chance to impart knowledge about CAM systems, modalities, diagnostics and opportunities for referral. Doctors drawn to the subject already have a sense of biomedicine's incompleteness; GPs learn the hard way that it takes more than a prescription pad and a referral letter to deal with everyday anguish. For doctors seeking ways of working more holistically CTs may not be the final destination, but they can often be an important signpost on this journey. Doctors are after all applied scientists, and there's the rub, because CTs are often based on world views quite different to those of scientific medicine. Of course, that's their attraction and possible strength too, but because they are shaped by other traditions and rooted in vitalism they illuminate an unfamiliar and alien psychosomatic territory. Entering this landscape doctors are taken to the roots of medicine, a place where they have to ask what motivates their work and must confront unavoidable issues about attitudes, ethics and diverse questions about the human condition. For their part, CPs coming into contact with doctors like these have to grasp what general practice is, for they have usually mistaken it for the stereotypical biomedicine we all tend to reject.

As you may imagine, scouts at the collaborative frontier all too easily plummet into an attitudinal and paradigm gap. Even those who don't fall over the edge suffer from time to time a sort of interdisciplinary vertigo that vexes communication. But real cooperation between conventional and CPs means tolerating this discomfort for the sake of exploring our rich potential for working together. No one told us integration would be easy!

When working with CPs, the following points should be borne in mind.

• The *authority* in any system where doctors hold ultimate medicolegal responsibility for patients and determine which of them is referred clearly rests with the medics. Nonetheless, this does not necessarily confer greater knowledge, insight or clinical experience.

• The expectations patients and their medical practitioners might have of CAM, and the beliefs doctors and CPs have about one another, will influence communication and determine how they might share clinical care.

• If appropriate ways of collaborating and sharing responsibility are to be developed, we need to understand that some practitioners see their work as underpinned by a *complete system* on which internally consistent aetiology, diagnosis and therapeutics are based: for example TCM, homeopathy, osteopathy, naturopathy or chiropractic.

• Such *alternative systems* of medicine are actually the preserve of autonomous practitioners who represent an expertise radically unlike that of doctors. *Therapeutic techniques* such as manipulation or dry needling do not constitute a system, and some doctors find they can easily incorporate them into their daily work. However, it is a greater challenge for conventional practice to integrate alternative therapeutic systems, mainly because their worldview and knowledge base are so very different from those of conventional medicine. Though these alternative systems of medicine are CAM's very core, it is not entirely clear how they complement conventional medicine.

In November 2000 the UK House of Lords Select Committee published a report on CAM that raised a number of concerns. Amongst its conclusions was the need to distinguish between CTs on the basis of evidence, training and regulation. Its recommendations on the future delivery of CAM were as follows:[33]

9.20 We recommend that those practising privately accessed CAM therapies should work towards integration between CAM and conventional medicine, and CAM therapists should encourage patients with conditions that have not been previously discussed with a medical practitioner to see their GP. We also urge CAM practitioners and GPs to keep an open mind about each other's ability to help their patients, to make patients feel comfortable about integrating their healthcare provision and to exchange information about treatment programmes and their perceptions of the healthcare needs of patients.

9.37 We recommend that all NHS provision of CAM should continue to be through GP referral (or by referral from doctors or other healthcare professionals working in primary, secondary or tertiary care).

9.46 We recommend that only those CAM therapies which are statutorily regulated, or have a powerful mechanism of voluntary self-regulation, should be made available, by reference from doctors and other healthcare professionals working in primary, secondary or tertiary care, on the NHS.

(A summary of all its findings and recommendations is included as Appendix I to this book (p. 317).)

KEY ISSUES TO BE ADDRESSED

The idea of providing complementary care within a framework of evidence-based medicine, NHS reorganizations and healthcare rationing raises various questions and concerns for the different parties involved. These need to be addressed properly before moving towards further integration into conventional healthcare. The most important questions are:

- what reasons might doctors have for wishing to introduce CTs into their practice—for instance, can CTs be used to fulfil perceived unmet needs?
- what concerns do doctors have about introducing CTs?
- are unreasonable assumptions being made about CTs?
- what is the evidence base for their effectiveness?
- which CTs might be particularly useful for particular conditions and for particular patients?
- are CTs safe?
- what are the clinical governance issues, including regulation, training and quality assurance?
- can CTs be used cost effectively in mainstream healthcare?

Unmet needs?

Why should there be a growing wish amongst doctors—especially GPs—for more collaboration between conventional medicine and CAM? Health professionals seek out new approaches for many reasons and many find innovation acceptable even though effectiveness has not been demonstrated by formal research. Some exploration of the reasons for CAM's popularity and wide acceptance by health professionals is a necessary background for understanding collaboration between doctors and CPs.

Clearly patient demand has been an important factor and CAM's popularity has been attributed to consumerism, to the emergence of the human potential movement,[34] to rejection of governance, and increasing prevalence of antiscientific attitudes, to paradigm shift and even to a return to occultism.[35] Whatever the reason, we may safely assume that society's views on health and healthcare are changing, and that because people feel their needs are not adequately met by mainstream provision they are looking elsewhere.

Do people think they have been let down by conventional medicine? Biomedicine (implying medicine as applied biology) has been a very effective approach to infectious and deficiency diseases; it has given us aseptic surgery, life-support technology and anaesthesia. But although life expectancy rises year by year (the swings of wealth?) even so medicine has not (yet) delivered on the promise of curing the West's new epidemic diseases (the roundabouts of affluence?): stress-, environment- and lifestyle-mediated disease, addictions and psychological disorders seem to respond partially if at all. But these conditions are the GP's bread and butter, and the levels of risk associated with drug treatment of even quite common conventional treatments are quite frighteningly high.

The biomedical model has little to say to GPs about ordinary unwellness and the sorts of 'undifferentiated disease' they encounter every day. Nor can strict biomedicine make sense of the complex way that learning, behaviour and lifestyle interact—even though they are central considerations in primary care. It is here that practitioners struggle to comprehend not only the disease as pathology but also individual patients and their predicament. Biomedicine gives an impression of concreteness and certainty, a sense that health can be reduced to biologically determinable elements. In reality, however, healthcare—and most especially primary healthcare—is, far from having sure solutions, actually riven with uncertainties about causes and cures.

This complexity is reflected in the ideas and beliefs people express about their own health problems and is revealed in their ambivalent and sceptical attitudes about modern medicine. Increasingly, as medicine's once-unquestioned authority seeps away, it seems that people feel free to adopt a 'pick-and-mix' approach. They use the ideas and treatments they find relevant to their own particular needs at any one time. And there may be no avoiding this sort of postmodern 'multiple narrative' approach to health and healthcare. Whether professionals or patients, in an ever more information-rich culture this trend is unlikely to change.

So it is not surprising that in primary care, where people manage their own health problems or seek advice about common and chronic diseases from a wide range of professionals, complementary medicine has had its biggest impact. GPs' clinical time is mostly spent dealing with acute self-limiting diseases (e.g. viral illness, chest infections), with chronic or terminal structural disease (e.g. osteoarthritis, heart disease) and with long-term relapsing disorders, such as asthma, menstrual disorders, gut dysfunction and skin problems. Patients not only present because they have a well-defined disease; they also bring their experience—of illness, stress and an inability to cope. For instance, a significant component of 'stress' and 'coping ability' is relevant in many encounters between GPs and patients, particularly in the last group, and, in addition, patients also bring to their GP problems of daily living, and their social crises.[36] Only a small proportion of contact is concerned with primary prevention and health promotion; more often this is done opportunistically and over long periods of time, because the time-scale of family medicine can be measured in generations. GPs see patients and their families for decades. Faced with this range of need, GPs understand better than hospital specialists, who deal more with acute, end-stage and uncommon diseases, that healthcare is only partly a matter of science. They know only too well that biomedicine has no 'cures' for ordinary unwellness and distress even though many patients expect doctors to provide them.

Conventional treatments often seem inappropriate, unsatisfactory or unacceptable in chronic, relapsing, functional and stress-related conditions. Yet, even though these are predominantly the conditions that CPs treat, it has not yet been properly established that CTs fare any better. And, unfortunately, CTs can often encourage high (and sometimes unrealistic) expectations and they also can appear antiscientific, individualistic and apolitical. These attributes resonate with a section of public feeling, but they could be the very reasons why the wider use of CTs in the mainstream might prove difficult. In fact, though, our own experience over the last 10 years of integrating CTs into the Marylebone Health Centre (MHC) suggests they can be rationally and effectively employed and audited.

Quite apart from any specific effects of particular therapies, which may account for a proportion of patient satisfaction, surveys and qualitative research indicate that many patients also value some of the general attributes of complementary medicine. These may include the relationship with the practitioner, the often non-technical ways in which illness is explained and the environment in which treatment is given. When these augment the therapeutic outcome, they contribute to what is sometimes called 'the human effect'.[37] Some CPs at least may be better than their conventional colleagues at maximizing these non-specific healing effects, which, although these are not unique to complementary medicine, are probably enhanced by the non-institutional settings in which many CPs work.

Concerns doctors have about CTs

Doctors commonly have concerns about CTs, which may include any of the following[38]:

- if patients are seen by unqualified practitioners there is a risk of a missed or delayed diagnosis
- patients may waste money on ineffective treatments, whilst discontinuing or declining effective conventional treatment
- conflicting loyalty (to practitioners, ideas, treatment regimens and expectations) may increase a sense of conflict between patients and doctors
- there may be adverse effects from the complementary treatment
- the claimed mechanisms of some complementary treatments are implausible
- the claimed benefits of many CTs are scientifically unproven.

These are understandable, since in the absence of inter-professional contact many questions will arise about the

working practices of those in the 'other' group. Whereas all CPs born and brought up in the UK will have had the experience of primary care from infancy, doctors may not have had any experience or contact with CPs. However, some of the more commonly held concerns need to be examined in the light of the increasing professionalization and training of CPs and the continuing development of CP professional bodies.

Will the CP suggest taking patients off their medication?

There is a fear amongst doctors that CPs will ask patients to withdraw medicines. This may have been the case with a small group of CPs historically but is largely no longer the case. Training courses for CPs emphasize the importance of working together with a patient's doctor and the actions, benefits, side-effects and dangers of withdrawing medication are known. A distinction is very clearly drawn between those drugs that a patient may safely cut down on (e.g. self-prescribed paracetamol for pain relief) and those that a patient may not (e.g. prednisolone). The average CP is suitably horrified when, on very rare occasions, a new patient presents and states 'I've come to see you so I've stopped taking my medication'. Those CPs who wish to find work within public medicine will by definition be those who have an interest in joint patient care.

Will the CP undertake a thorough diagnosis including taking into account the psychosocial background?

Many CPs, especially women, enter their profession because they have not been satisfied with their own conventional treatment and certainly in the past this would have included their experience of the doctor–patient relationship. This is not to say that just because practitioners may recognize how they would like to be treated that they can produce this behaviour themselves. There is a recognition now within CT training that just because the theory of the therapy practised may take the body, mind and spirit into account, this does not mean that the CP will automatically work in a patient-centred way. As a rule of thumb, practitioners of all descriptions will prioritize asking the patient for information that is directly useful for making a diagnosis. Some CPs need to ask patients questions about their psychosocial background including those related directly to their emotional life; others may not. There is a growing appreciation and evidence that communication skills can be taught and learnt. Both medical and CT trainings recognize this. The BSc Complementary Therapies course at the University of Westminster (website: http://www.westminster.ac), for example, has a pathway called 'practitioner development'. Running throughout the 3-year course, this programme not only presents skills for conducting a consultation, medical sociology and psychology but it also engages the students in a process of self-development where they reflect on what it actually takes to become a practitioner. This is a responsibility that colleges of CT take seriously as often their students can end up working in isolation from their colleagues, much like the single-handed GP. A CP with the skills to create good patient–practitioner relationships will work in a similar way as a doctor with the same skills.

Will the CP raise patient expectation?

There is a common perception that CPs may expect to cure their patients whilst doctors may hold a more realistic view of the prognosis for a patient with, say, a degenerative disease with a known developmental pattern. CPs themselves have undoubtedly contributed to doctors holding this view of them, which needs to be put into an historical context. Before CP training became available through higher education, taking CP education into the mainstream, small private colleges were run by highly committed and sometimes extraordinary individuals. At the time they learnt their craft they would have been

---

● *'Therapists may be poorly trained and are not adequately regulated.'* Although CPs (other than osteopaths and chiropractors) can legally practise without any training whatsoever, most have undergone an extended period of education in their discipline. Currently, in addition to osteopathy and chiropractic, which have had state registration and regulation for some time, a number of other CTs are going through a similar process (e.g. homeopathy, herbal medicine, acupuncture and hypnotherapy).
● *'They are not provided by the NHS.'* Complementary medicine is increasingly available on the NHS, including 39% of general practices.
● *'Unconventional, not taught in medical schools.'* 'Conventional' disciplines such as physiotherapy and chiropody are also not taught in medical schools; conversely some medical school curricula do now include some CT component.
● *'Unproved.'* Many conventional healthcare practices are also not supported by the results of controlled clinical trials; conversely, a growing body of evidence points to the effectiveness of some CTs in particular conditions.
● *'Irrational—no scientific basis.'* Scientific research is starting to suggest possible mechanisms of, for instance, acupuncture and hypnosis.
● *'Natural.'* Complementary medicine sometimes involves unnatural practices such as inserting needles into the skin; conversely, good conventional practice includes 'natural' advice—sufficient rest and exercise and eating healthily.
● *'Harmless.'* Adverse effects, some serious, have been reported with several types of CT, including acupuncture and herbalism.
● *'Alternative.'* This implies use of CTs *instead of* conventional treatment. However, most users of complementary medicine seem also to continue with conventional medicine.
● *'Holistic—treats the whole person.'* Many conventional healthcare professionals work in a holistic manner; conversely, some complementary therapists can adopt a narrow and reductionist approach in practice (see discussion below).

Adapted from Zollman & Vickers.[46]

---

seen, at best, as benign oddballs and, at worst, as dangerous charlatans. This marginalization led CTs to be regarded as either wholly good or wholly bad. CT students would have had a natural tendency to see them as wholly good, especially as a lot of people choose to study a CT because of the benefits they received as patients. As the acceptablity of CTs increases CPs can afford to relax into a more critical analysis of their work knowing that if they find that certain conditions do not respond as readily as others to their therapy that does not mean that the whole of their therapy is brought into disrepute. Furthermore, some of the vitalistic 'energy'-based therapies do not embrace the concept of cure. Within TCM the concept of Qi is that it is always moving and changing and can become imbalanced as it gets affected by pathogenic factors. If this imbalance is not corrected early in a disease process the condition can become progressively worse. When this imbalance is corrected and the patient perceives a 'cure' the practitioner does not understand it in this way. The Qi is still moving and changing and what happens next in the life of the patient will affect what happens to their Qi. If patients have a history of back pain aggravated by overwork in a manual trade and if they can't change their working life then treatment will not be as long lasting as if they could make the change. Practitioners can make a realistic prognosis based on whether there are ongoing factors in the patient's life (e.g. diet, lifestyle, overwork, poor housing, poor relationships with others) that will hinder the patient's attempts to stay well.

Some other concerns are discussed in Chapter 2.

Assumptions about CTs

Both members of the public and doctors make assumptions about CTs, which can be inaccurate and generally unhelpful. They include the following.

Are CTs holistic?

CTs generally conceive of the body and mind as a single informational entity, and practitioners tend towards a multifactorial view of illness as caused by disturbances at physical, biomechanical, psychosocial and spiritual levels. Diagnosis generally involves looking at the patient in context, relies largely on patients' own account of their experience and views them as having agency and choices. CPs frequently use a 'package of care' approach: modifying lifestyle, diet change, exercise as well as a specific treatment such as homeopathy. They often state that they rely on allowing or stimulating the person's capacity for self-repair, and see their role as largely providing the conditions for this to occur. Generally, the CT therapeutic intervention is supposed to restore balance and catalyse self-healing responses. Yet there are obvious examples of CT approaches where explanations and treatment can appear highly reductionist. For instance, a CP might ignore complex psychosocial factors in a case of depression and simply offer a nutritional supplement as an antidepressant or a homeopathic remedy; or prescribe antioxidants in high dosage to someone with cancer while ignoring the person's anguish and the family dynamics.

In diagnosis also, different CPs use diverse methods. Although generally they avoid hi-tech diagnosis in favour of using hand and eye, guided by unconventional theory, some use mechanical and recognizably scientific methods. For instance, most homeopaths base their prescriptions on an extensive history of symptoms, but some use a computer to analyse these symptom complexes and match them to particular remedies. Similarly, though TCM acupuncturists usually diagnose from history, pulse and tongue appearance, a few use electrical point locators or even complex computer applications to detect channels and 'organ disorders'.

If CAM can include reductionist and mechanistic elements, use synthetic medicines and incorporate fragments of technology then the case for its being inherently 'holistic' or 'natural' is not straightforward. The ideal of holism and whole person care is also not unique to CAM, as primary care at its best also adopts such a holistic approach. Clearly, then, holism relates more to the individual practitioner's outlook than to the type of medicine.

The evidence base

Both the public and a significant number of doctors[39] believe CTs to be effective. It is also widely believed, however, that the evidence for CTs is poor. In fact, more research now exists than is commonly recognized. Although early studies were poorly designed, for a number of reasons (see below), there are now more than 5000 RCTs published in peer-reviewed journals, which have already provided information about clinical outcomes.[22,40] At the same time, qualitative and pragmatic research studies have begun to clarify why patients seek CTs and to define models of provision.[21,41] New research designs have also been developed with the aim of taking into account the 'whole person' approach of CTs:[42]

The focus on the whole person as a unique individual provides new challenges to the scientific measurement of the healing encounter. Mobilizing the resources of each individual to stay healthy and get well also provides new opportunities to move healthcare toward a model of wellness and toward new models for helping solve our current healthcare crisis, which is largely driven by costs.

However, there is still a dearth of research compared with conventional medicine. In particular, too few cost-effectiveness studies are available. NHS decision makers want persuasive evidence that complementary medicine can deliver safe, cost-effective alternatives to problems that are expensive or difficult to manage with conventional treatment and at present such evidence is scarce and equivocal. Only very few reliable economic analyses of CTs have been performed to date, whilst no systematic process has yet been set up for collecting data on safety, adverse events and possible interactions.

The situation is slowing changing, however, as CPs are becoming increasingly aware of the importance of research, and research skills now form a part of many training courses. At the same time, conventional sources of research funds have become more sympathetic to proposals from researchers in CTs. However, until the much-needed evidence is gathered, the debate about more widespread integration of complementary medicine will be held back.

Specific and non-specific effects

Another question asked about CTs is the *nature* of their effects. In the past, the medical profession has tended to write off any perceived benefits of CTs as being almost entirely due to their non-specific effects (being frequently labelled as simply an example of the 'placebo effect'). Owing to the mounting weight of research on specific effects of particular therapies, however, the medical establishment has begun to change its attitude. The question of how 'human effects' influence treatment outcomes of all kinds nevertheless remains an important question, since their contribution to any perceived benefits is clearly significant. Why else would the RCT be so essential a tool for bracketing them off in a clinical trial? Specific effects of particular CTs—the right acupuncture point, the correct homeopathic remedy, the appropriate manipulation—probably account for a proportion of patient satisfaction, but only a great deal more research will allow us to say with any certainty. However, many patients also value the general attributes of complementary medicine because they help create a therapeutic relationship through time, touch and attention, the ways in which illness is explained and the environment in which the treatment is given. The relative therapeutic importance of specific and non-specific effects will vary from patient to patient and from practitioner to practitioner, but many CTs do appear to deliver these elements to a greater extent than is common in mainstream medicine.

Suitability of CTs for particular conditions

Over three-quarters of patients approaching practitioners of the major complementary disciplines have a musculoskeletal problem as their main complaint. Users of complementary medicine are more likely to have chronic, relapsing and remitting complaints, such as eczema, and neurological, psychological and allergic disorders are also common. Still others present with problems that are difficult to label conventionally, such as lack of energy. Some people come with no specific problems but simply want to improve or maintain, a level of general 'wellness'.[43]

Some differences have been identified amongst different therapies.[44] For instance, acupuncture patients often have the most chronic medical history and tend to be least satisfied with their conventional treatment; homeopaths and herbalists tend to treat conditions such as eczema, menstrual problems or headaches rather than the musculoskeletal and pain problems seen frequently by manipulative therapists and acupuncturists.

(The possible benefits of specific therapies for certain conditions are considered in detail in Chapter 2.)

Suitability of CTs for particular patients

Although myths and stereotypes abound about people who use CTs (e.g. that they have an alternative world-view that rejects conventional medicine on principle or that they are lured by exaggerated advertising claims), these are not supported by the research evidence. Both qualitative and quantitative studies indicate that users tend to have long-standing conditions for which they believe conventional medicine has not proved satisfactory. For example, they may perceive it as insufficiently effective or causing adverse effects or be dissatisfied with the amount of contact they can have with their GP. Patients have generally already consulted a conventional healthcare practitioner for their problem, and many continue to use the two systems concurrently. Some people will tend to 'pick and mix' between the two, considering that for some of their problems their GP is the better option, whereas for others a complementary treatment will be of more benefit. Most users arrive at the door of their CPs through personal recommendation.

Some surveys suggest that users of complementary medicine tend to have more psychological difficulties, are more sceptical about conventional medicine and have had more problems with conventional treatment, than users of conventional medicine. However, this finding probably indicates not that personality differences explain their choice, but rather that more people with persistent health problems resort to complementary medicine after conventional treatments have proven unsatisfactory. (The question of CTs with complex and 'heartsink' patients is discussed at length in Chapter 5.)

Users of CTs have been broadly classified into the following four categories[43].

- *Earnest seekers.* These often suffer an intractable health problem and may try many different treatment modalities searching for the one of significant benefit.
- *Stable users.* These may either use a particular type of therapy consistently for a variety of problems or have established the use of a regular blend of CTs for their particular problem.
- *Eclectic users.* These may select different forms of therapy according to their problems and circumstances at any particular time.
- *One-off users.* These often stop their complementary treatment after only a limited period.

Patients' choice of CTs may not always be well justified, particularly if initial expectations were unrealistic; media reports and popular myths about CTs no doubt contribute to this overoptimism. This is a cause for concern in serious or chronic disease when a patient is having difficulty accepting the diagnosis. Another aspect of this 'bargaining' can drive a patient to persist hopefully with multiple potentially expensive treatments for a condition even when it is not improving. The practitioner may collude, whether or not there are financial incentives, with patients' unwillingness to admit they are not improving or because one (or both) of them feels guilty about this. There is no doubt that, for some patients, the sense that they must search every avenue for a cure and be seen to 'take responsibility for their condition' can become a burden and a reason for self-blame. The limits and potential of CTs can be best explored where practitioners can collaborate and reflect on the intake and outcome of integrating approaches.

Safety

The evidence for the effectiveness of CTs has grown along with their popularity and availability, but the number of reports of adverse effects have increased too.[40, 45] In general, CTs appear *relatively* safe; for instance, a recent US study found that claims against practitioners of CTs occurred less frequently and typically involved less severe injury than did those against conventional practitioners in the same period.[46] CPs' own insurance payments are a fraction of what doctors pay.

In conventional medicine, before a treatment is advised a risk–benefit evaluation should be considered. The high levels of medicine-related harm suggest that if this is happening then it is being done badly. One consequence is the public's perception that modern medicine can be risky and is now something to avoid—hence, in part, CTs' growing credibility. But the potential benefits of CTs need to be evaluated in relation to potential risks in order to establish their relevance. There are two kinds of risk: direct effects, related directly to the therapy, including toxicity, adverse reactions and structural injury; and indirect effects, relating to practitioners and advice they may give about discontinuing vitally necessary conventional treatment. This problem does not arise in collaborative practice and is more likely when CPs are poorly trained, so it may be more prevalent where there is no legal requirement for practitioners to be trained, registered with a professional body or insured (see Regulation and training below). This is still regrettably the case in the UK where as a consequence no reliable system yet exists for reporting adverse events. The scale of risk from CTs is therefore certainly underestimated.

Direct risks

Although many CTs have been popularly considered 'safe', because they are believed to be 'natural' (see above discussion on Assumptions), a number of reports have noted toxic or other adverse effects. A growing body of research has started to focus on this.

Some therapies such as acupuncture, herbalism, homeopathy, chiropractic and osteopathy have specific risks, although their incidence is low. (Specific safety issues associated with individual therapies are detailed in Chapter 2.) In addition there is the question of interaction of effects, resulting from either using different CTs, remedies or supplements concurrently or using them together with conventional drugs, for instance. Some herbal remedies can interfere with a number of conventional drugs or heighten their effect,[47] and these were presumed to be uncommon, but the recent realization that St John's wort—a common OTC herbal antidepressant—interacts with the cytochrome-50 pathway has raised new levels of suspicion.[48] The risk of all CTs compared with conventional drugs of every kind is still most likely to be very low, but as systems for reporting adverse reactions and interactions are still in their in-fancy we cannot be sure.

Indirect risks

Indirect risks include misdiagnosis of treatable conditions, use of unproven therapies (rather than conventional treatment of proven efficacy), practitioners' disregard of interactions and contraindications and encouragement to ignore medical advice, and fragmentation of patient care.[45]

People who use CTs may not let their doctors know. Yet the risk of adverse effects means that patients should be properly advised that GPs need to be informed. Delayed diagnosis of a serious disease is perhaps the main concern, though actually most patients will already have seen their GP before they decide to try CT. Also, well-trained CPs are taught which symptoms ought to ring alarm bells (see Red flags, p. 117) and would send patients for medical advice appropriately.

Extreme dietary regimens can cause problems. In common with many people, CPs perhaps overestimate the potential for harm from antibiotics and immunization; this is one area of common disagreement between CPs and doctors. However, the great majority of well-trained CPs would be happy to work alongside GPs, communicating with them and discussing options for treatment.

The potential risk of further fragmenting patient care is clear, and that of contradictory advice obvious. Where CPs and doctors are not working under the same roof, there will be a greater need to ensure good communication in order to minimize risk and optimize outcomes.[49]

Regulation and training

Training

Despite recent moves towards establishing common standards, there is still considerable variation in the standard of CP training. Increasingly, accredited training in the major therapies—osteopathy, chiropractic, acupuncture, herbal medicine and homeopathy—involves extensive training; some courses are now offered at university level (see Ch. 3 for details of these). The less invasive therapies (such as massage, reflexology and aromatherapy) usually entail limited training; some may not even be recognized by the main registering bodies of the therapy. Some courses still have highly variable curricula and standards, with little time for clinical contact. Most CPs fund their own training, part time over several years, although degree-level programmes or equivalent now set the standard. Separate training courses in the main therapies are available for doctors and nurses.

Regulation

Recent Acts of Parliament have established the General Osteopathic Council and General Chiropractic Council for the statutory self-regulation of these professions. These bodies have stricter controls than the General Medical Council and only registered practitioners may use the titles Osteopath and Chiropractor. Other official registers are likely to follow: acupuncture and herbal medicine already have a single main regulatory body and homeopathy is working in that direction. All therapies may take steps towards statutory self-regulation. The support being given by Foundation for Integrated Medicine (FIM) (website: http://www.FIM) will be crucial to achieving success in this area. The more 'supportive' and less 'invasive' therapies (e.g. massage, reflexology, healing and aromatherapy) have various 'registering' organizations, whose published registers are linked to the diverse training programmes they recognize or accredit. Although there are now some 200 such organizations,[12] unified regulatory bodies will eventually develop for each discipline. Such bodies need published criteria for entry, to agree and to enforce codes of conduct, and require insurance cover. These requirements will, for now, be sufficient to protect patients and, although statutory self-regulation may perhaps develop in the long term, the expensive parliamentary legislation and ongoing administration entailed will be beyond the reach of most practitioner groups.

Quality assurance and clinical governance

Quality control can be broken down into three parts. The first is setting standards, through national service frameworks and paying attention to the questions of regulation and training. The second is delivering standards, through paying attention to good service design and delivery. The third is measuring standards, and for this the most appropriate methods of measurement need to be determined.

Clinical governance is a 'catch-all' term that brings together aspects of working that can best contribute to a high-quality, accountable health service, 'creating an environment in which excellence in clinical care will flourish' and 'aiming to create a working environment which is open and participative, where ideas and good practice are shared, where education and research are valued'.[50] It uses ideas developed in the field of management to achieve quality assurance and quality improvement[51] (i.e. being able to give an assurance about the quality of services provided[52]). Components of these processes are already familiar to primary healthcare workers, and will involve all clinical and administrative members of an integrated primary healthcare team as well as patients. The components of developing clinical quality assurance include:

• accountability (practitioner and practice)
• leadership and responsibility (individual and corporate)
• continuing professional development
• clinical audit
• teamwork and communication
• partnership with patients and carers
• management policies
• risk management
• performance monitoring
• sharing good practice.

These components will be discussed in detail in Chapters 3 and 4.

Cost effectiveness

Patients are spending their own money on CTs, so they must think the benefits are worth it. (The figure for private spending on CTs is in the region of a billion pounds, compared with the overall NHS expenditure of £40 billion.) However, in publicly funded medicine the limited nature of resources must be taken into account, hence economic analysis of any intervention needs to be undertaken.

An essential question is whether CTs are going to be an additional expense or whether they will be a substitute. Cost-effectiveness analyses must also take into account both short-term and long-term and both direct and indirect costs. For instance, an initially expensive therapy may save money in the long term compared with an initially less expensive treatment if the latter needs to be used indefinitely or produces complications that may be expensive to treat.

One major problem is exactly how to evaluate the benefits of CTs.[28] Although savings in terms of reductions in drug costs, referral rates, repeat visits to the GP and adverse effects can be costed, many benefits claimed by CT practitioners or patients are less tangible and difficult to assess with conventional measures. These include patient preference, patients' feelings of empowerment, the benefits of the consultation process itself, the quality of life (improved stress management, etc.), delayed health benefits from lifestyle changes and the value of having extra options when conventional treatment appears unsatisfactory.

Because only a few cost-effectiveness studies on CTs exist, it is difficult to form an overall picture and there are contradictions. For example, there is some evidence for the cost effectiveness of chiropractic in lower back pain, yet although one recent trial from the UK suggested that chiropractic might save expense,[53] another in the USA found that it was not good value.[54] There are emerging doubts that CAM will eventually save money, and some growing suspicions (even if it were to improve patients' quality of service experience or actually add to quality of life) that greater public sector access to CAM is likely to increase overall short-term expenditure in public healthcare systems,[15,54–56] which hardly seems surprising. But, because healthcare rationing is now regrettably a widespread necessity, rigorous studies on the total cost of CTs will be required if they are to find a place within financially constrained public sector systems. In the independent sector too, insurers have a similar need to establish whether and how CTs add value to private medical policies. More than ever before, with the growing public expectation that CTs should be made more widely available, there needs to be an effective demonstration that patients are being treated not only with a therapy that is effective and safe but also that it is more acceptable and cost effective than the conventional medical alternatives.[57]

HOW CAN CTs BE INTEGRATED INTO PRIMARY CARE?

Existing approaches

National strategies have begun to promote a 'primary care environment in which excellence in clinical care will flourish'.[58] Primary care currently has a leading role in the delivery of national healthcare systems,[59] and this emphasis on a primary care-driven health service[60] has opened up opportunities for GPs to commission and offer an extended range of services to patients[61] in primary care settings. During the 1990s there was a remarkable increase internationally in mainstream availability of CTs. The market-forces model that led to UK GPs being offered control of their own budgets meant that many GPs bought in CT services because they felt they offered good value. Consequently the wider availability of CTs through the public sector in the UK mirrored the growing access in other countries where a greater proportion of privately funded medical care has allowed systems to respond to changing patient demand. In the UK, however, these services were not evenly distributed, and recent reorganizations of the NHS have scrapped the internal market and abolished GP fundholding.

A number of different approaches to delivery have also developed in the UK. For instance the homeopathic hospitals are older than the NHS; others, like those developed during general practice fundholding, have come and gone. Currently, locality commissioning is the way forward. In the recent past in several areas (see References, p. 22) initiatives have been encouraged as part of waiting list reduction and primary care development projects. These are likely to be valuable ways of creating future services.

Integration implies the appropriate use of CTs alongside conventional care. Generally, successful integration is more likely to succeed where there is:

- demand from patients
- commitment from high-level staff in the organization
- protected time for education and communication
- ongoing evaluation of the service (which may help to defend service in the face of financial threat)
- good linkage with other conventional establishments integrating complementary medicine
- realism and good will from all parties
- jointly agreed guidelines or protocols between complementary and conventional practitioners
- support from senior management or health authority
- careful selection and supervision for CPs
- funding from the charitable or voluntary sector.

Problems are likely if there is:

- financial insecurity
- time pressure
- a lack of appropriate premises
- unrealistic expectation
- overwhelming demand
- inappropriate referral
- unresolved difference of perspective between complementary and conventional practitioners
- real or perceived lack of evidence of effectiveness
- lack of resources and time for reflection and evaluation
- a lack of respect.

A number of different approaches to integration have been employed to date. These are briefly reviewed in this section.

Direct versus indirect provision in primary care

Complementary medicine in the NHS is delivered mostly in primary care, usually by conventional healthcare professionals as part of everyday NHS services. In 1987 a regional survey of GPs revealed that 16% practised a CT, and this trend increased during the 1980s and 90s. Perhaps as many as 4000 doctors in the UK now have some sort of training in a CT—mainly medical acupuncture or homeopathy. In a 1995 national survey, around 30% of all general practices were found to offer NHS access to complementary medicine, and a further 10% had made private referrals to CPs.[21] By the mid 1990s at least 20% of primary healthcare teams were providing CTs directly in some form (e.g. homeopathy by GPs, or aromatherapy, reflexology or relaxation by nurses).

There are both advantages and disadvantages to this approach. On the plus side, only minimal financial investment is required, and GPs can retain control of case management and monitoring. This must be weighed against the disadvantages: generally appointments will be shorter, there will be less time for non-specific benefits to develop (see above) and team members will usually have undertaken only basic CT training. Consequently, with this kind of direct provision, the issue of team members' competence and effectiveness as CPs and the appropriate limitation of case mix must be kept under review.

Although PNMQPs usually work privately, they have been subcontracted as part-time staff in some units. In the mid 1990s, PNMQPs (most commonly osteopaths) were working in some 20% of UK primary care practices. However, this pattern of integration has more recently declined with the demise of fundholding (unpublished GostC survey 2000). In a minority of practices CT treatment may also be offered indirectly, through referral to PNMQPs working outside the practice. The advantage of having CPs work in-house are that the practice can be certain of practitioners' credentials, and will be in a position to develop clear guidelines for referral and to agree quality measures for collaborative CT services. However, levels of integration often fall short of the ideal, because, inevitably, the degree of communication varies. According to Luff and Thomas,[62] authentic integration is has so far been the exception.

In specialist provider units

In the UK, GPs have, since before the inception of the NHS, been able to refer patients to five regional NHS homeopathic hospitals (www.trusthomeopathy.org). These units make a range of CTs available free at the point of care, provided by conventionally trained health professionals. However, recently, because of ongoing NHS reorganization in England and Wales, such referrals have become more difficult to make. Meanwhile a few NHS purchasers have established contracts with independent complementary medicine centres to provide CTs for an agreed range of medical conditions. Also, with the reorganization of primary care, some primary care organizations (PCOs) have lately begun to pilot community-based musculoskeletal clinics that include osteopathy and acupuncture to referring GPs. A recent survey of the UK consultant physicians revealed that almost 10% of respondents used CTs in their practice.[63] Increasingly, pain clinics, oncology units and rehabilitation wards make provision for CTs, and a survey of hospices indicated that around 90% offered complementary treatments such as aromatherapy, massage and reflexology.[64]

A schema of current CT provision in the NHS is given in Figure 1.3.

Pilot schemes

In the last 10 years some health authorities and NHS hospital trusts have developed pilot units to make complementary medicine available either directly or indirectly. Unfortunately, such centres have always been a low priority and financially vulnerable. Two important examples are the Liverpool Centre for Health, which has barely survived through some 10 fruitful years of work in a deprived community, and the former Lewisham Complementary Therapy Centre, which closed because the NHS hospital trust had to reduce its overspend.[11,65,66]

CT service development tends to be demand led and almost totally dependent on local enthusiasts and product champions who have been so fortunate as to grasp an opportunity to resource an innovation. Some formal evaluations or audit reports of these services have been published (see the Glastonbury study in Ch. 4, p. 138). Some show benefits such as high patient satisfaction, significant improvements on validated health questionnaires compared with waiting list controls, and suggestions of reduced prescribing and referrals. However, data from others are less clear, and many have not been formally evaluated. The various pilot projects have also identified factors that influence the integration of complementary medicine practitioners within NHS settings (see below).

This book looks at several examples of pilot projects, and in particular the project with which the authors have been personally involved, the Marylebone Health Centre in central London. The MHC was, in 1988, one of the first general practices to offer multidisciplinary CTs to NHS patients and it still provides osteopathy, acupuncture, massage, naturopathy and homeopathy. In the rest of

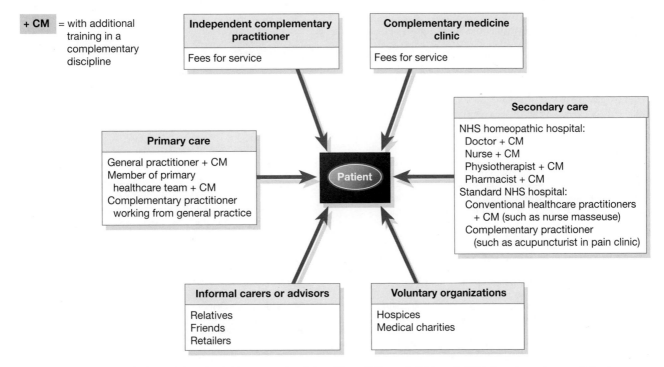

Figure 1.3 Approaches to NHS provision of complementary medicine. (From Zollman C, Vickers A 1999 Complementary medicine in conventional practice. British Medical Journal 319: 901–904, with permission of the authors and the British Medical Journal.)

this book, details of the authors' experience at the MHC are used to illustrate in concrete terms the issues that are likely to arise in the course of CT integration, in the light of our experience and the feedback generated by the project.

SUMMARY

The growing demand for CAM:
- the public popularity of CAM has grown rapidly over the last 20 years
- 75% of the public surveyed would use CAM if there were NHS access
- mid 1990s surveys showed about 40% of family doctors had provided some sort of access to CAM.

Why are CTs so popular?
- continuing media optimism and support for CAM
- the appeal of time and touch
- increased public wish for a wider range of healthcare choices
- CPs deal with high proportion of musculoskeletal problems (about 60%)
- CPs deal with high proportion of stress-related illness
- the majority of clients have already had conventional treatment for the same problems
- new consultations are mainly prompted by recommendation.

Medicine's attitude to CAM is changing. There is an increase in the use of CAM in NHS primary care:
- CAM was quackery in the 1950s and 1960s
- CAM was 'fringe' in the 1970s
- 'alternative' in the 1980s
- 'complementary' in the 1990s
- will it be 'integrated' into the 21st century mainstream?

The growing professional interest:
- is driven by concern for consumer choice, patient interest and client-centredness
- medical attitudes to CAM are increasingly positive, e.g. BMA supports good practice in cooperation, education and research
- in the UK, the GMC has clarified that doctors may delegate treatment to non-medical complementary practitioners if satisfied of their competence and if they maintain overall clinical responsibility.

Complementary therapies in Europe:
- there are huge national variations in: law, market, medical attitude, state funding, health beliefs and practices (e.g. Kur)
- also in regulation, e.g. in the UK, Germany, Scandinavia and France
- policy and legal reforms are under way (e.g. in the UK, Netherlands, Belgium)
- Brussels influence: harmonizing standards and regulation?
- growing popularity
- a booming market in herbals, homeopathics, nutriceuticals
- medical attitudes changing—'alternative' . . . 'complementary'
- but rising costs of health care
- evidence-based medicine: where will it take CAM?

REFERENCES

1. Tonkin R D 1987 Role of research in the rapproachement between conventional medicine and complementary therapies: discussion paper. Royal Society of Medicine 80: 361–363
2. Murray J, Shepherd S 1988 Alternative or additional medicine? A new dilemma for doctors. Journal of the Royal College of General Practice 38: 511–514
3. British Medical Association 1993 Complementary medicine—new approaches to good practice. Oxford University Press, Oxford
4. Zollman C, Vickers A 1999 ABC of complementary medicine: Users and practitioners of complementary medicine. British Medical Journal 319: 836–838/bmj.com
5. Zollman C, Vickers A 1999 ABC of complementary medicine: What is complementary medicine? British Medical Journal 319: 693–696/bmj.com
6. Coates X et al 1998 Integrated healthcare: a way forward for the next five years (a discussion document from the Prince of Wales' Initiative, the Foundation for Integrated Medicine). Journal of Alternative and Complementary Medicine 4: 2
7. RCCM 1997 Public usage of complementary medicine: an overview. Research Council for Complementary Medicine, London
8. MORI poll. The Times, 13 November 1989
9. Thomas K J, Nicholl J P, Coleman P 2001 Use and expenditure on complementary medicine in England: a population based survey. Complementary Therapies in Medicine 9(1): 2–11
10. NHS Alliance 1999 Primary care groups and complementary discussion: issues for local discussion. nhsalliance.org
11. Donnelly D 1995 Integrating complementary medicine within the NHS: therapist's view of the Liverpool Centre for Health. Complementary Therapies in Medicine 3: 84–87
12. Mills S, Budd S 2000 Professional organisation of complementary and alternative medicine in the United Kingdom. Centre for Complementary Health Studies, University of Exeter

13. Harris P, Rees R 2000 The prevalence of complementary and alternative medicine use among the general population: a systematic review of the literature. Complementary Therapies in Medicine 8: 88–96
14. Eisenberg D M et al 1993 Unconventional medicine in the United States. Prevalence, costs and patterns of use. New England Journal of Medicine 328: 246–252
15. Maclennan A H, Wilson D H, Taylor A W 1996 Prevalence and cost of alternative medicine in Australia. Lancet 347: 569–573
16. Eisenberg D M, Davis R B, Ettner S L et al 1998 Trends in alternative medicine use in the United States, 1990–1997. Journal of the American Medical Association 280: 1569–1575
17. Fisher P, Ward A 1994 Complementary medicine in Europe. British Medical Journal 309: 107–111
18. Consumers Association. Survey of CA members. Which? October 1986
19. Linde K, Clausius N, Ramirez G et al 1997 Are the clinical effects of homeopathy placebo effects? A meta-analysis of placebo-controlled trials. Lancet 350: 834–843
20. Wearn A M, Greenfield S 1998 Access to CM in GP; survey in one UK HA. Journal of the Royal Society of Medicine 91: 465–470
21. Thomas K, Fall M, Parry G, Nicoll J 1995 National survey of access to complementary healthcare via general practice. Report to Dept of Health. Medical Care Research Unit, SCHARR, University of Sheffield
22. CISCOM database. Research Council for Complementary Medicine, 60 Gt Ormond St, London WC1 NJF
23. Clinical Services Advisory Group 1994 Back pain. HMSO, London
24. BMA General Medical Services Committee 1991 Choices for the future. BMA, London
25. Cameron-Blackie G, Mouncer M 1993 Complementary therapies in the HNS. NAHAT, London

26. Donnelly D 1995 Integrating complementary medicine within the NHS: a therapist's view of the Liverpool Centre for Health. Complementary Therapies in Medicine 3(2):84–87
27. June 2000 Complementary medicine: information pack for primary care groups. www.doh.gov.uk; www.nhsalliance.org; www.fimed.org; www.primarycare.co.uk
28. White AR, Ernst E 2000 Economic analysis of complementary medicine: a systematic review. Complementary Therapies in Medicine 8(2): 111–118
29. Jewell D 1997 Supporting diversity in primary care. British Medical Journal 314: 1706–1707
30. Pietroni C 1996 Innovations in primary care. Churchill Livingstone, New York
31. Richardson J 1995 Complementary therapies on the NHS: the experience of a new service. Complementary Therapies in Medicine 3: 153–157
32. Department of Health 2000 A health service of all the talents: Developing the NHS workforce. Consultation document on the review of workforce planning. DoH, London
33. House of Lords Select Committee on Science and Technology 2000 Sixth report, 21 November 2000: Complementary and alternative medicine. HMSO, London
34. Callan J P 1979 Holistic health or holistic hoax? (editorial). Journal of the American Medical Association 241(11):1156
35. Avina R L, Schneiderman L J 1978 Why patients choose homoeopathy (commentary). Western Journal of Medicine 128(4):366–369
36. Fry J 1983 Common diseases, their nature, incidence and care. MTP Press, Guildford
37. Peters D (ed) 2001 Understanding the placebo effect in complementary therapies. Churchill Livingstone, Edinburgh
38. Zollman C, Vickers A 1999 Complementary medicine and the doctor. British Medical Journal 319: 1558–1561/bmj.com
39. Ernst E, Resch K L, White A R 1995 Complementary medicine. What physicians think of it: a meta-analysis. Archives of Internal Medicine 155: 2405–2408
40. Parkside Trust 1999 The evidence base of complementary medicine. Royal London Homoeopathic Hospital Academic Unit, London
41. Hills D, Welford R 1998 Complementary therapy in general practice: an evaluation of the Glastonbury Health Centre Complementary Medicine Service. Somerset Trust for Integrated healthcare, Glastonbury
42. Micozzi M 1996 Fundamentals of complementary and alternative medicine. Churchill Livingstone, New York
43. Sharma U 1995 Complementary medicine today: practitioners and patients. Routledge, London
44. Furnham A 1998 Why do patients chose and use complementary therapies? In: Ernst E, ed. Complementary medicine and objective appraisal. Butterworth-Heinemann, Oxford, pp. 71–88
45. Ernst E, Fugh-Berman A 1999 Complementary medicine—a critical review of acupuncture, homeopathy and chiropractic. Paper presented at NHS/Department of Medicine Exeter conference on complementary therapies in primary care, University of Exeter, September 1999
46. Studdert D M, Eisenberg D M, Miller F H et al 1998 Medical malpractice implications of alternative medicine. Journal of the American Medical Association 280: 1610–1615
47. Zollman C, Vickers A 1999 Herbal medicine. British Medical Journal 319: 1050–1053/bmj.com
48. McIntyre M 2000 A review of the benefits, adverse events, drug interactions, and safety of St John's wort (*Hypericum perforatum*): the implications with regard to the regulation of herbal medicines. Journal of Alternative and Complementary Medicine 6(2): 115–124
49. Murray J, Shepherd S 1988 Alternative or additional medicine? A new dilemma for doctors. Journal of the Royal College of General Practitioners 38: 511–514
50. Scally D, Donaldson J 1998 Clinical governance and the drive for quality improvement in the new NHS in England. British Medical Journal 317: 61–65
51. Koch H 1992 Implementing and sustaining total quality management in healthcare. Sage, London
52. van Zwanenberg T 1999 Clinical governance in primary care. Radcliffe Medical Press, Oxford
53. Meade T W, Dyer S, Browne W, Frank A O 1995 Randomized comparison of chiropractic and hospital outpatient management for low back pain: results from extended follow up. British Medical Journal 311: 349–351
54. Carey T S, Garrett J, Jackman A, McLaughlin C, Fryer J, Smucker D R 1995 The outcome and costs of care for acute low back pain among patients seen by primary care practitioners, chiropractors, and orthopaedic surgeons. New England Journal of Medicine 333: 913–917
55. Brugi M, Sommer J H, Theiss R 1996 Alternative Heilmethoden Verbreitungsmuster in der Schweiz. Rueger, Zurich
56. Assendelft W J J, Bouter L M 1993 Does the goose really lay the golden eggs? A methodological review of workmen's compensation studies. Journal of Manipulative Physiology and Therapeutics 16: 161–168
57. Ernst E 1996 The ethics of complementary medicine. Journal of Medical Ethics 22: 197–198
58. DoH 1997 The new NHS—modern, dependable. Stationery Office, London
59. DoH 1998 Modernising health and social services: national priorities guidance 2000/01–2002/3
60. Reith W 1996 Statement on a primary care led NHS. Royal College of General Practitioners, London
61. Pietroni C, Pietroni P (eds) 1996 Innovation in community care and primary health: the Marylebone experiment. Churchill Livingstone, New York
62. Luff D, Thomas KJ 2000 Sustaining complementary therapy provision in primary care: lessons from existing services. Complementary Therapies in Medicine 8: 173–179
63. George Lewith, personal communication
64. Wilkes E 1992 Complementary therapies in hospice and palliative care. Trent Palliative Care Centre, Abbey Lane, Sheffield S11 9NE
65. Donnelly D 1995 Integrating complementary medicine within the NHS: therapist's view of the Liverpool Centre for Health. Complementary Therapies in Medicine 3: 84–87
66. Richardson J 1995 Complementary therapy on the NHS: a service evaluation of the first year of an outpatient service in a local district general hospital. Lewisham Hospital NHS Trust, London

FURTHER READING

Bonnet J 2000 Complementary medicine in primary care—what are the key issues? NHS Executive, London

Brooks R, with the EuroQol Group 1996 EuroQol: the current state of play. Health Policy 37: 53–72

NHS Primary Care Group Alliance 1999 Primary care groups and complementary medicine: Issues for local discussion. NHS PCG Alliance, London

Scottish Office Departmen of Health 1996 Complementary medicine and the National Health Service. An examination of acupuncture, homeopathy, chiropractic and osteopathy. Scottish Office, Edinburgh

Thomas K, Fell M, Parry G, Nicholl J 1995 National survey of access to complementary healthcare via general practice. Medical Care Research Unit, University of Sheffield

Zollman C, Vickers A 1999 ABC of complementary medicine. British Medical Association, London

Chapter 1 REFLECTIVE LEARNING CYCLE AUDIT

1. **What did you need to know?** *(clarify learning objectives)*

2. **What did you notice?** *(key points)*

3. **What have you learned?** *(learning evaluation)*

4. **How will you apply it to practice?** *(clinical relevance)*

5. **What do I need to do next?** *(reflective educational audit)*

6. **Proceed to next area of interest / section you have identified.**

2

Models and research in CTs

INTRODUCTION

The natural mainstream home of CTs in the NHS is general practice:

there is clearly a bias towards primary care . . . it is firmly on the primary care agenda already. I think also psychologically there is an empathy there ... both general practice, primary care and complementary medicine are holistic from their point of view, they are taking the whole person not just the constituent bits. Secondly they are both very committed to the whole idea of self-care which secondary care often is not . . . Thirdly I think the whole concept of the therapeutic relationship is much stronger in primary than secondary care . . .

(*Dr Michael Dixon, the Chair of the NHS Alliance**)

If CTs are to become an integral part of mainstream health care then conceptual bridges have to be built. Because integration depends on effective lines of communication and the ability to complete learning loops, a good enough common language is an essential foundation. And, whether or not integration entails conventional and complementary practitioners working together, new working practices must encourage appropriate use of CTs and allow their evaluation. This chapter, which presents a theoretical basis for integration, includes a discussion of an integrative model of medicine, an approach for exploring CTs' relevance (including evidence available for different CTs in a range of common health problems) and basic information about the most prominent CTs.

CPs tend to adjust patterns of therapy to the unique individual being treated and, in theory, CTs aim to promote wellness through individual or group effort. Their focus on person-centredness and health promotion is consistent with current health beliefs. Common ground with conventional theory and practice may be hard to

---

* House of Lords Select Committee on Science and Technology 2000. Report on Complementary Medicine, para 9.15. The Stationery Office, London.

find nonetheless. Yet parallels between CPs' ideas about their approaches and conventional health care have to be found. And, even though CT treatments tend not to be standardized, research methods allowing their rigorous evaluation will certainly be needed to rationalize and justify their introduction.

Finding a scientific explanation for the principles behind some of the therapies is one challenge. There is, for instance, no anatomical basis for the existence of acupuncture meridians; nor do we have a biochemical explanation for how homeopathic remedies work. However, although these theoretical objections appear to be barriers to integration within primary care, there should be no absolute objection to the pragmatic use of some CTs. After all, aspirin was used for decades before pro-staglandins were discovered, and it was only with the advent of the endorphins and pain-gate theory that a scientifically coherent explanation for the acupuncture treatment of pain became possible.

MODELS AND THEORIES OF HEALING

Defining common ground

It seems that new science provides support for the idea of 'whole person care' and 'holistic medicine' and, moreover, they are now by-words for good mainstream practice. This convergence between conventional and traditional systems of medicine has provided the common ground for practitioners in our own team at the MHC and consequently we had to define this shared theoretical territory.

If intelligence is the capacity to adapt to challenging circumstances then the central nervous system and the immune system manifest this ability beyond all others. It would be remarkable if each of these supreme exemplars of rapid and subtle adaptation did not tap the other's almost limitless potential for variation.

(*Norman Geschwind*)

The highly focused biomedical model is fundamentally unlike any CT model. This raises interdisciplinary issues whose undercurrents are not unlike those that beset relationships between men and women. Here too as in many situations where the different approaches to health care work together—despite the potential one might have for complementing the other—a sense of difference and unequal power relations can incite polarization and separateness. The biomedical approach to the body is analytical and positivist. It deals with the body as an object with the aim of categorizing its disorders in order to predict and control their outcome. This approach has met with enormous success even though important cornerstones of a rapidly changing scientific worldview have not been incorporated into the biomedical framework—in particular, mind–body interactivity, homeostasis and

organismic biology. This contributes to a growing sense of biomedicine's inadequacy, but can CT approaches truly address this lack? Complementary medicine systems, it is true, rely on subjective and synthetic methods, and describe the body in terms of its qualities, processes and feelings; they view the body as a dynamic interconnected whole. If these attributes are in tune with current health beliefs they might allow individuals to express themselves and make better sense of their experience. Such congruence could also help build the therapeutic relationship. Could CT models of disease and recovery perhaps help people with long-term health problems deal more appropriately with their condition? It would be important to seek answers to these questions alongside the necessary inquiry into CT effectiveness.

The biomedical and the biopsychosocial models

An emerging view called the 'biopsychosocial model' of medicine is a framework widely acknowledged in family medicine and in nursing. It aims to take account of the influence of social, psychological and physical factors on self-regulatory processes: how psychosocial pressures are met by physiological and potentially pathophysiological responses. A person's psychosocial predicament, their knowledge, beliefs and emotional repertoire will largely determine how they cope with life's pressures and adapt to a change in their health. Research suggests that interactions between mind and body influence health outcomes: perhaps the best example is hostility as a risk factor for developing coronary heart disease. Lifestyle factors are the major risk factor for cardiovascular disease and nutrition is the most significant determinant for cancer. Dietary factors apparently contribute to a wide range of common chronic diseases. Stress is a popular explanation for ill health and improving a person's ability to relax has been shown to improve some outcomes. The discovery of biochemical pathways intertwining psyche and physiology implies that, in future, clinical science will apply this 'inner pharmacy'.

The fundamental ideas of the biopsychosocial model are summarized in Figure 2.1. In this, the person is composed of smaller component parts which influence the whole and from which regulatory processes of greater complexity than the constituent parts are emergent. The person therefore exists in relationship to others and to larger systems whose stability and meaningfulness in turn contribute to (or may interfere with) the individual's ability to self-regulate.

Basic theory and fundamental mechanisms

We have found that the most fundamental element in successful collaboration is for practitioners from different

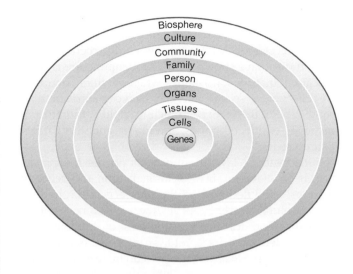

Biosphere
Culture
Community
Family
Person
Organs
Tissues
Cells
Genes

Figure 2.1 Biopsychosocial medicine.

disciplines to find ways of communicating. This takes time, and implies the need for developing a common language, and at least a basic understanding of one another's concepts of health and disease. Therefore, if integration is to come about, GPs will need to understand CP colleagues' ideas and beliefs; complementary personnel in turn have to grasp medical terminology and, importantly, the nature of family medicine as distinct from hi-tech biomedicine. Fortunately our disciplines share some extant common ground. For instance, anatomy, physiology and pathophysiology now form a large part of modern training in the major CT disciplines (acupuncture, herbal medicine, homeopathy, therapeutic bodywork, naturopathy, osteopathy and chiropractic). Doctors, however, are unlikely to have come across the type of 'vitalistic' notions expressed by CPs. CT treatment methods are obviously diverse, yet important common theoretical themes form a kind of 'ecology of ideas' common to all complementary disciplines. Some of these ideas have parallels in conventional disciplines whereas others apparently do not and so they become a focus of contention in an extended care team. We have found that primary care medicine and CTs nevertheless share important underlying ideas and aims that, although couched in unfamiliar terms, provide the basis of a common language for health care. In order to speak this language, an extended team has to demystify its own professional jargons. The aim, however, is not to level out this territory into some meaningless conceptual no man's land, but rather to value its diverse features and explore how they might expand our understanding of health, patients' needs and our capacity to deal with them.

A multifactorial and multilevel view

CT models tend to take a multifactorial view of health and intervention. They see illness and ultimately disease as having not only physical causes, but also causes due to underlying psychological, social–environmental, spiritual and 'energetic' disturbances. CT systems often describe disease and dysfunction as signs of 'imbalance' or 'disharmony' in body–mind states. They might attribute this dysregulation to *biochemical* (e.g. genetic, nutritional, environmental toxins), to *biomechanical* or to *psychosocial* influences. Some systems suggest that primary underlying 'energetic' disturbances are to blame. The idea that the 'flow of life forces' (however that is conceived) regulates and gives coherence to the organism is a central (though increasingly among 'modern' CPs a disowned) notion. Our integral model combines these three categories and includes (contingently) the 'energetic' as a fourth. We have done this because we believe it allows the model to embrace a significant set of unknowns. Many primary care workers will recognize that indeterminacy and uncertainties (about patients' illness and recovery) colour their daily experience. They will, we hope, agree on the need for a category that can include influences and processes that we do not yet fully understand.

The body's capacity for self-repair

CT models view the body–mind (under normal circumstances and given appropriate conditions) as self-regulating and self-healing. The aim of facilitating the body's own healing responses could be expressed as 'restoring balance'. Treatments stimulate more effective self-regulation, either by enhancing function or by removing obstacles to self-regulation, whether structural, biochemical or psychological. If they can in fact achieve it this would suggest their suitability as possible treatments for relapsing dysfunctional conditions where tissues are unharmed—for example in migraine, IBS, a large proportion of musculoskeletal pain, and gynaecological dysfunction (see Box 4.3, p. 121). However, conversely this begs the question of their relevance in established pathology, unless we concede that even in such cases the aim of improving health, resilience and quality of life is legitimate and quite possibly cost beneficial. However, this means being quite explicit about the limitations of various CTs: where they might be seen as legitimate alternatives to conventional management rather than as possible adjunctive (complementary) options.

Self-care, health promotion and packages of care

Whatever the particular CT, practitioners' typical advice can include lifestyle change (e.g. healthy diet and exercise) as well as a specific treatment. So a medical herbalist might suggest an exercise regimen, guidance on breathing and relaxation and dietary advice along with a specific herbal prescription. The collective intention is often described as 'improving homeostasis'. We have taken this as implying the totality of organic activities—including immune, digestive, respiratory, circulatory and eliminative functions—on which bodily well-being and individual integrity depend. A stress-coping model, though unstated, means CPs are likely to give advice aimed at reducing adaptive demands and enhancing resilience. Such health promotion advice is likely to involve diet, stress management or exercise and a GP would probably agree with their general objectives unless the suggested regimen were extreme and irrational. However, the explanation for the lifestyle advice might be offered in 'energetic' terms or be based on the CP's own discipline-specific theory, for instance about physiology or nutrition. An integrated team might therefore have to consider ways of reaching a consensus about advice on self-care and lifestyle change.

Significant doubts about positivist science

Few CPs have been concerned to find a scientific explanation of the underlying mechanism of their particular therapy. The traditional CT systems are based on a long empirical tradition of clinical observation, and make an assumption that a long tradition must necessarily be a reliable one. However, traditional teachings can be handed down in ways that either discourage questioning and the development of better practice or encourage reliance on practitioners' own and others' individual anecdotal experience or on 'intuition'. Within the context of public health care, however, CPs and doctors will definitely question one another's views and must be prepared to deal with the challenges this will present.

A conventional framework can comprehend the manipulative methods, nutrition and herbal medicine. Their clinical objectives can be explained and understood relatively easily. Both homeopathy and acupuncture require a more elastic and imaginative kind of thinking to accommodate them, based as they are on ideas of 'subtle energy'. Perhaps the term 'subtle energy' can be viewed as a way of describing the complex information flow that coordinates all the processes in a living organism. Although the idea has yet to penetrate mainstream science, chaos theory holds that coherence and self-regulation are 'emergent properties' in biological systems. Be that as it may, scientists' inability to detect and measure 'life forces' suggests that a certain leap of faith is necessary even so.

There is a modern scientific (usually characterized, sometimes disparagingly, as 'Western') explanation for acupuncture's clinical success; the 'gate' theory of pain control and acupuncture's ability to cause the release of endorphins are well known. This has encouraged medically trained practitioners—who do not generally accept traditional Chinese explanations, nor believe in its wider applications—to use acupuncture for treating pain. However,

there is irrevocable evidence for the effectiveness of acupuncture in treating nausea, and neither gate theory nor endorphins can account for this. Similarly, recent real-time brain studies have shown that 'real' acupuncture changes cortical circulation consistently whereas 'sham' acupuncture does not. So science may have to keep an open mind: a more general theory of acupuncture could yet confirm the functional reality of points, meridians and the Chinese 'organ systems'.

Homeopathy's 'law of similars' is not an insuperable obstacle to dialogue, but its insistence on the action of microdoses (diluted beyond the presence of single molecules of solute) clearly is. As yet, there is also no biophysical explanation for the effectiveness of homeopathy's highly diluted medicines. Yet a series of RCTs has found them to be more effective than placebo treatment. So it has been argued that this means either that RCT design does not work or that homeopathy does! And, although some researchers claim these solutions are different from water that has not been 'potentized', such work represents the borderline of what is currently scientifically accepted. It may be that new explanatory models are required; meanwhile there are good pragmatic grounds for using homeopathy in primary care for the treatment of several common conditions.

If a sense of antiscience prevails—even as an undercurrent in an extended team—practitioners with a conventional scientific background will feel alienated. This is another reason for developing a conceptual consensus, in order to allow coexistence and a mutual valuing of scientific and vitalistic approaches.

Symptoms as signs of self-regulation in action

Some CT systems view symptoms as indicating self-regulation in action and may even expect (and value) a brief exacerbation following treatment. Sometimes this is described in terms of toxins and their elimination. Searching for some familiar parallels, we find them in psychology: the notion of conversion symptoms as unconscious but necessary and purposeful ways of avoiding unacceptable feelings, memories or drives. However, while the conviction that bodily disease has psychological implications pervades complementary medicine (and may be a dogmatically held and generally insufficiently examined belief), the idea in question here is of a symptom as being functional rather than symbolic. At first it seems more difficult to point to similar processes at work in physical medicine, because this idea is so obviously at odds with conventional medicine and its approach to aetiology and treatment. Examples are available though: increased body temperature is hostile to infecting organisms; inflammation immobilizes an injured limb while a wound knits together and reorganizes. The purposive nature of such reactions is clearer in an acute condition (see Box 2.1, p. 33) but gets more obscure in relapsing and chronic disease. We have introduced the idea of 'downward spirals of dysfunction' in order to help make collective sense of this complex and rather counterintuitive idea (see Figures 2.2–2.4 below). We present here three examples each intended to illustrate the different implications.

Stress and the gut: symptoms due to toxins and their elimination Traditional medical theories emphasize the role of digestion, absorption, processes of detoxification and elimination in maintaining health. Chronic disease is commonly attributed to their poor functioning and the consequent accumulation of toxic metabolites. Symptoms develop as other tissues are irritated by them or as other organ systems become inappropriate pathways for their elimination—in particular the skin, mucosal or synovial membranes. Figure 2.2 illustrates some possible mechanisms and the potential for processes to feed back and become persistent.

Hyperventilation: symptoms due to sympathetic hyperarousal Misattribution of bodily sensations triggered by flight or fight reactions (in response to real or imaginary emergency) provokes further anxiety. Sympathetic overarousal dysregulates neuromuscular, cardiac, gut and respiratory function. This tendency to disturbed rhythmic activity (which the French call 'spas-

mophilia') includes inappropriate muscle tension, heart and peristaltic arrhythmias and overbreathing. Hyperventilation can cause a cascade of metabolic compensatory changes including calcium loss to the point of tetany. Dysfunctional symptoms involving all bodily systems may occur, as well as altered states of consciousness that may distort perception and cognition. Just as in the stress–gut–toxins cycle the tendency to self-perpetuate and become persistent is obvious. Figure 2.3 illustrates the mind–body vicious circle of hyperventilation.

Pain–tension cycles: symptoms due to inappropriate adaptive responses Musculoskeletal trauma or inflammation is usually painful. But must musculoskeletal pain imply damage or could primary muscular dysfunction exist? Osteopaths theorize that pain can be generated when a joint is hypomobile or when a muscle becomes habitually tense. Such stiffness or tension may have initially been appropriate, a response to continual postural or occupational overuse or overloading, or to a sudden loading or excessive stretching. In fact, such 'checkstrap' activity is partly responsible for maintaining joint movement within its appropriate range of movement and preventing loading. This is especially the case with the spinal facet joints, which may explain why the small muscles of the back are particularly prone to developing painful and self-perpetuating local spasm. The associated hypersensitivity, though it diminishes with time and may entirely

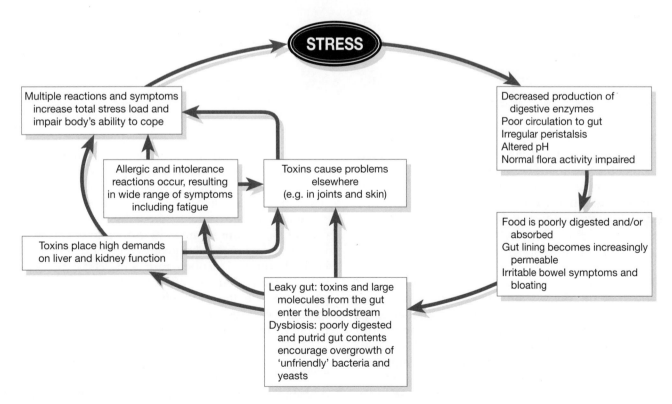

Figure 2.2 The vicious circle of stress and digestion.

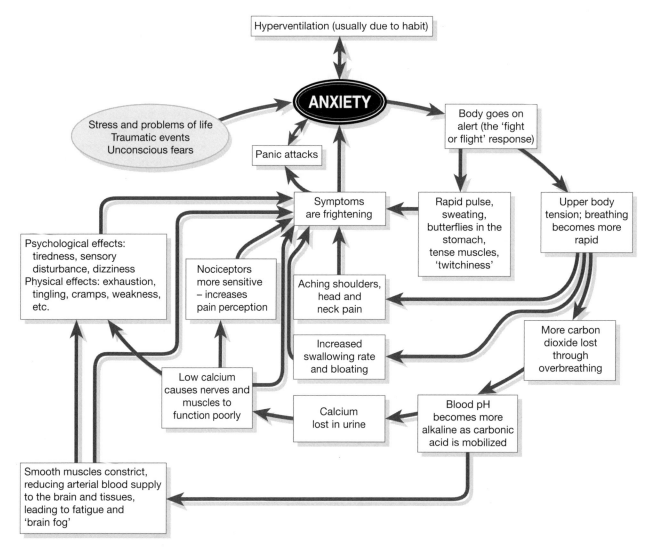

Figure 2.3 The mind–body vicious circle of hyperventilation.

remit, commonly persists at a level that leaves the affected segments prone to further spasm. The irritable muscles may then become once again tense and painful after even relatively mild overuse, overstretching or overload. Figure 2.4 illustrates the pain–tension vicious circle.

Reductionist or holistic: bottom up or top down?

If CPs have a typical view of conventional medicine then it would be of doctors targeting particular disease processes at a cellular level or simply eliminating (or 'suppressing') symptoms. In contrast to this 'bottom-up' ('treating the part') model of intervention, CTs value a more 'top-down' approach. CPs talk about large-scale influences on tissue health and use terms like 'treating the whole' or even 'dealing with the real cause' when they discuss aetiology and treatment.

Different therapies tend to focus on different levels of the organism. Osteopathy and chiropractic imply that a healthy musculoskeletal system supports other organ function and recovery; herbal medicine, complex homeopathy, nutritional therapy and naturopathy claim to stimulate organ function (for instance, by aiming to eliminate environmental and metabolic 'toxins' in order that tissues can heal); traditional acupuncture and 'classical' homeopathy—which claim to affect whole system regulatory processes—are the most obviously 'energetic' in their models of diagnosis and ways of speaking about treatment. Figure 2.5 (p. 34) characterizes the different approaches.

Differences in language and terms

A basic problem when complementary and conventional practitioners work together is that they often use very

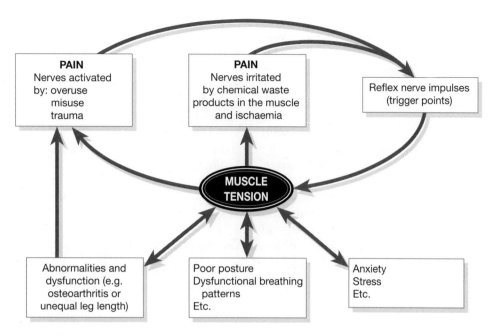

Figure 2.4   The pain–tension vicious circle.

different methods of assessing and diagnosing patients, and so they describe their findings and treatment in radically different terms. Sometimes familiar words are used but with a different meaning—for instance, acupuncturists may talk of 'taking the pulse', but they classify its characteristics using terms such as 'wiriness' or 'slipperiness', which are unrecognized in Western medicine. Similarly, the TCM understanding of terms such as the 'Spleen' and 'Kidney' is not confined to the organ itself, but rather relates to categories of processes and emotions that TCM associates with these organs: for example, the 'angry liver', the 'anxious heart', the 'melancholy spleen'. It is important, then, not to interpret terms used in complementary medicine too literally and to understand that they are sometimes used metaphorically or as a shorthand for signs, symptoms and syndromes that are not recognized (or not seen as of significance) in conventional medicine.

Vitalistic explanations of healing

A great variety of languages are used in health and community care; among them is the 'language of energy'. It is common parlance to speak about well-being as having to do with energy: we may lack it, have too much or an imbalance of it and we all know what it feels like 'to have too little'. In the CT world 'energy' may be described as being blocked or disordered, to be at work in social relations and emotional life, and as having spiritual as well as physical qualities.

This notion of 'energy' is part of the ecology of ideas in CTs—so much so that any therapy using this term can be classified as 'CT-like'. Used in this way the word 'energy' implies a subtle foundation of 'forces' that underpins and shapes our physiology. This vitalistic framework, the idea that living beings both depend on and create a sort of 'life force', is the notion that unifies the many disparate CTs. The 'energy' concept is often used by CPs as a way of explaining the basis of their work. For instance, 'vital force' is at the root of many CT systems, notably Eastern systems (TCM and ayurveda in particular), but also homeopathy. In TCM this is expressed as 'Qi'—a term usually translated simply (and inaccurately) as 'energy' or 'life energy'. In fact, the term is highly differentiated in the complex Eastern systems of medicine. Scientists, however, are bound to find such apparently inexact use of the word 'energy' hard to take: to someone with a conventional medical training the term recalls Newtonian billiard ball mechanics or the biochemical pathways of carbohydrate metabolism. 'Energy' is part of everyday speech now and in a post-Einstein world we are told we have to make sense of the world in new ways. Indeed because matter is empty space mysteriously bound up with 'energy' some pundits have used metaphors derived from quantum physics to help us understand holism, the subtle regulatory processes in the organism and the therapeutic relationship. Certainly this is a fashionable language but most people are as nonplussed by the quantum model as they are by notions of 'energy' as the mystical ground of being (another fashionable language set). If the same 'energy' is the object of both quantum reality and mysticism then it seems that for practical purposes the word is now too thinly stretched to be meaningful. Therefore we found it of little help as a way of explaining CTs' action and the basis of health in our multidisciplinary group.

On the other hand the 'energy metaphor' certainly hints at some sort of shared subjectivity. We have found that it can serve as a useful signifier for all that we do not yet understand about the mind–body–spirit–environment relationship, and the dimly perceived organizing principles involved. Perhaps when more is understood about self-organizing living systems and the interactions that sustain them then scientists will want to revisit the notion of 'life energy'. Meanwhile, a group trying to develop a common clinical language may find, as ours has, that when used carelessly the term 'energy' can be a noun that impedes the search for the adjectives and verbs needed to discuss qualities of lived experience. Our group had to confront this (and other kinds of) confusion, even at the cost of exploding comfortably shared but unexamined myths. We suspect any working group whose aim is integration will have to overcome the limitations inherent in its different professional languages and 'tribal' beliefs.

Vital energy and homeostasis: finding a basis for discussion

Because health depends on an optimal flow of materials, energy and information—between the organism and the environment and between the different parts of the organism itself—countless physiological processes must work in harmony to maintain the integrated form and function of the body–mind. This integration must occur at innumerable points and if it fails the living processes become dis-organized. Dysfunction, disease and death are the result. Yet even if cellular biology and genetics could provide a basis for an information system that was rapid and complex enough, how might such an information system coordinate function and shape structure? In order to understand homeostatic processes and why they fail, medical science is challenged to comprehend the organism as a whole system and to find ways of studying self-regulatory functions. The living body is, after all, a highly 'improbable' event—thermodynamically speaking. Because the organism is a very non-random kind of highly organized matter a great deal of information must be encoded in the organism if its form and function are to be preserved. Science already knows something of the information borne by DNA, in the immune system and in the electrical activity of the brain and has begun—for instance, using real-time brain studies—to reveal the dynamics of information and how

they could be encoded in the *whole* living organism. Homeostatic processes depend on the traffic of regulatory information, which has to be encoded, disseminated and processed by the organism in immeasurably complex ways. So we may have a parallel here between extremely subtle and dynamic regulatory information flow in the organism and what CT systems have described in diverse ways as 'subtle energy'. This makes a dialogue with science feasible; indeed only an interdisciplinary science of human vitality could comprehend the whole organism in such terms, for we did not evolve as separate organ systems and health is too big an idea for any one discipline to comprehend.

Stress, coping and an integrated medical science

Being alive entails continuous generation, growth and breaking down of cells, and the ever-changing environment and flux of feelings and thoughts. Life and awareness are inevitably dynamic and our bodies are well equipped to deal with everyday challenges, perpetually making the adjustments needed to maintain equilibrium. In order to do this, we draw on resources: biochemical and metabolic processes; structural and locomotor resources that support these processes; and our psychosocial capacity for thought and language, beliefs and desires, drives and emotions. When challenges are more intense, or too frequent, then the capacity to adapt is strained; there is simply not enough 'energy' and the struggle for 'balance' may be signalled by reversible metabolic, structural or psychological dysfunction. If the demands are too great or persistent then defence and repair systems begin to fail and pathological changes establish themselves.

Dr Hans Selye during the 1950s developed his theory of stress and the three stages of general adaptation. These are listed in Box 2.1.

Working models for collaboration

The idea that homeostasis, or our ability to maintain it, depends partly on how we react to external influences is relatively new to modern medicine (but is at the heart of traditional CT systems). It implies that individual internal factors (both physical and mental) determine a person's response to external demands, and that, although illness may be triggered by outside factors such as infections, environmental toxins and work crises, internal factors—biochemical (e.g. good diet, genetic constitution), structural (e.g. fitness, flexibility) and perhaps especially psychosocial (e.g. temperament, coping style)—will determine the outcome. Older holistic medical systems, such as TCM, ayurveda and naturopathy, have always recognized this. One possible reason why there has been such a swing towards these approaches is that they take

---

Box 2.1 Stress and the three stages of general adaptation

Stage one
This is the alarm stage, or the 'fight or flight' response. At a *biochemical* level, the stress hormones adrenaline (epinephrine) and cortisol pour from the endocrine glands. *Structurally*, muscles tense, especially around the head, neck, lower back, chest and abdomen; blood flows to the muscles and away from the gut. *Psychosocially*, thoughts and feelings focus around escape or attack: flight, fight or freeze. If there is a real cause, this emergency mode can make such urgent action possible. If there is not, then it feels like needless panic, but either way if the stressor is removed the body returns to normal functioning.

Stage two
If stress continues, the body copes but only by maintaining resistance reactions. Though this may feel normal at first, the adaptive effort is at a cost: 'energy' is used up by continual biochemical, structural and psychosocial strain. Dysregulation may be signalled by minor infections, clumsiness or discomfort, anxiety and psychological unease.

Stage three
Long-term biochemical, structural or psychosocial stress can lead to a deeper kind of exhaustion as reserves are depleted. Overall powers of recovery from any demand will be diminished and more severe health problems will develop. Whether this is expressed biochemically (e.g. as a chronic inflammatory disease), structurally (e.g. as persistent pain) or psychosocially (e.g. as serious problems with daily living) depends more on the individual than on the stressors involved.

---

account of this interplay between our inner and outer worlds. These approaches insist that prevention, and better coping, or rehabilitation and recovery can all be enhanced by mobilizing the self-regulation processes (and this is obviously in tune with the current wish to take a new kind of responsibility for one's health). An integrative model of susceptibility and resilience suggests that the three categories of adaptive processes are interdependent. Therefore an intervention that eases the strain or improves adaptive capacity in any one realm—biochemical, structural or psychosocial—will tend to increase resilience in another. This is thought to be the case irrespective of how, or where, the problem has manifested.

The effects of one category on another can be illustrated by a number of examples, for instance:

- effects of biochemistry on structure: diet (e.g. high fat intake) can lead to hardened arteries
- effects of biochemistry on psychology: diet (e.g. low blood sugar) can affect feelings and sense of well-being
- effects of structure on biochemistry: a narrowed artery causes ischaemia
- effects of structure on psychology: upper body tension and chest breathing can increase anxiety
- effects of psychology on biochemistry: stress makes diabetes more brittle
- effects of psychology on structure: anger, sadness or fear may be expressed as muscle tension and can determine pain distribution.

One implication of this integrated approach to 'psycho-somatics' is that we should re-examine the commonly held idea that if someone presents with psychosocial difficulties then the appropriate intervention must also be psychosocial. Working in a team that includes a naturopath, at the MHC we were challenged to consider new GP options for someone with problems of daily living (stressed, can't cope, tired all the time, aches and pains). Might they benefit at least as much by improving their diet, a simple exercise regimen or a relaxation technique as from counselling? The argument is that people will feel better and cope better if, for instance, their metabolism is relieved of the burden of food intolerance (biochemical), their circulation and muscle tone improve (structural) and they are taught the skill of relaxing their body (psychosocial) whose constant tension is making them so tired. In our team we have begun to allow the word 'vitality' back into our language of health care and we would like to find ways of making it stronger. We would never deny, however, that supporting a patient who feels 'tired all the time' through a lifestyle change is not easy; nor can we claim always to have been successful! Our team have found the practice's 'stress management groups' a very useful intervention (we suspect they are relevant in a wide range of long-term health problems) and we use leaflets and tapes as a cost-effective way to promote these approaches. They are an important element of integrated care and potentially highly cost effective.

A working classification of medical treatments and CTs

The three-categories model also provides a basis for classifying the effects of medical interventions, whether conventional and complementary, upon the organism. Any treatment can be categorized as working predominantly in one of the three. The fourth category embraces 'vitalistic' therapies whose practitioners use an entirely different rationale for diagnosing and prescribing. Their effects on the organism nevertheless depend on final pathways that must involve categories one to three.

1. *Biochemical/nutritional*—these affect how cells, tissues and organs work to keep metabolic processes (of building up/breaking down) in balance; examples include drugs, nutritional supplements, herbs and low-potency homeopathic remedies. These approaches act at the *cellular* level.

2. *Structural/biomechanical*—these affect how mechanical factors impact on transport, movement and support; examples include surgery, physiotherapy, massage and medical acupuncture. These approaches act at the *organ systems* level.

3. *Psycho/social*—these affect how ideas, knowledge, feelings, relationships, actions, etc. support or constrain the capacity to cope and adapt; examples include

psychotherapies, behavioural approaches, meditation, health promotion and social work. These approaches act at the *personal and interpersonal* level.

4. *Regulatory/vitalistic*—these affect how 'vital forces' shape and regulate all mind–body processes (i.e. systemic information flow or totality of emergent self-regulatory processes); examples include high-potency homeopathic remedies, traditional acupuncture and traditional Chinese herbal medicine and spiritual healing.

These are illustrated in Figure 2.5.

Summary

A common language will be crucial when cooperating in patient management. Our collaborative group has developed a modified biopsychosocial language of stress and coping. Our working model of the roles and relationships of CTs and their interface with conventional medicine can be summarized as follows:

- health is defined as successful adaptation of the organism
- this depends on three interdependent kinds of capacity (biochemical, structural, psychosocial)
- the person's 'internal milieu' and environment (biochemical, structural, psychosocial) can support or undermine adaptation
- to a degree the three categories can be dealt with as clinically separate
- some CPs postulate an emergent fourth category (which we imagine as implying a whole system regulatory influence)
- our agreed working model of CTs is that they influence adaptive processes in one of these four possible ways.

Summary

Some common features of CM approaches:

- CPs tend towards a multifactorial view of illness
- disease is caused not only by biochemical disturbances
- biomechanical, psychosocial and spiritual causes are important
- the body has a capacity for self-repair, given the appropriate conditions
- therapeutic intervention aims to restore balance and catalyse healing responses
- use a package of care—i.e. modify lifestyle, change diet, exercise, together with a specific treatment (e.g. homeopathy)
- an holistic approach is not unique to CT.

Do CTs have anything in common with conventional medicine?
How cells, tissues and organs work to keep metabolic processes (of building up/breaking down) in balance:

- drugs
- nutritional supplements
- diet
- herbal medicines
- low-potency homeopathics.

These approaches act at a cellular level.

How mechanical factors impact on organ systems, transport, movement, support:

- surgery
- physiotherapy
- massage
- osteopathy
- chiropractic
- medical acupuncture.

These approaches act at the organ systems level.

How ideas, knowledge, feelings, relationships, actions, etc. support or constrain capacity to cope and adapt:

- psychotherapies
- behavioural approaches
- health promotion information
- social work
- hypnotherapy
- meditation.

These approaches act at the personal and interpersonal level.

How 'vital forces' shape and regulate all mind–body processes (i.e. systemic information flow and totality of emergent self-regulatory processes):

- high-potency homeopathics
- spiritual healing
- traditional acupuncture
- traditional herbalism.

These approaches claim to effect some sort of whole-system coherence.

RESEARCH

The challenge inherent in researching CTs

If CTs help make effective use of resources compared with other treatment options, they should find their place in the mainstream and thrive. But, given the limitations on time and funding, CTs are likely to be rationed, which means we have to find ways of using them efficiently in mainstream health care. It will be the

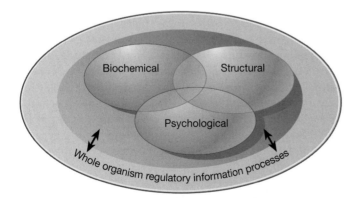

Figure 2.5 Whole-person health care.

'value for money' question that determines whether CT services continue to develop a role in relation to mainstream health care. How then are practitioners to establish whether CTs provide this? This section will explore this question.

Can CTs be used in an evidence-linked way?

Good research is an essential aspect of the integration process. Randomized clinical trials (RCT) are accepted as the gold standard for evidence. So if RCT results that are relevant to the questions an integrative team face are available then these would form an important part of their rationale. As yet though there are too few for, although at least 5000 have already been published, this is a tiny fraction of the numbers of drug RCTs conducted. Can the availability of RCTs be the key determinant for introducing CTs then? Probably not, but in the cause of evidence-based medicine we have to proceed 'using the best available evidence'. As the summary at the end of this chapter shows, relatively few RCTs of complementary therapies have been done. Therefore it is not yet possible to base absolute guidelines for using complementary therapies in common conditions on RCTs. We should take this as a lack of evidence *for* benefit rather than as evidence of *no* benefit.

The RCT approach has been criticized for a number of important reasons but RCTs undoubtedly do have their place (despite opinions expressed to the contrary) as well as their inadequacies. With careful design and painstaking application, ways of rigorously researching CTs while also taking account of individual variation and practitioner variability will emerge. However, such studies will be less straightforward to conduct than randomized drug trials and, rather than demonstrating objective change—whether biochemical or histological—they will often rely on what patients say about their improved well-being. A discussion of a parallel approach for gathering evidence—outcomes research—is given later in this section.

Evidence-based medicine (EBM) aims 'to eliminate the use of expensive, ineffective, or dangerous medical decision making'. Evidence-based practice (EBP) is currently being promoted in all areas of health care; it is an 'approach to health care that promotes the collection, interpretation and integration of valid, important and applicable patient-reported, clinician-observed, and research-derived evidence. The best available evidence, moderated by patient circumstance and preferences, is applied to improve the quality of clinical judgements.' Importantly, this definition does not make the RCT a mandatory element in EBM and it takes into account that much of what is done in conventional health care—most surgery and physiotherapy, for example, and counselling

therapy too—has hardly been the subject of RCTs. Moreover, it is estimated that only a quarter of what is published in the best professional journals is based on RCTs: clinical case studies, qualitative research and basic research all figure there too.

There is no treatment—conventional or other—that does not also entail non-specific effects: human factors, some of them disparagingly termed 'placebo effects'. And these may be crucial to the outcome of a healing encounter. Certainly, good communication will affect patients' adherence and determine whether they feel enabled by a consultation. Some practitioners believe that the biggest influence that CTs will have is in bringing these effects to the forefront of medicine. These elements include the therapeutic setting, the personality of the therapist, the amount of time given to patients, and even the very words spoken. They are also, however, the very elements that RCTs are usually designed to cancel out. CAM researchers argue, conversely, that rather than being lumped together in the placebo arm these elements should be disentangled and studied systematically, so as to understand and harness their therapeutic power for the benefit of all those involved in all health care provision. The 'complexity of caring', in David Reilly's words, is difficult but not impossible to quantify.

What then, constitutes good enough evidence on which to base the introduction of CTs into mainstream practice? Clinical impression is evidence of a sort, but all practitioners like to think they are effective: why else would we be practitioners? Therein lie several potential problems: first, we might be less effective than we like to think; secondly, therefore it will be difficult to reflect 'objectively' on our effectiveness; thirdly, even if a rigorous study did show a complementary practitioner was effective, to what extent would it have been determined by the presence of the CP rather than their technical skill in the therapy? Complementary therapies claim to catalyse regulatory processes, but how much of that increased resilience is due to a patient's own effort or changed circumstance rather than the technique used or the practitioner's presence? GPs face similar questions about their own field and effectiveness, for the effectiveness and comparative cost effectiveness of everyday health care would actually be extremely difficult to establish. It would mean evaluating the outcomes of all the complex, multidimensional (and often unknown) factors that impinge on real outcomes. Because of these complexities it may be more accurate to speak of *evidence-linked* CAM practice—that is, practice established with a reasonable expectation that it will meet a perceived need, practice that is reflective and incorporates an outcome measure, and practice that nevertheless mirrors a therapist's real way of working, unconstrained by the need to conform to an intricate research protocol. This has been our aim in the Marylebone project.

A view of CTs from the outside

Doctors often make criticisms about the claimed benefits of CTs. Some of these points are well made, but can be applied equally to conventional therapies. Some typical criticisms are listed in Box 2.2.

Potential research areas

Despite the above criticisms, there are a number of areas where CTs appear to be of benefit. Some have been revealed by existing studies; in others anecdotal

---

Box 2.2 Typical criticisms of CTs (from Bandolier)
• *Poor-quality research* Better-designed studies of CTs tend to have negative results, and only the lower-quality studies are positive. If experimenter bias exists in the usual clinical situation, it is particularly relevant for research done by CPs in whom belief in the therapy's value is high. • *Many diseases are naturally self-limiting* It is as well to remember that, unless rigorous study methods are ensured, it will be difficult to say whether an apparent benefit can be ascribed to the intervention or to the natural course of the disease. • *Many diseases have a cyclical history* In allergies, multiple sclerosis, arthritis and gastrointestinal problems like IBS where the natural course is up and down, patients tend to seek relief when the condition is particularly bad. So the apparent benefit can be ascribed to the natural course of the condition rather than to the therapy. Again, only rigorous study design can distinguish between the two. • *Mood improvement or cure?* CPs often have much more time to spend with their patient than a harassed GP loaded down with guidelines and tight budgets. Is it any wonder that they make patients feel better? That mood change is sometimes taken to be the cure. • *Psychological investment in alternatives* Alternative healing can involve a commitment of considerable financial expense, huge amounts of time, extensive family involvement and a large investment of belief that the treatment will have some effect. With such an investment, it is not surprising that many people will find some value in the treatment. • *Placebo effect* Both the above points contribute to the placebo effect, which can be seen as the natural course of things. There will always be some people who benefit without an intervention—for instance, some people need no pain relief after surgery—so making any intervention that claims to reduce pain after surgery will surely work in some people at least. • *Some patients will 'hedge' their bets* If a person is under the doctor for 6 months and then visits a homeopath, a condition that has been slowly resolving over the course of time may finally show results. The fact that the poor GP persevered with the patient for the previous 6 months is forgotten in the 'glamour of magic' of the homeopathic remedy. • *The original diagnosis may be wrong* Bandolier (see Further reading Websites) has highlighted the difficulty of diagnosis. If the original diagnosis (e.g. of cancer) was wrong, then claimed 'miraculous' cures may be less than miraculous.

---

reports suggest effectiveness. A third category of conditions—where conventional treatment is unsatisfactory, is inappropriate or is being awaited—offers opportunities for ethical studies to be developed even though we have no reason as yet to believe that CTs could help. The areas of potentially fruitful research are listed in Box 2.3.

Research methods and levels of evidence

In a cost-limited funding system like the NHS, available funds have to be directed towards the most effective treatments, whether conventional or complementary. Therefore a number of research methods are going to be needed if we are to explain the popularity of complementary medicine and their impact on the public health and health expenditure.

Essentially research evidence is hierarchical. There are grades of evidence and levels of complexity to research methods, but the foundation of research is everyday experience, so at its most basic it involves (clinical) observations and descriptions. Only through hunches do we first suspect something clinically significant is going on. At the MHC our hunch was that certain aspects of CT could be valuable additions to primary care practice. Some RCTs and systematic reviews backed this up but we clearly had to introduce some rigorous ways of confirming these hunches. So, in the initial phase of our project, we have tried to base our practice on a naturalistic, qualitative pragmatic approach. It is an approach that mirrors the ordinary process of referral and CT consultation in order to capture what happens in the real world of primary care.

Levels of evidence

Sackett's hierarchy of evidence has provoked much unresolved controversy about the kind of evidence that is actually most relevant to practice; for example, controlled

---

Box 2.3 Potential research areas
• Persistent or relapsing illness with little or no tissue damage: e.g. IBS, headache and migraine, fibromyalgia syndrome, insomnia, chronic fatigue and premenstrual syndrome (PMS) • Areas where no effective conventional treatment is available: e.g. viral illnesses, traumatic injuries, surgical wounds, hepatitis and neurological diseases • Areas where conventional treatment is unsatisfactory or requires continual use of conventional drugs: e.g. allergic and chronic inflammatory diseases of gut, joints, skin and respiratory tract • Areas where elective surgery has been proposed, but immediate attention is unnecessary: e.g. fibroid tumours, gallstones and haemorrhoids • Areas where conventional treatment is inappropriate, the nature of the disease intractable or the patient determinedly non-compliant

trials often restrict the kind of patients recruited, whereas cohort studies better reflect normal patterns of patient management. The hierarchy of levels of evidence is briefly:

1. A Systematic reviews/meta-analyses
   B Randomized controlled trials
   C Experimental designs
2. A Cohort control studies
   B Case–control studies
3. A Consensus conference
   B Expert opinion
   C Observational study
   D Other types of study, e.g. interview based, local audit
   E Quasiexperimental, qualitative design
4. Personal communication.

Reasons for the lack of research in CTs

There are many reasons for the yawning gaps in the evidence for and against complementary therapies. To start with, CPs have only recently begun to get involved in research and as yet those who do want to engage generally do not have the backing of university departments, statisticians, large databases and full-time research staff, which are all necessary elements in a research culture. As complementary therapists' professional bodies develop and academic groups form, coherent research programmes will develop. Funding is hard to find, however, and will remain so; for instance, pharmaceutical companies and commercial interests (who fund most of the clinical pharmaceutical trials) have no reason to fund CT research and there are few financially attractive patents to acquire in the CT field, even in herbal medicine.

Problems with RCTs of complementary therapies

We all welcome the clarity that RCTs provide about pharmacotherapies, and they have become the scientific foundation of modern clinical therapeutics. Yet they are relatively new and, before their advent in the 1940s, there was no structured way of determining a treatment's potential for cure or harm. However, though the precision such trials bring to drug prescribing is welcome, they were in an important sense specifically designed to throw the humanistic baby (i.e. the non-specific effects of the therapeutic relationship) out with the bath water of other confounding variables (e.g. regression to the mean, patient variability). Complementary therapies, in contrast, intentionally involve non-specific elements, depend on practitioner skill and generally entail multidimensional packages of care. Obviously they are quite different from just taking a pill. They also appear to be most relevant in

chronic diseases and for patients with relapsing dysfunction—the sorts of condition where conventional medicine is often unsatisfactory or relatively ineffective. Because it is difficult to establish hard end-points by which to determine objective outcomes, these health problems are also more difficult to evaluate using the conventional RCT.

Placebo-controlled randomized double-blind trials are valuable precisely because they can test for causality, determine effect size, assess risks and benefits of treatments, and because they minimize selection and measurement bias. Although many CAM interventions are difficult to blind or have no satisfactory placebos, CAM researchers have tried to address these methodological problems and overcome at least some of them. For instance, acupuncture researchers have developed a 'placebo needle' that looks exactly like an acupuncture needle, and causes the same dull pain sensation, but does not penetrate the skin. This might make it possible to explore the specific physiological effects of acupuncture.

Most of the available RCT studies have been done by doctors, who are only lately taking an interest in complementary medicine. Being hospital based, such medical researchers have usually focused on the sorts of condition commonly seen there. Take, as an example, the research into acupuncture for postoperative and chemotherapy nausea, a condition in fact rarely seen by CPs in typical practice. Because hospital-based researchers have access to large numbers of this kind of patient (who have the sorts of problem that are relatively easy to measure) they have been studied intensely. In contrast, chronic fatigue syndrome (CFS) or persistent back pain is something hospital doctors seldom see and so relatively little research has been done on the role of CT in conditions like these, even though they are the kind of problem CPs treat regularly.

An RCT will focus on a particular therapy and a particular disease in order to make a definite statement about this therapy and how it applies to this one condition. For instance, if a therapy were shown to be effective for IBS that would not mean it was necessarily helpful in any other condition. Can it therefore be appropriate to make generalized statements about research-derived evidence for complementary therapies as a whole? Clearly not. Questions like 'does acupuncture work?' or 'can IBS be treated with CTs?' are completely meaningless. Furthermore, CTs depend very much on the skills of individual practitioners. So, although a trial might show that acupuncture is a good treatment for migraine, practitioners of acupuncture actually operate on the basis of several different theories and practise in diverse ways.

Randomization and placebo control entail special problems when RCT methods are applied to CTs.

- The RCT was designed to investigate the effects of drugs. CT treatment is quite different (particularly bodywork and movement-oriented therapies) and the therapist's work is not at all like giving pills.

- Randomization neglects patients' right to choose, yet motivation towards CT is an important factor in real clients' help-seeking behaviour; conventional trials appear to be incompatible with patients' need to participate actively in the therapeutic process.

- Results of RCTs are often of limited practical usefulness in CAM; for example, patients in RCTs are often not like the patients CPs see in everyday practice—patients in real life often have multiple problems, whereas designers of RCTs usually use exclusion criteria that tailor a homogeneous sample.

- RCTs are costly; there are insufficient resources to use them widely to cover all the major CAM interventions in all the common conditions of interest.

- Publication bias is significant; funding for RCTs generally comes from the pharmaceutical industry, which has the power to suppress unwanted results, so evidence synthesized in meta-analyses and systematic reviews may be positively biased.

- An additional argument that may apply in rare instances is that the methodological soundness of 'blinded' RCTs can be challenged because the patients and doctors may easily guess the treatment group because of side-effects in the active treatment; these well-described methodological shortcomings are rarely addressed when evaluating the evidence for a treatment.

- Selection of a control treatment that can be blinded is difficult (e.g. how can you give placebo massage, placebo rolfing or placebo psychotherapy?).

- It can be difficult to turn the results of research into practice. For instance, a placebo-controlled trial of healing might show that real healing is more effective than sham for a certain condition, such as migraine. But that still would not tell you whether healing is preferable as a treatment over one of the other approaches researched and found to be effective for migraine (e.g. environmental medicine, herbal medicine, relaxation therapy, manipulation or acupuncture).

- Even though a single positive study can be significant, systematic reviews or meta-analyses are said to be better still. These methods have been criticized, particularly on the grounds of publication bias: the implication being that negative studies do not get published often enough to allow the systematic equation to include all the relevant evidence.

Until more trials of CT are available, opportunities for meta-analyses are few. Several such reviews have now been carried out but even they have reached different conclusions. These overviews do, however, appear to suggest that homeopathic treatments, acupuncture and manipulative therapies (osteopathy and chiropractic) have significant clinical benefits. Obviously, though, such reviews do not tell us whether therapy X works in condition Y, which is what practitioners really want to know.

The problem of non-specific factors

RCTs are intended to bracket off personal, interpersonal and contextual factors as unwanted variables. Therefore this experimental approach potentially distorts the ordinary processes of practice. At some point it may be highly desirable to do this when studying the effectiveness of a drug (especially when a treatment may involve potential risks); however, such a method is arguably inappropriate when studying any intervention that explicitly entails human skills and 'presence factors' as well as technical factors.

In real life, practitioners do much more than prescribe; they also counsel, facilitate, empathize, teach, advise and offer hope, give confrontation, support and sympathy—activities that do not conform to the RCT yardstick. These activities may therefore have come to be undervalued in a healthcare system ostensibly rooted in bioscience, but they are attributes that patients value very highly. In CTs it is difficult to separate the practitioner's 'art' (e.g. caring presence, conviction and communication skills) from the science (i.e. knowledge of, for example, technical specifics, points and prescriptions). Competent practice in nursing and in conventional medicine as well as in complementary medicine involves far more than a technical activity like prescribing. These aspects contribute to what has been called the 'therapeutic relationship' and it is difficult (though not impossible) to embrace the part played by these activities in an RCT study. However, because they are so intrinsic to good practice and enhance the benefit and improve outcomes of every kind of intervention, they have to be somehow accounted for in research designs.

It is because these potent 'non-specific factors' affect all forms of therapy that RCTs try to account for and subtract their influence from the total outcome—hence placebo control, blinding and randomization. Complementary therapies, however, profoundly blur all the distinctions that biomedicine has so carefully constructed: between subjective experience and objective reality, mind and body, practitioner and patient, therapy and therapist, the modern and the medieval. There can be no doubt that CTs and their practitioners are a powerful source of these non-specific factors: it would be naïve to suppose that the touch and time they entail—and the sense that the patient's problem is understood and can be treated—do not significantly contribute to positive outcome. Another essential influence on real-world outcomes is how a patient engages with and takes part in a treatment process—perhaps especially so in chronic illness, which is arguably the area where CPs do their best work. One of CAM's great strengths is its capacity to generate powerful beliefs and expectations in practitioners and clients. If in the future mainstream medicine reclaims these non-specific processes it will be largely because CAM research has made it possible to ignore their importance.

Outcomes research*

Although the validity and rigour of RCTs is undoubted, their status as the 'gold standard' of effectiveness in CAM is open to question for a number of reasons. For instance, rather like psychotherapy, CAM entails complex interventions. Early research in psychotherapy relied exclusively on RCTs. By focusing on specific aspects, this approach could be rigorous, but its internal validity was at the expense of real-world relevance. This is so because, rather like CTs, the practice and outcomes of psychotherapy depend on a complex package of human factors as well as technical skill. Inevitably, they involve various intrapersonal and interpersonal factors. Therefore, if research is to be true to such complex therapies, more naturalistic approaches have had to be developed.

Moreover, where complementary treatments for chronic disease are concerned, it can be difficult to conduct RCTs over long time periods, for the costs would be too great. Also, it is not generally practical to keep everyone blinded where treatments are physical (as in many types of CM), or when patients state a treatment preference or need to be actively involved in lifestyle change. These considerations suggest that CM research calls for a multistaged or 'mosaic' approach, which can augment the RCT.

Large-scale outcomes studies can be just as valid as RCTs as a way of assessing CTs, provided certain conditions are met. For instance, if effects are large and obvious, then RCTs are unnecessary. And, if the natural course of a disease is known and predictable or the baseline status is fairly stable, then clear effects observed over a long period can be very persuasive. Chronic, painful, atopic or inflammatory conditions, such as rheumatological diseases or irritable bowel syndrome (IBS), represent a large part of complementary practitioners' caseload. Such cases generally fit these criteria, for the patients usually have a long history and previous conventional treatment will often have been ineffective or even counterproductive.

A single observed case does not tell us much, but where a large number of cases can be observed for a long time in well-designed studies the results can be convincing, particularly if many different practitioners are involved. In such large-scale outcomes studies, evidence of effectiveness would actually be more real and useful than evidence from RCTs, which would anyway be quite impractical. Because State or independent medical insurance organizations have a strong interest in cost–effectiveness and demand management, they need to establish such large databases of treatment outcomes, for, unless they do so, questions about the overall effectiveness of most forms of chronic disease management will remain unanswered. Such research will call for new kinds of documentation systems that record activity and then allow reliable tracking and evaluation of long-term outcomes. With the cooperation of State and independent medical insurance organizations, such studies become easier and the further development of electronic records and intranets will make this kind of research increasingly practical.

Outcomes research in CAM can be an alternative to an RCT if certain conditions are met:

- The question is about general practical effectiveness rather than efficacy.
- The question of whether effects are specific or nonspecific is irrelevant (as it is when the intervention is patient oriented and practice guided, or involves patient cooperation and learning or individualization and variability).
- The natural course and prognosis of the condition are well described.
- The patients to be studied have a well-documented history of their previous treatments.
- Clinical experience leads us to expect the treatment effects to be large.
- A large number of patients can be entered over long time-periods (i.e. years).
- In recurrent or fluctuating diseases, the research period covers at least the period that is known, from the literature, to be representative of the average time to relapse.
- A well-known, widely used and valid outcome measure, such as a visual analogue scale (VAS) or the Short Form 36 (SF-36) scale, can be used so that results may be seen and interpreted in relation to other studies in both CAM and conventional medicine.

Given these conditions, observational outcomes studies are probably the best and most cost-effective option. Ultimately, as no single research methodology can deliver all we need to know about service use, effectiveness, efficacy, safety and treatment preferences, outcomes research should be just one facet of a multilevel strategy

---

* This section is based on a chapter by Walach H, Jonas W, Lewith G. The role of outcomes research in evaluating complementary and alternative medicine. In Lewith G 2002 Clinical research in complementary therapies, Churchill Livingstone, Edinburgh

for CAM research. This is because, even where there is evidence for specific efficacy from RCTs, the data will usually have been derived in what amounts to an artificial setting. Outcomes data can put RCT evidence into context and make it more practically useful. In fact, methods with high external validity (e.g. outcomes studies) but low internal validity (e.g. RCTs) actually complement one another. Ideally, RCTs and outcomes research should be executed together, perhaps by nesting one within the other or by following an RCT with a long-term observational phase.

Can outcomes studies be made to work?

Although long-term observational studies entail many challenges (e.g. handling patient attrition and missing data), the procedures required are no different from standard procedures in clinical trials. Such studies are difficult, entailing at least as much planning as an RCT; their statistical evaluation can be even more complicated and, in addition, initial research will be needed to establish the meaning and relevance of the outcomes chosen. Only a broad interdisciplinary approach can achieve all this. Perhaps this is why CAM research has, so far, almost completely neglected the non-randomized or quasiexperimental comparison, even though this type of research focuses on natural groups and stays close to clinical practice, therefore honouring patients' and doctors' preferences. Outcomes studies are also often rejected as a way forward for CM research because pure observation can distinguish the effects of treatment from the effects of time only indirectly. However, waiting list-controlled RCTs with open treatment can meet this objection, and such an approach has been used with positive results in a recent study of healing.

An example of a successful outcomes study is an ongoing study of 5000 patients who had sought acupuncture or homeopathy. Results so far reveal a patient-reported improvement rate of roughly 70% following acupuncture treatments in patients whose mean disease duration was 8 years. Benefit was reflected in a 10–20-point improvement in their SF-36. Whether or not these results will remain stable over the 4-year follow-up, this study already provides a strong case for the clinical usefulness of acupuncture and homeopathy. It cannot, however, tell us whether these methods have specific efficacy or only non-specific effectiveness. However, this is of little importance to patients seeking symptom relief for chronic illness when conventional medicine has proved relatively ineffective; nor would it matter to an individual purchaser, a State health service or insurance company, as long as the treatment actually reduces the demand for other items of treatment expenditure.

David Reilly and colleagues are using a mosaic approach in their research work on homeopathy. The research mosaic explores three overlapping profiles. The first was the narrow and highly specific question of whether homeopathic treatment effects vary from placebo. This was addressed by a sequence of RCTs. The second stage taught a group of GPs to prescribe homeopathic remedies in everyday practice, and then involved them in a series of 'action research' cycles following up more than 1000 prescriptions made by members of the group and analysing the results centrally. The third layer is an observational assessment of holistic care (which includes but is not dominated by homeopathy) followed by a prospective waiting-list-as-control study. This phase is linked to a qualitative research study evaluating the factors that make a consultation 'therapeutic' in its own right. Placed together, these jigsaw pieces build a multidimensional evidence profile that can begin to capture the complexities of real practice.

Evidence-linked CT practice: rigour and relevance

Outcomes research can be a valuable tool for evaluating CT interventions. Although it cannot replace controlled trials, it can and should complement them because it adds practical relevance and external validity to the otherwise detached rigour of RCTs. It is also an important instrument for gathering data that cannot be gleaned from RCTs: data on long-term effects, on patients who do not wish to be randomized, and on patients with strong preferences or with strong belief systems—in short, on typical users of CTs. We see our work at Marylebone on rapid clinical evaluation cycles as preparatory work for this.

What the CT field needs is a way of collecting and reviewing everyday practice and of putting together large sets of such outcomes data. However, we would never deny that outcomes research needs RCTs in order to strengthen and qualify its results. However, too few RCT studies have been done in this area to build a precise evidence base for using complementary therapies based on RCTs. Sackett's hierarchy of evidence puts RCTs near the top, but his definition of EBM emphasizes the need to use the best evidence available. So at MHC we have begun to develop evidence-based complementary medicine on the basis of 'research-derived evidence' as well as 'patient-reported, clinician-observed evidence'. On that basis there is enough evidence to justify their use in certain common conditions, and this chapter presents some options for exploring that evidence base. We have responded to Sackett's advice that the EBM process be 'moderated by patient circumstance and preference . . . to improve the quality of clinical judgements' by developing our own approach to evidence-*linked* complementary medicine practice that is connected to an evidence base and that strives continually to be reflective and re-evaluate itself. Later in this book we present our guidelines as a starting point for an action research process for using CTs in mainstream practice. This approach is justifiable given that CTs are low risk, patients are keen to have access to them and a great deal of primary care work is tentative. Day to day, it can be validated only by experience and is reshaped by patients' reports of their experience and preference, and by rigorous clinical judgement. With this aim in view we introduced a patient-centred measure, the Measure Your Own Medical Outcome Profile (MYMOP), to assess and monitor patients' experience of CT effects. MYMOP is a simple open-ended questionnaire designed for use in general practice, which allows a patient to choose the two symptoms they most want to see get better, to note how these symptoms interfere with one significant aspect of daily living and to record their sense of overall well-being. At the initial consultation the patient is carefully helped to identify the symptoms to be tracked and marks against these four items on a 0–6 Lickert scale. Thereafter, clinical change is tracked in terms of these four markers. Patterson's original study shows the form to be not only valid and responsive but also applicable to CT practice.

Action research

'Action research' is a term first used in the 1940s, and attributed to Kurt Lewin. It is more a style of research than a specific method. It entails cycles of: identifying a goal, devising a plan, carrying out plan, assessing outcomes, revising plan/changing the goal, and choosing a new goal. The term has come to be identified with research in which the researchers work with people rather than undertake research on them. Its focus is practical, getting practitioners to engage systematically in the research process—identifying problems, seeking and implementing practical solutions, and monitoring and reflecting on the process and outcomes of change. Although not synonymous with qualitative research, action research typically draws on qualitative methods such as interviews and observation. Participation is fundamental to this type of research as it demands that participants perceive the need to change and are willing to play an active part both in the research and in the process of change. Hence the level of commitment required goes beyond simply agreeing to answer questions or be observed. It is concerned with inquiry involving close integration of experience, action and reflection:

Action research methodologies aim to integrate action and reflection, so that the knowledge gained in the inquiry is directly relevant to the issues being studied. It aims at helping the individual practitioner develop skills of reflective practice. It also aims to help organizational members develop a culture of inquiry, learning organizations or communities of inquiry . . . The newer approaches to action research place emphasis on full integration of action and reflection and on increased collaboration between all those involved in the inquiry project . . .

> (Peter Reason, Centre for Action Research in Professional Practice School of Management, University of Bath)

This research style is particularly suited to identifying problems in clinical practice and helping develop potential solutions in order to improve practice. For this reason, it is increasingly being used in health-related settings.

RESEARCH INTO SPECIFIC CONDITIONS

One of the problems of basing evidence-linked complementary treatment exclusively on the available RCTs is the sparse number of such studies available in CAM. There are many reasons for this. Some of them are not confined to CTs but also apply to conventional disciplines. They include lack of funding, insufficient patient numbers, lack of research skills amongst CPs, frequently a lack of an academic organization with the accompanying resources, support and supervision, difficulty in undertaking meta-analyses and review owing to the poor quality of early studies, and lack of standardization of CT treatment, making responses to treatment hard to interpret. It has also been difficult to design appropriate controls for some CTs (e.g. acupuncture, manipulation) and conduct blinded studies. Currently RCTs do not cover the range of conditions and the range of therapies that primary care practitioners might want to consider in their planning. Hence at the present state of research it is necessary to cast the net wider. It makes sense to begin with those complementary health systems with the longest tradition, highest levels of training and professional organization within the vast body of 'alternative and complementary' medicine, as these currently provide the greatest potential for integration or collaboration with mainstream practitioners and institutions. They include:

- acupuncture/TCM
- herbal medicine
- homeopathy
- massage therapy
- naturopathy/nutritional therapy
- osteopathy/chiropractic
- stress management/hypnotherapy/relaxation.

When trawling for evidence one should also bear in mind that there may not be any research on a specific condition, for instance on acupuncture for carpal tunnel syndrome, but there may be research on a wider category, for example on acupuncture for pain. The research literature is also not representative of practice: just because a therapy has been researched in a particular condition this does not imply that this therapy should be used in preference to others.

So it is not always easy to advise or select a CT treatment for particular conditions; unlike conventional medicine CT is rarely a question of treatment X and condition Y. For instance, acupuncture treatment has been shown by research to be valuable in such diverse and unrelated conditions as chemotherapy nausea, angina pain, stroke rehabilitation and persistent back pain (chronic back pain can be effectively treated with manipulation, relaxation therapy or acupuncture).

Box 2.4 gives some general guidance on interpretation of the research evidence.

Research can also be difficult to turn into practice. For example, a placebo-controlled trial gives information about whether real homeopathy is better than placebo, but it does not show whether a homeopath, acupuncturist, GP or a psychotherapist would be the best choice of therapist. The choice instead has to rely on:

- patients' preferences (and aversions)
- patients' health beliefs
- patients' motivation and ability to engage in and adhere to advice the CP might give (e.g. lifestyle change and dietary regimen, etc.)
- patients' convictions about what is most likely to work
- the available published evidence
- the availability of an appropriate practitioner who is properly trained, qualified and accredited.

Having said this, there has been a considerable amount of research on CAM in recent years, so increasingly an indication of the potential benefit of CTs in certain conditions will become part of evidence-based practice.

Cardiovascular conditions

Angina

There is evidence that acupuncture improves workload, pain and use of nitroglycerine; however, there may be no difference between true and sham acupuncture.

Heart disease

The Ornish regimen—a multifactorial approach (diet, exercise, relaxation and support group)—reduces stenosis as measured by heart scans. But there is no research on whether this leads to improved survival.

A Cretan Mediterranean diet adapted to a Western population protects against coronary heart disease much more efficiently than does a prudent diet. Thus, it appears that the favourable life expectancy of the Cretans could be largely due to their diet.

Certain simple changes to diet (e.g. essential fatty acid supplementation) may not be of benefit, however. The type of fatty acid is likely to be of importance here.

Clinical trials support the use of hawthorn (*Crataegus* spp.) in congestive heart disease due to ischaemia or hypertension, and cardiac insufficiency (particularly that relating to NYHA stages I and II), and of ginseng (*Panax ginseng*) for congestive heart failure. Other trials indicate the usefulness of grapeseed (*Vitis vinifera*) and the Italian or Mediterranean cypress (*Cupressus sempervirens*), which are also rich in similar antioxidants, for their angioprotective qualities.

Good evidence exists that psychosocial interventions (e.g. relaxation) given during rehabilitation improve quantity and quality of life.

Hypertension

Homeopathy shows no effect here. The nutritional recommendations (e.g. lose weight, eat less salt) are well known, and some vegetarian diets may be of additional benefit.

Box 2.4 Interpretation of research evidence

When you read or listen to views and research on complementary or alternative medicine, bear the following in mind.

- Don't jump to conclusions.
- Try to distinguish between promising advances, reported as scientific news, and public health recommendations.
- Keep your scepticism in working order.
- Notice where the information is coming from.
- Use your own logic and common sense.
- Be wary when studies are cited to sell you a product.

Beware words commonly—and erroneously—used to report scientific studies.

breakthrough	so overworked it is meaningless
contributes to/is linked to/ is associated with	none of these terms means 'causes'
doubles the risk	may or may not be meaningful: are you told what your risk was in the first place? If your risk is 1 in 1 000 000 and you double it, that is still only 1 in 500 000. If your risk is 1 in 100 and increases by 25%, that is 1 in 80, which may be cause for concern
proves	scientific studies gather evidence in a systematic way but they seldom prove anything
dramatic proof	probably neither dramatic, nor proof
indicates/suggests	does not mean 'proves'
in some people	does not mean 'in all people'
may	does not mean 'will'

Adapted from *The Wellness Encyclopedia 1991 University of California, Berkeley, published by Houghton Mifflin, Boston.*

Data on psychological interventions (including cognitive–behavioural therapy (CBT), hypnosis, relaxation and meditation) are complex. The best review found the methodological quality of studies variable; interventions were better than waiting-list control groups but not placebo controls.

Raynaud's disease

There are no research data on CISCOM for the use of CTs in this condition. However, clinical trials support the use of bilberry (*Vacinium myrtillus*) extract and of *Ginkgo biloba* in this and other peripheral vascular disorders.

Venous insufficiency

Systematic reviews support the use of *Ginkgo biloba* for cerebral insufficiency, peripheral arterial disease and disorders caused by reduced retinal blood flow, of ginseng for cerebrovascular deficit, and of horse chestnut (*Aesculus hippocastanum*), melilotus (*Melilotus officinalis*) and witchhazel (*Hamamelis virginiana*) for general venous insufficiency—for instance, varicose veins, haemorrhoids and oedema of the lower limbs.

Dermatological conditions

Warts

Some evidence indicates that hypnosis speeds wart regression. Although we have not seen this data and feel unable to comment on its validity, the research was conducted by Nick Spanos, a well-known and highly respected researcher.

A large, high-quality trial of homeopathy found no effect. Individualized treatment was not attempted, but three homeopathic doctors were consulted about the right complex of remedies to be used.

Acne

Tea tree (*Melaleuca alternifolia*) oil is a widely used therapy and appears to be effective. It has been found to be comparable in effect, slower in action but causing fewer adverse effects than conventional topical treatment. Though this is only one trial, it is complemented by other data showing an effect of tea tree oil on skin conditions.

Clinical trials also support the topical use of hawthorn for acne.

Eczema

The studies on traditional Chinese herbs in this condition are well known (see report in the Therapies section).

There is also some evidence that fatty acid supplementation is of benefit, and elimination dieting is of benefit for some. Some evidence exists that: (i) hypnosis can modify responses to allergic challenge, and (ii) relaxation and hypnosis are of clinical benefit.

Psoriasis

There is conflicting evidence on whether fatty acid supplementation is of benefit here.

Skin infections

Trials on tea tree oil have also been conducted in athlete's foot and onychomycosis (a fungal disease of the nails). In the onychomycosis trial, tea tree oil was as effective as clotrimazole, a topical antifungal, but it is not entirely clear that clotrimazole has been shown to affect the natural course of this condition. The athlete's foot trial is particularly interesting: tea tree oil has been shown to be active against tinea pedis infection in the lab but was no better than placebo at effecting a mycological cure. However, it was the most effective treatment for relieving clinical symptoms. Tea tree oil appears to be a good example of a herbal product for which it is difficult to ascribe an active principle or mode of action (e.g. antifungal).

Urticaria, hives

Urticaria has been successfully treated by the Chinese herb *Rehmannia glutinosa* (rehmannia or Chinese foxglove) in Chinese studies; However, data from clinical trials are as yet absent. There are no other data of interest in these conditions.

Gastrointestinal conditions

Crohn's disease and ulcerative colitis

It is fairly widely accepted conventionally that these are related to food intolerance in some cases. It seems that essential fatty acid supplementation is of no great benefit. Clinical trials support the use of German chamomile (*Matricaria recutita*) for spasm or ulceration of the gastrointestinal tract.

Relaxation therapies have been shown to reduce symptoms.

Dyspepsia

Fennel seed (*Foeniculum vulgare*) and peppermint (*Mentha X piperita*) have been shown by clinical trials to be of benefit for dyspeptic conditions of the upper gastrointestinal tract, including pain, nausea, belching and heartburn, and chronic colitis with diarrhoea or constipation, including infantile colic.

Infections

Clinical trials support the use of citrus seed extract to reduce infectious organisms in the gastrointestinal tract, including *Candida, Geotrichum* and haemolytic *Escherichia coli*.

Irritable bowel syndrome

Hypnosis is beneficial for those with persistent disease. Apparently it is more effective in those with classic disease and aged under 50. Psychotherapy is of benefit—as are relaxation techniques, but it is unclear whether they are as effective as hypnosis.

Food intolerance is implicated in some individuals. Fennel seed is of benefit for nausea, belching and heartburn. Traditional Chinese herbs have been shown to be effective.

Liver imbalance

There is evidence from clinical trials of the benefits of St Mary's thistle (*Silybum marianum*) and globe artichoke (*Cynara scolymus*) in hepatic insufficiency, gall bladder conditions, dyspepsia, constipation, hyperlipidaemia and bowel disorders. There is also evidence for the benefits of greater celandine (*Chelidonium majus*) for gall bladder disease, gallstones, hepatic congestion, toxic conditions and jaundice.

Nausea

Considerable evidence exists that stimulation of the P-6 acupuncture point on the inner wrist is of benefit in nausea generally. A systematic review showed that 11 of 12 high-quality trials and 9 of 13 subsequent trials were positive for acupuncture in this condition.

There is also good evidence that ginger is an effective antiemetic. Clinical trials support the use of globe artichoke in nausea associated with hepatic insufficiency and gall bladder conditions (see above), and of fennel seed for nausea, belching and heartburn.

Hypnosis and CBT are effective interventions in chemotherapy nausea.

Gynaecological conditions

Cystitis

There are no research data for this condition on CISCOM, other than isolated studies. Some trials support the use of

bearberry (*Arctostaphylos uva ursi*) and the Chinese herb *Andrographis paniculata* for urinary tract infections.

Herpes

There are no research data for this condition on CISCOM, other than isolated studies. Several studies do, however, concur that a diet rich in the amino acid lysine and low in arginine discourages herpes. The Chinese herb *Astragalus membranaceus* (astragalus or milk vetch) has also been shown to be of benefit for cervical erosion associated with herpes simplex viral infection.

Menopausal problems

There are no research data for this condition on CISCOM, other than isolated studies. Some clinical trials provide evidence for the benefits of the North American herb black cohosh (*Cimifuga racemosa*) in treatment of climacteric symptoms and ovarian insufficiency.

Menstrual symptoms

There is moderate evidence that acupuncture is of benefit for menstrual pain and PMS, and that manipulation is also of benefit for menstrual pain. One trial found reflexology or acupressure to be beneficial for PMS.

The widely used herbal remedy chaste tree (*Vitex agnus-castus*) was found in one multicentre trial to have no greater activity than placebo. However, the herb has been shown to have dopaminergic activity and effects on excessive prolactin release and corpus luteum insufficiency, and other trials have found a positive effect in menstruation disorders and MS.

Vaginal infection

There are no research data for this condition on CISCOM, other than isolated studies.

Immune-related conditions

AIDS/HIV

There is very little evidence for effect on AIDS directly, but many AIDS-related symptoms (e.g. pain, nausea) have been researched (see also under Gastrointestinal conditions). There is also contradictory evidence from two small trials as to whether relaxation techniques improve immune function. There are a number of studies indicating the following herbs to be of benefit: garlic, astragalus, liquorice, St John's wort (*Hypericum perforatum*) and the lichen *Usnea barbata*.

Research on supplementing with antioxidants such as *N*-acetyl cysteine (NAC) in AIDS cases has been widely reported as beneficial. According to Dr Luc Montagnier, the discoverer of HIV:

In HIV patients the glutathione system is depressed even at the early stages. I am convinced that oxidative stress is involved in the progression from HIV infection to AIDS.

I believe that antioxidants are necessary in the treatment but are not sufficient by themselves. Patient treatment may include several antioxidants such as NAC, beta carotene, vitamins A, C and E, the enzymes superoxide dismutase (SOD) and catalase, proteins such as metallothionine, plant extracts and other nutrients as indicated.

Cancer

Specialist centres such as Bristol or the Bernie Siegel programmme have been investigated but though remarkable case studies are quoted there is no generalizable evidence that they improve survival or quality of life.

Many herbs have been used to treat cancer, but there is little evidence that any are effective, whereas some such as Laetrile are probably harmful. An exception appears to be Sho-saiko-to (TJ-9) a Japanese drug for which there is evidence of an effect in liver cancer. There is also some evidence that extracts of St John's wort show antitumour and antimutagenic activity in vitro, though it is premature to conclude that it will prove useful in clinical trials. A number of studies demonstrate antitumour effects of green tea (*Camellia sinensis*), in addition to epidemiological studies showing a protective effect; research is currently underway to establish whether it is of benefit to cancer patients. Clinical trials also support the use of the Chinese herbs astragalus and ginseng or Siberian ginseng (*Eleutherococcus senticosus*) as an adjunct in cancer treatment, and melilotus particularly to prevent recurrence of metastases.

There is some evidence that a variety of different interventions can improve pain, anxiety and nausea associated with cancer diagnosis or treatment. (See the relevant sections of each of these symptoms.)

There is also evidence that counselling and group support extend survival times in breast cancer.

Neurological conditions

Bell's palsy

Acupuncture is a widely used modality here. However, no trials have been undertaken that compare acupuncture with placebo or control intervention. Two trials from China compare different forms of acupuncture, but one is an uncontrolled trial. We do not believe that these form a reliable basis for action.

Carpal tunnel syndrome

Various chiropractic/osteopathic techniques are used, but the only evidence is from a non-randomized trial.

Migraine and headache

There is evidence from double-blind controlled trials for the effectiveness of feverfew (*Tanacetum parthenium*) in migraine prevention, and of nutritional therapy to cut out food allergens.

A placebo-controlled trial in 1989 showed a significant difference between acupuncture and sham treatment, so acupuncture is at least partially effective here.

Homeopathy, biofeedback, relaxation and hypnotherapy and manipulation can also show good results.

Neuralgia/neuropathy/peripheral nerve diseases

There are conflicting data on the usefulness of acupuncture here: two trials have been undertaken, one with a positive result, one with a negative result, but both were very small.

Pain

A large number of studies on the effect of acupuncture on pain have shown there is good evidence for its effectiveness in postsurgical pain and some evidence for effectiveness in chronic pain. One study comparing acupuncture with sham treatment in molar extraction also found a significant difference between the two.

As well as lifting mood, St John's wort is anti-inflammatory and has pain-relieving properties, as does a cream containing capsaicin, the active ingredient in chili peppers.

(Back, neck and head pains are discussed below under Rheumatological conditions.)

Pregnancy

Research has consistently shown that P-6 acupressure is of moderate benefit in prevention of morning sickness (see under Gastrointestinal symptoms).

Acupuncture before labour has not been shown to aid birth; similarly, it is unlikely that acupuncture is a good method of pain relief during labour. However, it may be used to induce uterine contractions and shorten labour. Moxibustion has been shown to vert breech presentation.

Oil of lavender (*Lavandula* spp.), commonly considered to be a relaxant, was not shown to be effective at aiding perineal pain and healing when added to bath water, whereas the presence of a supportive companion at the time of birth has been demonstrated to be of benefit.

Prostate conditions

There have been a number of uncontrolled trials, and many randomized, double-blind placebo-controlled trials, on the use of extracts of *Serenoa repens*, or saw pal-metto ('Permixon', 'Cerniton') for a variety of prostate symptoms. These have provided compelling, though not yet incontrovertible, evidence that it is of benefit.

Psychological conditions

Addiction

Acupuncture has been shown to be a useful adjunct in heroin, cocaine and alcohol addiction, but seems to be of only minor benefit in smoking. A Cochrane review of acupuncture effects on smoking cessation showed that cessation rates were not high with acupuncture, with no apparent difference between acupuncture and placebo treatment.

Anxiety

Massage has a short-term effect, but it is unclear whether use of essential oils is of additional benefit.

Clinical trials indicate the herb kava kava (*Piper methysticum*) reduces anxiety, nervous tension and restlessness. St John's wort has also been shown to be of benefit here.

Depression

An extract of St John's wort has been found to be effective compared with both placebo and conventional antidepressants in mild to moderate depression, and has fewer adverse effects than imipramine. Kava kava has also been indicated to improve mild depression.

There is also some evidence that relaxation and meditation techniques are of benefit, but are probably not as effective as, say, CBT.

Hyperactivity

This appears to be related to food intolerance in some children.

Sleep problems

Hypnosis and relaxation therapy are helpful here. In one trial, massage improved sleep in psychiatric inpatients.

Valerian is a sedative herb that reduces sleep latency. Clinical trials have also indicated Californian poppy (*Eschscholtzia californica*) and *Corydalis cava* to be of benefit.

Bedwetting

Acupuncture is of some benefit in this condition.

Respiratory conditions

Asthma

The evidence on the use of acupuncture in this condition is very mixed.

Relaxation techniques including yoga, meditation, relaxation and hypnosis seem to be of benefit, but it is not clear which technique is to be recommended or which patients respond best.

Clinical trials give evidence for the benefits of peppermint. The Chinese herb rehmannia has also been shown to be of benefit, though no data from clinical trials are as yet available.

Hay fever

Two single homeopathic remedies have been found to have a moderate effect on symptoms: isopathic grass pollen and *Galphimia glauca*.

Infections

A homeopathic remedy called Oscillococcinum has been shown to shorten the duration of flu, but does not prevent it. Individualized homeopathy is also of moderate benefit in recurrent upper respiratory tract infection in children.

There is some evidence that *Echinacea angustifolia* aids immune function, as do the herbs garlic (*Allium sativum*), astragalus, liquorice (*Glycyrrhiza* spp.), golden seal (*Hydrastis canadensis*), St John's wort and the lichen *Usnea barbata* (which has some antitubercular activity).

Vitamin C supplementation probably does not prevent the common cold but does reduce severity and duration of symptoms. Vitamin C may be useful for those in particular need (e.g. chronically sick older people). Zinc lozenges apparently shorten cold duration.

Rheumatological and musculoskeletal conditions

Back, neck and head pain

Some studies show spinal manipulation to be of benefit here, though others contradict this and it is also unclear whether efficacy depends on type of manipulation (osteopathic, chiropractic, Maitland, etc.).

There is more limited evidence, though still positive, for acupuncture.

Persistent back pain can also be helped by relaxation, exercises such as yoga and hypnotherapy.

Bruises and sprains

There is some evidence that a proprietary homeopathic ointment containing a mixture of remedies, including *Arnica montana* tincture, is of value.

Fibromyalgia

Electroacupuncture has been found to be of benefit in one well-known trial. Soft tissue manipulation can reduce trigger point pain and improve sleep. One study found that massage was more helpful than TENS in this condition.

Clinical trials also support the use of *Arnica montana* for muscle ache. Mind–body therapies and hypnotherapy can be useful in chronic pain with no apparent organic cause.

Mouth ulcers

LongoVital, a herb-based tablet enriched with recommended doses of vitamins, is shown to be of benefit for mouth ulcer. Clinical trials also support the topical use of liquorice for recurrent mouth ulcers.

Osteoarthritis (OA)

There are mixed results for the benefits of acupuncture in osteoarthritis. The balance of evidence, however, is that it is of benefit for pain.

Clinical trials have shown nettle (*Urtica* spp.) and turmeric (*Curcuma longa*) to have some effect. Devil's claw (*Harpagophytum procumbens*) is effective in reducing inflammation.

A long-term RCT of glucosamine has shown it to be effective in reducing symptoms and modifying the course of OA.

Rheumatoid arthritis (RA)

Some patients with RA are food intolerant and benefit from exclusion dieting. There is also evidence that supplementation with omega-3 essential fatty acids and a low-fat diet are of benefit.

Green-lipped mussel extract was shown to be ineffective in two trials, although both of these had small numbers. Devil's claw is effective in reducing inflammation. Turmeric has also been shown in clinical trials to have some effect.

Temporomandibular joint (TMJ) dysfunction

There is limited evidence that acupuncture is of benefit.

Tennis elbow

Acupuncture but not laser acupuncture improves short-term outcome here.

Tiredness and fatigue

In persistent fatigue syndrome there may be some food intolerance, in which case nutritional therapy is of benefit.

Fatigue may also be postviral: high levels of antibodies to viruses such as Epstein–Barr virus are sometimes found in chronic fatigue syndrome (CFS) patients, so immune-boosting herbs such as *Echinacea angustifolia*, astragalus and golden seal (*Hydrastis canadensis*) are appropriate. Also, St John's wort is effective against enveloped viruses such as Epstein–Barr virus, and improves the mood, Siberian ginseng increases stress resistance and *Ginkgo biloba* boosts circulation.

CBT and graduated exercise work for some kinds of CFS; recent evidence indicates that exercise should be of low to moderate rather than high intensity.

MODELS AND RESEARCH IN INDIVIDUAL THERAPIES

At the time when we began our integration project in the late 1980s, the evidence base for complementary therapies was even less developed and hard to track down than it is now. However, by the mid 1990s, when we began more deliberately to link our practice to an existing evidence base, there was still relatively little we could rely on. The previous section of this chapter summarized an evidence report we were able to commission from the Research Council for Complementary Medicine's CISCOM database in 1997. This useful source, now available on-line, can be found at: http://www.rccm.org.uk. Requests for searches of the database can be submitted to this site. We recommend it to colleagues attempting to link their practice to research-derived evidence.

Yet, in reality, our own practice development was based on our experience of using CTs when faced with health problems that are difficult to treat conventionally; and on doctors' and CPs' experience of what appeared to them to have been effective approaches. It was not research-derived evidence that made us explore the role of CTs, but rather our own experience as practitioners and the wishes of our patients that persuaded us. For our group, research-derived evidence from RCTs took second place; and, while it provided something of a rationale for using CTs, our project was not primarily evidence driven. It has, however, become evidence linked, because we have tried continually to collect data about clinical activity and outcomes. We hope that colleagues using CAM will be interested in employing a similar approach and thereby add to a growing data set about patient-centred outcomes.

The Further Reading section of this chapter includes some relevant books and papers. It is intended to be indicative, and we offer it for the reader who wants to explore CAM in more depth. At the end of the chapter there is a summary of the RCT-derived evidence relating to our use of CAM at the Marylebone Health Centre (see Table 2.2). Practitioners who want to access research-derived evidence from RCTs will have a much easier task than we did, for a number of books condensing the evidence have appeared since 1996.

A notable trend in the medical world has been a growing determination to establish the validity of any and all forms of treatment according to evidence derived from randomized controlled trials (RCTs) and to aggregate the results of these trials by systematic review. Anyone concerned for the future of CAM should be aware of how systematic reviews and meta-analyses aim to apply strict criteria for research quality in order to summarize and evaluate the existing evidence. This research method is not without its critics, who, for instance, declare that RCTs gain their rigour at the expense of any real relevance because they distort everyday practice and so their results are unreliable. The value and validity of systematic reviews is, if anything, even more hotly disputed, yet they have appeared in ever-increasing numbers over the past 10 years and there is no doubt that the emergence of a Cochrane field for CAM presents an opportunity to show that these very exacting methods do support aspects of CAM practice.

However, many practitioners also perceive RCTs and their systematic review as a threat because their findings run counter to practitioners' experience and traditional beliefs about what works. The most notable source of systematic reviews of research-derived evidence about CAM comes from Professor Ernst's unit at the University of Exeter. Ernst's recently published overview of the evidence base 'The desktop guide to complementary and alternative medicine—an evidence-based approach', is the most comprehensive available collection of reviews and citation for RCTs in CAM. Although interpretation of the evidence may seem as much an art as a science, this book is thorough and wide ranging, so colleagues who want to see how this approach can be used should look there first. In addition, there are now websites that focus on complementary therapies and the evidence for their effectiveness. The internet now offers unprecedented access to research papers and libraries where even the most obscure publications can now be tracked down.

Therefore we considered it inappropriate for this book to go into great depth about the definitive RCT-derived evidence, partly because the evidence is not static and neither this nor any other paper publication can keep up with the latest findings. Furthermore, we believe that colleagues intending to explore the potential for integrating CTs ought to develop their own perspective on research-derived evidence—an increasingly easy undertaking and a necessary part of the process of developing integrated practice. One thing we would add, though, is that RCT-derived evidence inevitably lags behind practitioners' and patients' own experience-based hunches. It may also fail to validate their deeply held convictions that certain complementary therapy treatments are useful and effective. Practitioners should bear in mind, then, that every RCT study of CAM ever done was preceded by hunches, tradition and clinical experience of a treatment's effectiveness, for that is where the research process begins.

Models and modes of action

The following section is our attempt to present some ideas about the modes of action of CTs. In this exercise, we have had to use conventional scientific terms even though we understand that this creates difficulties. The most important among these difficulties is that this language is likely to distort the meaning of a therapy's underpinning theories, for they are inevitably bound up with more traditional, qualitative, vitalistic concepts. We are aware of the conceptual dangers of squeezing CT models into boxes made by reductionistic science, and even more conscious that it could seem to imply that traditional systems are an unfit explanatory model for practitioners' findings and interpretations. That is not our intention, so we hope that colleagues will not feel colonized or disempowered by our attempts at a clumsy translation of their languages, whose aim is to build bridges for doctors and scientists.

We included this section for three reasons, firstly because in many cases there *are* examples of scientific evidence for physiological and therapeutic effects of complementary therapy treatments. While this by no means constitutes the whole story about a therapeutic system, we offer it to doctors and scientists to help them take an open-minded attitude to the potential effectiveness of CTs. Secondly, we see our model-making as forming connections between scientific thinking and vitalistic imagination and, that if undertaken with good will, this can invite a mutual exploration of one another's approaches. Thirdly, there is a real need to address the issue of the safety of CTs. Therefore, even though this subject, too, can look like an implicit criticism of complementary practice if taken out of context, we have included the topic because doctors understandably need to be reassured about this aspect of CTs.

Models, evidence, safety: we want to address these problematic topics and encourage a healthy dialogue between conventional and complementary fields—but certainly not because we want to offer ammunition to those who would interpret integration as colonization or to others who would argue that CTs are ineffective and even unsafe. Some integrators might not question the effectiveness and safety of CTs, or feel the need to build theoretical models that link science and the art of complementary practice. However, we believe that integration will be best served by an open mind that can remain critically alert to the potential shortcomings and hazards of *every* kind of intervention. How else could we practise reflectively?

Acupuncture

Model

Traditional acupuncture is based on the concept of Qi (pronounced 'chi'), loosely translated as 'vital energy' or 'life energy'. This is something thought to be present in all living organisms and which also finds expression in the surrounding world. When Qi is 'in balance' the person is healthy, but if it becomes deficient, is present in excess or 'stagnates' then illness will eventually manifest. According to TCM theory, Qi travels along pathways called meridians, along which are certain points (called acupuncture points or acupoints) at which Qi may be brought back into balance by various physical methods.

Neurophysiological processes help to explain *some* aspects of acupuncture. In particular, its effects on pain are at least partially explicable within the conventional medical model. For example, acupuncture stimulates A-delta nerve fibres and thereby closes pain gates through spinal cord pathways. Needling also stimulates the release of endorphins, serotonin and other neurotransmitters. Perhaps these findings throw some light on how needling in one part of the body can influence pain sensation elsewhere. Consequently, many doctors, physiotherapists and nurses, as well as some chiropractors and osteopaths, use 'dry needling techniques', generally at myofascial trigger points. Indeed there is a high degree of correspondence between 70–80% of acupuncture points and the sites where myofascial trigger points most commonly develop. 'Medical acupuncturists' make their diagnosis conventionally, often having dispensed with traditional concepts entirely. Some even dispute the existence of meridians and points, although there is evidence that there may be patterned functional relationships that connect peripheral nerve junctions and trigger points. Although our team does not dispute the value of medical acupuncture, we believe that it constitutes only a small part of what acupuncture as a whole can offer. We have found traditional diagnosis and treatment to be useful in ways that the available research-derived evidence does not yet adequately reflect.

Clinical evidence

Acupuncture is one of the most popular therapies amongst doctors and it has been subjected to more research than almost any other therapy. However, methodological quality in this area, as throughout the field of CT research, has gradually had to improve because there are many problems concerning trials of this and all CTs. A recent review of almost 3000 trials concluded that the quality of trials of TCM must be improved urgently. Nonetheless, many good studies on pain as well as others on nausea have found real acupuncture to be more effective than a 'sham' procedure. And, in general, research shows that needling actual acupuncture points is more effective than with false points. Acupuncture has an effect in anaesthetized animals, so its effects clearly cannot be dismissed as purely psychological. There is obviously something as yet inexplicable going on here, but research is still equivocal as to whether these effects are really useful to patients even though clinically there would appear to be little doubt. For example, studies have generally been too short term to tell us whether there is lasting benefit in people with chronic pain, although on the whole they support the use of acupuncture in the treatment of pain. Systematic reviews and RCTs have not shown acupuncture to be of benefit for stopping smoking, tinnitus or obesity, although other studies say it may help asthma, stroke, alcoholism and some skin conditions. There is still too little definitive research on these conditions, and on fatigue, digestive disorders and anxiety. For a summary of these and other research-derived evidence on a range of CTs we recommend the CISCOM site and the Ernst (2001) book (see Further Reading, research evidence summaries).

Safety

The overall safety of CTs cannot be evaluated without a formal reporting system for adverse events. However, serious adverse acupuncture events are rare, even though it is one of the more invasive CTs. Acupuncture, then, seems to be relatively safe. However, needle pain, dizziness and discomfort are not unusual, and minor adverse effects, such as fainting, local skin infections and transitorily increased pain, although not uncommon are easily avoidable. More serious events (e.g. internal injuries to the pleura, kidney or spinal cord) are reported very occasionally and, although systemic infection is rare, it can be extremely serious. A worldwide systematic review found a total of 395 serious reported cases in 20 years, the most common being hepatitis. Relatively few of these events were recorded in the UK. The figure should be seen in the context of the huge number of acupuncture encounters that took place. To put this into context, a Norwegian study estimated that the average acupuncturist would have to work full time for a total of 120 years before encountering a pneumothorax, and the predicted gap between adverse events would be 4–5 years. All the more serious events are avoidable, provided that disposable needles are used and the practitioner is competent.

Herbal medicine

Model

Traditional herbalism is based on an essentially holistic model which is physiological in its approach. The different herbs are used for their effect on particular body systems (e.g. to help the liver detoxify or the kidney excrete better), and the synergistic effects of herbs or herb mixtures is considered to be of prime importance. However, a herbalist will prescribe individually for each patient, rather than select for a named condition, and will vary the exact prescription over time as the condition changes. Most clinical trials of herbal medicine have looked at whether a single herb or mixture affects a specific disease, but even on this basis many traditional uses seem to be justified.

Clinical evidence

Many medical drugs are still extracted from or based on traditional herbal remedies, and drug companies continue to screen new kinds of plant material for active ingredients. Most of these laboratory-based studies consider the effects of plant extracts on animals, and show clearly that plant medicines have wide-ranging pharmacological effects. The research-derived clinical evidence is less clear, and neither is it obvious just which components of a whole plant are the most pharmacologically significant. For instance, it was thought that the water-soluble component called hypericin was the active ingredient in St John's wort (*Hypericum perforatum*), until more recent studies found fat-soluble hyperforin to be equally important. St John's wort was assumed to be a kind of monoamine oxidase inhibitor, but is now thought to be a serotonin uptake inhibitor.

Increasingly, systematic reviews of RCTs suggest that many herbal medicines are effective. However, not all traditional herbal therapies have clearly been shown to be of benefit under trial conditions—as elsewhere in the CT field, studies often contradict one another or are equivocal. One big RCT found that chaste tree (*Vitex agnus-castus*) was indistinguishable from placebo as a treatment for premenstrual syndrome, although other studies have disagreed. Feverfew does not appear to be effective for rheumatoid arthritis, but used regularly as fresh plant it can prevent migraine.

The demand for St John's wort boomed after the press reported a meta-analysis of patients with mild or moderate depression, which found *Hypericum* extracts to be significantly superior to placebo and as effective as conventional antidepressants such as amitriptyline and imipramine but with fewer side-effects. Since this article was published, at least nine further randomized trials of the herb have appeared, all confirming its efficacy. There is, on the other hand, no shortage of RCTs that say otherwise, including the most recent large-scale trial.

More systematic reviews or meta-analyses of herbal drugs are continually appearing. A list can be found on the BMJ website: http://www.bmj.com/cgi/collection/com-plementary medicine. Box 2.5 Lists eight herbal remedies that have a research-derived evidence base.

Safety

An ever-growing range of freeze-dried herbs prepared as film-coated, foil-packed tablets is available over the counter. Increasingly popular with the public, they are also likely to become an attractive prescribing option for doctors, given the publicity around the effectiveness of St John's wort. On the other hand, this herb's interaction with drugs that are detoxified by the C50 hepatic pathway has alarmed officials as well as health professionals. Even though its significance may have been wildly exaggerated, this realization has been an important reminder that natural does not inevitably mean safe. Reporting systems are being developed and will eventually tell us whether side effects and interactions are commoner than we thought. Interactions with other medicines and foods, although probably a minor risk, are likely, but the great majority of herbs are relatively safe. Some are highly toxic, however, and there are real problems overall in regulating the quality, identity, contamination and adulteration of herbal medicines.

The indirect risks from poorly trained practitioners are considerable. The National Institute of Medical Herbalists and the University of Exeter are piloting a 'yellow card' reporting system on adverse events, and the National Poisons Unit has a database of adverse events and interactions. Most reports of serious adverse events involve herbs that were self-prescribed or

---

Box 2.5 Some herbal medicines with a strong research-derived evidence base

- *Maidenhair tree (Ginkgo biloba)*. A review of nine RCTs confirmed its benefit in delaying the clinical course of dementia. It also improves circulation, particularly to the head, and helps short-term memory loss. It is useful for tinnitus.
- *Horse chestnut (Aesculus hippocastanum) seed extracts*. A systematic review showed it to benefit chronic venous insufficiency.
- *Saw palmetto (Serenoa repens)*. A meta-analysis of 18 RCTs found it to be as effective as finasteride for symptomatic treatment of benign prostate hyperplasia (with fewer adverse effects).
- *St John's wort (Hydrastis)* is useful for long-term, low-grade depression and mild to moderate major depression; it is also an immune system enhancer
- *Echinacea (purple cone flower)* is an immune enhancer with antifungal, antiviral and antibacterial properties; it improves white blood cell production and mobility.
- *Dong quai (Angelica sinensis)* is good for dysmenorrhoea. RCTs have not found that it helps menopausal symptoms.
- *Pygeum africanum*. Numerous experimental double-blind studies show benefits in terms of all major symptoms of benign prostatic hypertrophy, with minimal side-effects (such as mild gastrointestinal irritation).
- *Bromelain (pineapple stem extract)* contains high levels of proteolytic enzymes which can reduce most forms of inflammation (e.g. in arthritis, trauma and surgery) without side-effects.

obtained from an unqualified or unregulated source. For instance, Chinese herbal tea used for eczema caused two cases of severe nephropathy; eight of 11 Chinese herbal creams for eczema were found on analysis to contain dexamethasone, and patients in a Belgian weight loss clinic were given, in error, a poisonous Chinese herb, *Aristolochia fangchi*, which has been linked to kidney failure and cancer.

Herb–drug interactions are important and under-researched. Some interactions are well known, and any competent medical herbalist will take a detailed drug history to avoid them. As yet unknown interactions exist, so, while we should bear in mind the relatively low risk of such medicines as these and not overreact, doctors ought to be alert for adverse events and be more curious about their patients' use of this and other CTs. Nonetheless in properly trained hands, traceable high-quality herbal medicines can—despite some recent negative publicity—be highly effective. Their use will become much more widely integrated into the mainstream in future and, in order to learn more about their use, doctors would be well advised to learn from properly qualified herbalists.

Interactions between herbal remedies and synthetic drugs are more than theoretically likely:

- *Echinacea angustifolia* might affect the liver if used beyond 8 weeks, especially if taken with drugs associated with liver toxicity (e.g. anabolic steroids).

- Evening primrose oil (*Oenothera biennis*) and borage oil (*Borago officinalis*) can decrease the effectiveness of anticonvulsants.
- Ginseng can increase the effect of oestrogens and corticosteroids; it may affect blood glucose levels, so diabetics should not take it. Ginseng and liquorice can interfere with digoxin levels.
- Kelp may interfere with thyroid replacement therapy.
- St John's wort is an effective mild antidepressant. However, it may increase the side-effects of other antidepressants and can interfere with certain drugs, in particular cyclosporin, warfarin, digoxin or theophylline, or oral contraception.
- The sedative effects of barbiturates may be increased by Valerian (*Valeriana officinalis*).
- The effects of warfarin can be unpredictable if taken with feverfew, *Ginkgo biloba*, garlic, ginseng or Chinese angelica (dong quai).

Table 2.1 lists potential interactions to be aware of.

Homeopathy

Model

Homeopathy is based on three main principles:

1. *The law of similars.* This is the idea that 'like should be cured with like': that a substance that would produce

Table 2.1 Important potential interactions between herbal preparations and conventional drugs

Herb	Conventional drug	Potential problem
Echinacea used for > 8 weeks	Anabolic steroids, methotrexate, amiodarone, ketoconazole	Hepatotoxicity
Feverfew	Non-steroidal anti-inflammatory drugs	Inhibition of herbal effect
Feverfew, garlic, ginseng, gingko, ginger	Warfarin	Altered bleeding time
Ginseng	Phenelzine sulphate	Headache, tremulousness, manic episodes
Ginseng	Oestrogens, corticosteroids	Additive effects
St John's wort	Monoamine oxidase inhibitor and serotonin reuptake inhibitor antidepressants	Mechanism of herbal effect uncertain. Insufficient evidence of safety with concomitant use therefore not advised
Valerian	Barbiturates	Additive effects, excessive sedation
Kyushin, liquorice, plantain, uzara root, hawthorn, ginseng	Digoxin	Interference with pharmacodynamics and drug level monitoring
Evening primrose oil, borage	Anticonvulsants	Lowered seizure threshold
Shankapulshpi (ayurvedic preparation)	Phenytoin	Reduced drug levels, inhibition of drug effect
Kava	Benzodiazepines	Additive sedative effects, coma
Echinacea, zinc (immunostimulants)	Immunosuppressants (such as corticosteroids, cyclosporin)	Antagonistic effects
St John's wort, saw palmetto	Iron	Tannic acid content of herbs may limit iron absorption
Kelp	Thyroxine	Iodine content of herb may interfere with thyroid replacement
Liquorice	Spironolactone	Antagonism of diuretic effect
Karela, ginseng	Insulin, sulphonylureas, biguanides	Altered glucose concentrations. These herbs should not be prescribed in diabetic patients

From Vickers A, Zollman C 2000 ABC of complementary medicine: herbal medicine. BMJ, London. Data from: Miller L G 1998 Herbal medicinals: selected clinical considerations focusing on known or potential drug–herb interactions. Archives of Internal Medicine 158: 2200–2211 symptoms similar to those being experienced by the patient can be used to treat these symptoms.

2. *The minimum dose* should be used in order to stimulate the body's adaptive responses and promote the processes needed for recovery, but without provoking any toxicity.

3. *The principle of potentization* demands that 'remedies' are prepared by a process of serial dilution and succussion (which involves vigorous shaking). The more times this process is repeated, the greater is said to be the 'potency' of the remedy. This implies a greater specificity to treat a particular complex of symptoms

A growing number of double-blind randomized trials have demonstrated significant benefits of homeopathic treatment over and above placebo, yet the scientific community generally dismisses homeopathy's mode of action as simply a 'placebo effect'. For conventional medicine, the ideas of like treating with like and of using the minimum dose are less of a problem than the principle of potentization. Examples of drugs that treat the symptoms they cause in higher doses are obvious enough—consider digoxin and heart failure, for instance. Homeopathic medicines are commonly so diluted that they contain few or even no molecules of the active ingredient. Some homeopaths believe the remedies contain a 'vital force'. One biophysical model for this notion is that potentization alters the complex molecular lattices in the solvent (water) so that it retains an electromagnetic 'memory' of the original active ingredient. Using in vitro models, the French immunologist Jacques Benveniste found strong evidence for the physiological activity of homeopathic dilutions even when no material trace was present. However, he was controversially accused of fraud and scientific misconduct after his findings were published in the journal Nature. Consequently, scientists' enthusiasm for further research into such basic mechanisms appears to have (temporarily) damped down.

Homeopaths consider disease to be the result of a deep-seated imbalance affecting the whole person. Initially, the vital force would have been disturbed by, for instance, exposure to environmental strain, lack of sleep, continuous psychological stress, previous disease or genetic susceptibility. The intensity of these symptoms is related to the body's ability or inability to adjust to change. If this disorder persists, then symptoms will localize in specific areas (e.g. tonsils or throat). Homeopaths see this localization as the 'result' of the underlying disease and possibly as the vitality's attempt to reorganize itself. Disease is understood as a response of the body–mind to several factors, but it is not seen as something separate from the sick person. A homeopathic remedy is intended to stimulate the vitality, increase the body's own resistance to disease and stimulate the organism's own capacity to heal itself.

This is why homeopaths say they treat the individual and the 'whole person', and why they see cure as entailing more than simply removing the local problem.

After a remedy is administered, homeopaths expect the disease to get better from the inside out. Patients may feel better in themselves initially, with an increase in energy and well-being before an improvement in specific physical symptoms. Homeopaths believe that a deep-seated cure starts in the upper body and proceeds downwards (i.e. a rash will clear up on the face before the feet); that recent symptoms improve as older ones recur; and that deeper-seated problems improve (e.g. asthma) as more superficial ones may recur or be provoked (e.g. eczema).

A conceptual division—a schism perhaps—exists between the classical single-remedy approach and the selection of remedies in complex homeopathy—rather like the difference between traditional and medical acupuncture. The selection of a remedy in classical homeopathy is based on the main complaint and an assessment of the mental, emotional and physical condition of the patient. Complex homeopathy incorporates a combination of remedies that are mixed together and focus on a variety of complaints. These remedies are low potency and are not specific to the person, but to the disease. This is not considered by classical homeopaths to be good practice; however, many practitioners do use this approach successfully with their patients.

Because the homeopathic model of causes and cures is far less focused on disease labels, homeopaths may find it easier than a doctor (who relies on a pathological identifier to guide prescription) to cope with ill-defined distress, functional disorders and health problems with a strong psychological component.

Clinical evidence

The British Medical Journal published a review of all trials of homeopathy in 1991. It was one of the first such reviews to appear. The reviewers, sceptical epidemiologists, had previously described homeopathy as 'incomprehensible', yet they decided that 'the evidence of clinical trials is positive but not sufficient to draw definitive conclusions' as many of the studies were of only moderate quality. In the 22 most rigorous trials, 15 found homeopathy superior to placebo; a typical example was a double-blind study of Oscillococcinum for influenza in which 17% of patients recovered within 48 hours compared with 10% of controls. A meta-analysis of 100 RCTs concluded that placebo could not explain their overall positive findings. Laboratory experiments showing effects of homeopathic medicines on animals also provide evidence that they are not due entirely to placebo.

So, even though homeopathy's basic mechanism remains unknown, many high-quality randomized double-blind placebo-controlled clinical trials suggest its effectiveness is over and above that of a placebo. This has caught science in a cleft stick between two unacceptable conclusions: either homeopathic dilutions have a physiological effect or RCTs are an ineffective research tool.

The evidence is less clear, however, on just how effectively everyday homeopathy treats the conditions that homeopaths commonly see. Trials investigating acute conditions treated with a single remedy are easy to complete but do not reflect real clinical practice. When treating one named condition, classical homeopaths would give different remedies on the basis of the individual symptom picture. Rigorous research methods can deal with this, but few of the complex trials needed have yet been done.

Safety

The idea that homeopathy (like other forms of natural medicine) must be harmless is widespread. Given the infinitestimal quantities involved, serious unexpected adverse events must be very rare, although, as with herbal preparations, there have been cases of remedies being adulterated with drugs. A flare-up of symptoms (the predicted 'aggravation reaction' which homeopaths say indicates the body's initial favourable response to a homeopathic treatment) is said to be common; therefore, patients and their doctors should appreciate the possibility of such transient events and be willing to interpret them as a positive prognostic sign. Most reactions are mild and transient: headaches, tiredness, skin eruptions, dizziness, diarrhoea or loose stools. However, because these are all symptoms commonly provoked by placebo, whether they are actually caused by homeopathic treatment is unclear. It has been said that some PNMQPs tell patients to reduce conventional and prescribed drugs or advise strongly against vaccination. Some offer untested alternatives to vaccination. Well-qualified and experienced PNMQP homeopaths would deplore such advice.

The manipulative therapies: osteopathy and chiropractic

Model

Although osteopathy and chiropractic differ in their ideas about the homeostatic role of the nervous system, and originally in the type of manipulations, they share common ground. Both consider the body to be self-healing, unless structural and biomechanical factors undermine this capacity by reducing functional efficiency. For example, a round-shouldered kyphotic posture (structure) constrains free and efficient breathing (function), and spinal musculoskeletal restrictions in particular interfere with nerve and blood supply, which in turn many influence visceral and circulatory function. Therefore, these therapies aim to restore normal function.

Clinical evidence

Whereas the research-derived evidence for the effectiveness of most CTs in specific conditions is relatively sparse, many RCTs suggest osteopathy and chiropractic are effective for low back pain. Several national guidelines on the treatment of low back pain recommend spinal manipulation as a symptomatic treatment if acute, uncomplicated cases of pain fail to resolve spontaneously within a few weeks. The evidence base for these recommendations has recently been called into question. More than 50 reviews of RCTs of spinal manipulation have been published, but it has been difficult for these studies to exclude non-specific effects. Nor is it clear whether one form of manipulation is any more or less effective than another. However, there are many approaches and it would be surprising if individual effectiveness did not depend on practitioner skill.

So, how consistent or generalizable could studies in this area be? One recent study concluded that spinal manipulation for back pain is no more effective than specialized physiotherapy and only slightly better than doing nothing at all. Moreover, when results like these seem to be so at odds with clinical experience, how should we interpret them and how much should we allow them to influence ordinary practice? Reviews tend to lump different forms of manipulation and diverse conditions together, making interpretation impossible. One systematic review of RCTs of chiropractic for low back pain considered all the trials as flawed. These difficulties with research into manipulation have many obvious parallels in other CT disciplines.

Manipulators sometimes treat non-musculoskeletal problems, although there is almost no reliable evidence for effectiveness apart from in dysmenorrhoea. Despite patients' accounts of benefit in childhood asthma, one study of chiropractic groups found no added improvement over and above sham treatment. On the other hand, outcomes data from 18 hospitals using osteopathic manipulative treatment (OMT) suggest that it can be an important adjunctive treatment even in psychosis, cerebrovascular diseases, infections and some gut disorders.

Many studies suggest a benefit from spinal manipulation:

- low back pain (not established beyond reasonable doubt)
- symptoms of chronic fibromyalgia

- early developmental problems in neonates (cranial osteopathy)
- significantly reduced use of drugs in otitis media
- in infectious and postsurgical settings.

Safety

The risk of severe complications is low. Manipulation of the lower spine appears to be less risky than that of the neck and upper spine. The incidence of vertebral artery damage is probably less than one per 1 million neck manipulations, and that of cauda equina injury less than one per 1 million treatments. Manipulation (even cervical manipulation for neck pain) is much safer than using non-steroidal anti-inflammatory drugs, the usual 'conventional' first-line treatment for similar musculoskeletal conditions. The potential indirect risk due to the possible overuse of radiography by some chiropractors may have been overestimated.

Exercise systems—tai chi, qigong and yoga

Models

Tai chi and qigong are exercise systems based on Qi and meridians. Yoga is rooted in traditional Indian medicine. The traditional aim of the exercises, postures and breathing exercises is to increase the flow of life energy (perhaps this can be interpreted as adaptive capacity, or homeostatic regulatory information) throughout the body. Some practitioners take a more conventional biomechanical view, interpreting their effects as due to muscle stretching, mental relaxation and circulatory stimulation.

Clinical evidence

Tai chi researchers have studied its benefits with regard to general health, particularly in older people. One study of healthy older people aged between 70 and 80 years doing twice-weekly tai chi classes found evidence of psychological and physical improvement compared with a control group. Regular practitioners have above-average cardiovascular fitness levels and people with rheumatoid arthritis improve their flexibility. Research on the effects of qigong is still in its infancy. One study showed that yoga breathing increased feelings of energy, alertness and enthusiasm more than in control groups using relaxation or visualization. Some trials of yoga for elderly people found psychological benefits; others did not. Several researchers have shown that yoga (even yoga breathing alone) improves lung function, and in a controlled trial of people with asthma, those practising yoga regularly had fewer attacks and used less medication.

Research is less clear as to whether yoga helps to improve arthritic pain and stiffness, or whether yoga definitely reduces blood pressure in hypertension (see Hypnosis and relaxation therapies).

Safety

Yoga, tai chi and qigong should be properly taught by qualified instructors. Breathing exercises can provoke hyperventilatory symptoms. Yoga postures, if forced, can cause musculoskeletal strain and possibly even joint dysfunction.

Healing

Model

Healers believe a benign source of 'energy' is available for well-being and that they can tap into this source. Some interpret the source in religious or overtly spiritual ways; others see their actions simply as triggering self-healing processes. They are the natural successors of the 19th century 'magnetic' healers who believed their powers were explicable from a scientific point of view. As yet, however, there is no such explanation, although some studies have suggested that increased feelings of well-being and even immunochemical changes might be attributable to entrained rythmicity detectable in cardiac and EEG traces.

Clinical evidence

There is no doubt that some patients experience general health improvements, reduced anxiety and reduced feelings of hopelessness after healing. These effects have been confirmed in numerous research studies comparing 'real healing' with 'placebo healing'. It is not clear that healing produces specific biological changes, although in one experimental study on skin wounds, 'healed' patients' wounds improved more rapidly than those who did not receive healing. Although many studies using plant and animal models are said to demonstrate biological effects of healing, critics point to flaws in their design and cast doubt on the results.

Hypnosis and relaxation therapies

Model

Conventional medicine is very familiar with cognitive and behavioural techniques such as relaxation, 'stress management', biofeedback and hypnosis. Midbrain–autonomic interconnectivity has long provided one possible mainstream explanatory model. More recently, aspects of research in psychoneuroimmunology (PNI), and the discovery that nervous and immune systems both bear receptor sites for a similar spectrum of neurotransmitters, have suggested even more complex psychosomatic unity. The potential for using these therapies in an even wider variety of illnesses is still too little explored.

Clinical evidence

There is strong evidence that hypnosis and relaxation can reduce state-anxiety of every kind. No one technique is superior, although combined cognitive–behavioural therapy (CBT) programmes can also be effective in panic disorders and insomnia, while hypnosis plus CBT improves phobia, obesity and anxiety. Relaxation techniques can help problems that are caused or made worse by stress. Pain is the best example—not only pain caused directly by tension (e.g. headache) but also pain due to physical damage (e.g. rheumatoid arthritis), presumably because stress and anxiety intensify the experience of pain. Relaxation techniques are an essential part of conventional pain management. RCTs provide good evidence for these techniques in acute as well as chronic pain. Hypnosis may be of benefit for headache and migraine, but the evidence is not as clear. Randomized trials show that imagery techniques help patients with cancer to relax and that hypnosis can help relieve their anxiety, pain, nausea and vomiting, particularly in children. In one famous RCT that involved teaching imagery and relaxation to women with fairly advanced breast cancer, survival time was significantly increased in the intervention group.

Regular home practice of relaxation techniques improves asthma, an effect widely recognized ever since the 1960s when the British Medical Journal published two big trials. It is interesting that, despite this, further research has been slow to take off, and medical practice has not integrated these findings. This raises important issues for those who believe that integration of CTs into the mainstream will have to be levered by RCT-derived evidence. This example suggests that impressive research studies do not necessarily produce changes in everyday practice and that it is perfectly possible to ignore a potentially cost-effective, empowering and simple approach.

Hypnosis can be of benefit, even for patients with severe, persistent, irritable bowel syndrome, but—surprisingly perhaps—it is of limited value in hypertension. Some pilot trials have suggested that hypnosis can help obese people to lose weight, but it appears to be no more effective than a health education class for smoking cessation or substance misuse.

Safety

In some susceptible people, hypnosis, deep relaxation or prolonged meditation may possibly trigger epileptic attacks or latent psychosis, post-traumatic stress disorder (PTSD) or 'false memory syndrome'. Although the research evidence is not conclusive, clinical experience suggests the need for caution and a high index of suspicion because these simple techniques can sometimes be surprisingly powerful.

Massage and touch-based therapies

Models

Touch and manually applied pressure have biomechanical and psychological effects: vigorous massage improves the circulation of the blood and lymph and produces powerfully relaxing effects by stimulating the parasympathetic nervous system; psychological effects of massage include reduction in anxiety and improvement in self-image. A growing number of touch-based and massage therapies are rooted in non-European systems (e.g. tuina, acupressure, shiatsu, based on TCM theory) or are idiosyncratic systems developed from the ideas of a particular individual (e.g. Alexander technique, rolfing, Feldenkrais technique, reflexology, tragerwork), or combining massage with the effect of active plant substances (e.g. aromatherapy). All, however, believe that both mind and body may derive benefits.

Clinical evidence

Most people find massage relaxing, so it is surprising how little good-quality evidence there is for this effect (Box 2.6). In the better studies of massage, a typical outcome would be reduced anxiety levels compared with an equivalent period of rest. In various settings randomized trials suggest that massage improves short-term anxiety scores in healthy students—intensive care units, psychiatric institutions, hospices and occupational health. However, there is limited evidence for any long-term benefit. Neither has there been much investigation of

---

Box 2.6 Summary of research-derived evidence on effectiveness of massage

- Massage can reduce anxiety and improve the perceived quality of life of patients with cancer.
- Massage therapy (30 minutes, twice weekly for 1 month) significantly decreased anxiety and depression in women who had been sexually abused.
- Adult patients with multiple sclerosis who had massage twice weekly for 45 minutes for 5 weeks reported improved function and self-image, reduced anxiety and depression.
- Circulatory benefits include the ability to enhance lymphatic drainage as well as improved tissue oxygenation.
- Asthmatics receiving massage therapy report improved respiratory function.
- Massage can reduce pain and stiffness, even in chronic inflammatory conditions such as rheumatoid arthritis.

massage effects on musculoskeletal pain, except for sports massage where some research exists. However, surprisingly, massage has not been shown to improve performance, muscle soreness or recovery time. It is entirely feasible that massage could relieve pain through endorphin release and by closing pain gates (see Acupuncture, p. 49). Many effects on well-being have also been claimed and patients speak of them, but as yet these effects have not been studied rigorously. Circumstantial evidence for a wider-ranging and profound impact of touch comes from randomized trials of massage for premature infants, which found that it produced more rapid weight gain and development.

Acupressure and shiatsu. Acupuncture has been shown almost certainly to be effective for nausea. Trials also show that finger pressure on the same PE-6 acupuncture point may have an effect on vomiting and nausea. True acupressure was highly significantly more effective than either placebo acupressure or no intervention, in a trial on pregnant women with morning sickness, and halved the rate of severe sickness. A number of well-designed studies of acupressure for various sorts of nausea have found it effective in adults, but not in children. Rigorous research has shown that manual pressure on acupuncture points has significant effects, but we are far from understanding the mechanism or scope of acupressure, nor whether it is a valid and more wide-ranging approach to treatment.

Aromatherapy. Aromatherapists say that essential oils contain pharmacologically active substances that enter the bloodstream during a massage and that the sense of smell affects feelings and behaviour. In most studies, patients massaged do better than those who are not, whether or not aromatherapy oil or plain massage oil was used. However, the existing trials on, for instance, lavender oil drops in the bath have shown no difference to pain or perineal wound infection rates compared with placebo oil. Therefore, even though there are good reasons to accept that aromatherapy may be beneficial, there is as yet little hard evidence that it is.

Reflexology. Very few RCTs have tested reflexology; however, in a recent well-designed study of reflexology for premenstrual syndrome, women receiving 'true reflexology' reported much greater improvements in symptoms than those having 'pretend reflexology'.

Safety

Very vigorous massage techniques are uncommon in the UK, but in the USA there have been very rare reports of their causing adverse events. The safety of aromatherapy has been called into question, because the essential oils used are highly concentrated and in some cases would, if swallowed, be potentially toxic. However, when used for aromatherapy massage they are well diluted (estimated

as less than 3%) in a carrier oil and used only externally. Although direct adverse events must be extremely rare, until a formal reporting scheme has been developed and more research has established both the benefits and risks of essential oil massage, the current (slight) uncertainly about essential oil massage safety will continue. As things stand, caution about the use of some oils is advised during pregnancy and in people susceptible to dermatitis.

Naturopathy

Naturopathy grew out of the 'nature cures' practised in 19th-century Austrian and German health spas, and was introduced to the USA by a German, Benedict Lust, who founded the American School of Naturopathy in 1896. John Kellogg famously used natural therapies at his sanatorium in Battle Creek, Michigan. Advances in surgery and pharmaceuticals overshadowed natural methods, however, and it was not until the 1960s that interest revived. In some US states, naturopaths are licensed as GPs, and Germany has several thousand state-licensed naturopaths called *Heilpraktiker* ('health practitioners').

Model

According to naturopaths, the organism has to process a complex flow of information ('the vital force') in order to self-regulate and maintain homeostasis. Naturopaths conceive anything to which the organism is required to respond or adapt as a potential stressor. The ageing process, maladaptation and an unhealthy lifestyle all tend to disrupt this capacity, so this is said to 'weaken the vital force'. With the inevitable decline of vitality, metabolic and environmental 'toxins'—the removal of which depends on adequate nutrition, fluid transport and elimination—tend to accumulate. In the long term, as these defence processes fail to cope, chronic manifestations of disease result. Practitioners look for underlying causes of maladaptation and use natural resources, such as whole foods, medicinal herbs, fresh air and water, to stimulate the body's self-healing processes. Naturopathy is practised throughout the Western world, and there is an increasing convergence between many of its ideas (the importance of a high-fibre, low-fat diet, the value of exercise and relaxation) and conventional biopsychosocial medicine. Key ideas are outlined in Box 2.7.

Clinical evidence

Studies mentioned under the headings of herbal medicine, acupuncture, homeopathy, nutritional therapy,

Box 2.7 Key naturopathic ideas

- Naturopaths conceive ill health as due to three broad categories of dysfunction, which interact, impacting on an individual's inborn and acquired characteristics:
  - *biochemical* (toxicity, deficiency, allergy and infection)
  - *biomechanical* (postural, respiratory, and inadequate or excessive exercise)
  - *psychosocial* (emotions, stress levels and coping abilities).
- Rather than treating symptoms, naturopaths aim to build up underlying vital reserves.
- Inborn and acquired biochemical, biomechanical and psychosocial factors will determine an individual's vulnerability, susceptibility and 'vital reserves'.
- An individual's basic 'vital reserves' will largely determine the effectiveness of their adaptive processes.
- The naturopath's central issue is to decide which stage of general adaptation a patient is in: acute, adaptative or exhausted.
- Are the symptoms evidence of active homeostatic processes? (acute stage and adaptation).
- Are the symptoms evidence of depleted adaptation resources (stage of exhaustion)?
- If so, then how much residual vitality remains?
- Can homeostatic and adaptive capacities be enhanced (by attending to structural/physical, psychosocial, biochemical, other factors)?
- Can the 'stress' load (whether physical, psychosocial, biochemical, other) be reduced?
- Interventions that suppress normal defence functions encourage inappropriate adaptive responses.
- Ideally, therapeutic interventions should enhance coping and elimination without suppressing normal adaptive and defensive responses.

manipulation, massage and relaxation all relate to naturopathy, as these (amongst others) are the methods it employs. In addition, naturopaths might advise hydrotherapy and fasting. Some specific studies of the last two methods have been conducted. Medical students at Hanover Medical School were divided into two groups, and for 6 months they took either a 5-minute cold or a 5-minute warm shower each morning. After 6 months those taking the cold shower had half the number of colds of those having warm showers. This study seems to confirm the naturopathic conviction that cold water bathing can be a way of enhancing immune function.

Numerous studies have shown that controlled therapeutic fasting (a key intervention in naturopathy) can improve immune and general function. The work of Bastyr University in Seattle, USA (one of the centres with federal funding to research into CM) includes developing a number of RCTs on general naturopathic approach to chronic disease.

Nutritional therapies

Model

Nutritional science is part of mainstream medicine, but there are diverse unconventional nutritional and dietary interventions relating the many aspects of CM. For instance, Chinese and Indian traditional medical systems have their own dietary theories. The use of diet and nutritional supplements as a primary treatment for disease is known as nutritional medicine. A variety of approaches fall under this general heading, including orthomolecular medicine (the use of high-dose nutrients for their pharmacological effects), certain nutritional aspects of naturopathy, which emphasizes the value of fasting and of mono-diets, and clinical ecology (also confusingly called environmental medicine).

The over-arching concept in this field is that the body's self-healing ability is compromised by diet (inadequate levels of essential nutrients and dietary components that are allergenic or in some way biochemically irritant) and that dietary modification may therefore be helpful. Certain foods may be advised or eliminated; perhaps various food supplements (e.g. vitamins, minerals, fatty acids, enzymes, amino acids, etc.) may be recommended for restoring normal biochemical function. Most practitioners use dietary questionnaires to determine deficiencies or food intolerances; some are guided by blood, stool and urine tests, whereas others use even less conventional tests (including methods derived from electroacupuncture) for which there is as yet no reliable evidence.

Clinical evidence

There is some RCT-derived evidence for certain aspects of high-dose vitamin and mineral treatments: vitamin C and zinc may be an effective way of treating the common cold, vitamin B6 apparently helps premenstrual syndrome and autism, and vitamin E has been shown to reduce angina. Also, an increase of polyunsaturated acids and/or reduction of saturated acids in the diet has beneficial effects in patients with hypertriglyceridaemia, rheumatoid arthritis or IBS. The RCT evidence for many of nutritional therapy's interventions is generally sparse, however, although vegetarian and oligo-antigenic diets are known to be valuable, for instance in some cases of RA, eczema and asthma. Nutritional influences on chronic disease are probably far more important than the available evidence has demonstrated. The examples of atherosclerosis and perimenopausal symptoms (Boxes 2.8 and 2.9) provide a snapshot of the emerging evidence available.

Safety

Some nutritional supplements can have mild adverse effects, for example diarrhoea after high doses of vitamin C and flushing after taking niacin. Because excess water-soluble vitamins leave the body in the urine, adverse events are rarer with water-soluble vitamins. Nevertheless, water-soluble vitamin B6 in high doses

---

Box 2.8 Nutritional influences on atherosclerosis

- *Diet* should be rich in complex carbohydrates and low in saturated fats.
- *Vitamin E.* Supplementation (600 IU three times daily) may reduce oxidation of low-density lipoproteins and is inversely correlated to risk of death from ischaemic heart disease.
- *Chromium.* Regression of atherosclerotic plaques and reduction of total and low-density lipoproteins have been demonstrated.
- *Omega-3 fatty acids.* Supplementation (3 g daily, or eating oily fish several times weekly) produces a reduction in serum triglycerides, fibrinogen, blood viscosity, red blood cell rigidity, total cholesterol, low-density-lipoprotein (LDL) cholesterol and systolic blood pressure.
- *Omega-6 fatty acids.* Evening primrose oil (and/or borage oil) (3 g daily) lowers LDL and very low-density-lipoprotein (VLDL) cholesterol plasma concentrations.
- *Magnesium.* Apart from the well-documented value of intravenous magnesium after myocardial infarction, oral supplementation (400 mg elemental magnesium daily) has been shown experimentally to reduce plasma LDL and VLDL cholesterol levels safely and significantly.
- *Coenzyme Q10.* Preliminary evidence strongly suggests cardiovascular benefits for CoQ10 supplementation (not less than 90 mg daily).
- *Garlic and onion.* A meta-analysis based on five randomized placebo-controlled studies of patients with high cholesterol levels showed that garlic (200 mg daily; equivalent to half a clove per day) decreases total serum levels by approximately 9%.

Box 2.9 Perimenopausal conditions

Nutritional strategies for perimenopausal symptoms include:

- *Vitamin A.* Supplementation with 5000 IU daily increases progesterone levels substantially.
- *Gamma-oryzanol (rice bran oil, ferulic acid).* Supplementation with 300 mg daily reduces hot flushes and other perimenopausal symptoms without side-effects.
- *Plant oestrogens* can be used safely to raise oestrogen levels.
- *Calcium.* Supplementation (1.5 g postmenopausal, 1 g premenopausal) and reduced meat intake for osteoporotic prophylaxis.
- Caffeine increases urinary and faecal calcium loss; a lacto-ovo-vegetarian diet reduces bone density loss, increases prolactin levels and reduces progesterone levels.

---

may produce a reversible neuropathy. Oil-soluble vitamins can be stored in the body. Excess vitamin A causes birth defects and irreversible bone and liver damage, and excess vitamin D leads to hypercalcaemia. Many of these nutritional supplements compete for absorption or assimilation, so a dietary excess of one vitamin or element will result in a deficiency of another. Consequently, taking single vitamins of the B group may cause deficient uptake of the others and of zinc and copper, or amino acids. Iron competes with zinc; zinc itself or selenium in excess can cause immune suppression. It has been reported that evening primrose oil can trigger temporal lobe epilepsy. Certain diets (e.g. vegan or macrobiotic) that restrict animal products have been linked with reduced growth in children, and with anaemia.

Summary

Research:

- the Cochrane Library lists over 4000 randomized trials
- the CAM field is still poorly researched compared with conventional medicine.
- CAM practitioners are now more aware of value of research
- many CM training courses include research modules
- conventional sources of funding (e.g. NHS R&D programme and major research charities) are becoming more open to CAM research proposals
- in the USA NCCAM has $70 m annual federal funding
- mainstream scientists (therefore) have a growing interest in doing CAM research.

Research types:

Randomized controlled trials:

- have high rigour
- preclude all bias
- test for specific efficacy
- have internal validity

but:

- are problematic in chronic disease
- are less generalizable to the real world of practice.

Outcomes research:

- has high relevance
- can complement RCTs
- tests general outcomes
- has external validity
- uses an evidence mosaic
- has large numbers
- is applicable to actual effects of ordinary treatment in everyday practice.

Ideally CT research should combine the two streams: the rigour of RCTs (including randomized comparative trials) plus outcome studies relevant to real-world practice to help explore the value of integrating CT into mainstream health care. Pragmatic, participative and action research methods can help us understand the role and relevance of CT in mainstream medicine.

Directions for future CAM research

- developing infrastructure for CAM research in primary care
- developing pragmatic studies that mirror everyday practice: outcomes, comparative observational and outcome studies
- creating large datasets: pooling clinical outcome studies
- generating relevant questions: collaborative research, CT training colleges, CPs, PCG/Ts, patients groups
- collaboration between university departments to develop relevant research projects
- collaboration between universities and with research organizations
- cost-effectiveness studies: collaboration with health economists
- collaborate with PCG/Ts: develop models for mainstream CAM access
- developing clinical governance of CAM: procedures and guidelines.

RESEARCH EVIDENCE

The available RCT-derived evidence, though patchy, can be used to sketch out an impression of the likely benefit of the different therapies in a wide range of common conditions. The evidence for specific therapies is summarized as an 'evidence grid' in Table 2.2. The numbers on the table indicate how the emerging evidence maps on to everyday practice. At one extreme a treatment might have been shown to be ineffective (1 = rumour); at the other extreme a treatment might have been researched in such depth that meta-analysis allows us to say with some certainty that it should be effective (5 = definitely). In the majority of cases, however, the jury is still out, as the large number of 3s (possibly) bears witness.

Table 2.2 A summary of the current research evidence for CTs in common conditions

	Acupuncture	Homeopathy	Manual therapies	Nutritional therapies	Herbal medicine	Mind–body methods & hypnotherapy
asthma	3[1] subjectively	3[2]	1 chiro[3] 3 yoga[4]	3 diet strategies[5] 3 Mg, Sn, antiox[6]	3 various herbs[7]	4 hypnotherapy[8] 4 autogenic training[9]
rhinitis and hay fever	2 prevention?	4[10,11] hay fever		2 exclusion diets?	3[12] urtica	3 hypnotherapy
headache	3[13]	2[14]	3 ost/chiro[15]		3[16] apply peppermint oil	3 relaxation[17] 3 hypnotherapy[18]
migraine	3 prevention[19] 3 treat attacks[20]	3[21]	1 chiropractic[22]	4 exclusion diet[23,24,25] 2 Mg? B2?	3[25] feverfew prevents	4 biofeedb/relaxn[26]
eczema		2		3 exclusion diets[27] 4 evening prim[28]	3 TCM[29]	4 hypnotherapy[30]
colds and flu		3[31]		3 Zn lozenges[32] 3 high-dose vit C[33]	4 echinacaea[34]	evidence that 'stress' decreases mucosal IgA
IBS	3[35]	2		3 exclusion diet[36]	3 p'mint oil[37] 3 TCM herbs[38]	4 hypnotherapy[39]
inflammatory bowel disease				3 exclusion diet Crohns[40] 3 fish oil u colitis[41]		3 biofeedback for pain[42]
mild–moderate hypertension			3 tai chi[43]	3 Mg supp[44] 3 veg diet[45]	3 garlic[46]	3[47] meditation, relaxation biofeedback & exercise
ischaemic heart disease	3[48] reduces pain		3 tai chi[49]	3 CoQ10[50] < 3 gly 3 monascus[51] < 3 gly	3 garlic[52] < 3 gly 3 guar[53] < 3 gly	4 Ornish CBT package[54] (< fats, exercise, relaxn)
intermittent claudication					4 ginkgo[55]	
dementia					4 gingko[56]	
back pain	4 (chronic)[57]		4 ost/chi (acute)[58]		4 devil's claw[59]	4 exercise progs[60] 4 yoga[61]
neck pain	3[62]		3[63]			
osteoarthritis	4 knee[64] 2 hip	3[65]	4 ost/chi (back/neck)[66] 3 yoga (hands)[67]	4 glucosamine[68] 4 chondroitin[69] 4 avocado unsap[70]	4 devil's claw[71] 4 phytodolor[72]	
rheumatoid arthritis	3[73]	3[74]	2 massage	4 veg diet[75] 4 fasting[76] 4 fish oil suppls[77]	4 devil's claw[78] 4 phytodolor[79]	4 relaxation < pain[80]
fibromyalgia	3[81]	3[82]	3 massage[83]		3 capsaicin oint > grip[84]	3 hypnotherapy[85] 3 meditation[86] 4 exercise[87]
premenstrual syndrome	2	2	3 reflexology[88]	3 B6[89] 4 calcium		4 aerobic exercise[90]
period pain	3[91]	2	3 chiropractic[92]			
perimenopausal problems	4[93]	2		3 dietary phyto-oestrogens[94]	3 St J wort[95] 3 bl cohosh[96]	3 exercise > bone mass[97]
benign prostatic hyperplasia					4 s palmetto[98]	
chronic fatigue syndrome	2	3[99]	2 (if hyper-ventilation?)	2 (if food intolerance?)	3 St J wort[100] (depression?)	4 CBT and exercise progs[101]

Table 2.2 (*cont.*)

	Acupuncture	Homeopathy	Manual therapies	Nutritional therapies	Herbal medicine	Mind–body methods & hypnotherapy
anxiety		2	3 massage[102] 4 aromatherapy[103]	3 if hypoglycaemic	4 kava[104]	4 relaxation[105] 4 meditation[106]
insomnia			3 aromatherapy[107]	3 melatonin[108]	3 valerian[109]	4 hypnotherapy[110] 4 relaxation[111]
mild to moderate depression	3 electro-acu[112]	2	3 massage[113] 3 yoga[114]		5 St J Wort[115]	3 exercise[116]
smoking cessation	1[117]					
cancer-related problems	5 chemo-nausea[118]		3 massage[119,120]	4 allium and veg diets prevent[121]		4 > quality of life & survival in Ca breast[122]
persistent pain	3[123]					4 meditation prog[124]

Evidence-linked practice must include a hierarchy of evidence from clinical case reports through to systematic reviews.
5 = DEFINITELY—good evidence from systematic reviews or meta-analyses
4 = PROBABLY—evidence from one or more sound randomized and/or controlled trials
3 = POSSIBLY—some evidence from RCTs available: results inconclusive, studies conflicting or methods open to question
2 = OPINION—practitioner conviction, expert opinion or clinical experience, but no reliable research
1 = RUMOUR—'traditional use', but effectiveness doubted or research suggesting CT ineffective

REFERENCES

1. Cochrane Library. Systematic review: acupuncture for asthma. 1998
2. Reilly D, Taylor M, Beattie N G M et al. Is evidence for homeopathy reproducible? Lancet 1994; 344: 1601–1606
3. Balon J, Aker P D, Crowther E R et al. A comparison of active and simulated chiropractic manipulation as adjunctive treatment for childhood asthma. N Engl J Med 1998; 339: 1013–1020
4. Fluge T, Richter J, Fabel H, Zysno E, Weller E, Wagner T O. Long-term effects of breathing exercises and yoga in patients with bronchial asthma. Pneumologie 1994; 48: 484–490
5. Monteleone C A, Sherman A R. Nutrition and asthma. Arch Intern Med 1997; 157: 23–34
6. Baker J C, Tunnicliffe W S, Duncanson R C, Ayres J G. Reduced dietary intakes of magnesium, selenium and vitamins A, C and E in patients with brittle asthma. Thorax 1995; 50(suppl 2): A75
7. Huntley A, Ernst E. Herbal medicine for asthma: systematic review. Thorax 2000; 55: 925–929
8. Ewer T C, Stewart D E. Improvement in bronchial hyper-responsiveness in patients with moderate asthma after treatment with a hypnotic technique: a randomised controlled trial. BMJ (Clin Res) 1986; 293: 1129–1132
9. Henry M, De Rivera J L G, Gonzalez-Martin I J, Abreu J. Improvement of respiratory function in chronic asthmatic patients with autogenic therapy. J Psychosom Res 1993; 17: 265–270
10. Taylor Reilly D, McSharry C, Taylor M A, Aitchison T. Is homoeopathy a placebo response? Controlled trial of homoeopathic potency, with pollen in hayfever as a model. Lancet 1986; ii: 881–885
11. Wiesenauer M, Ludtke R. The treatment of pollinosis with Galphimia glauca D4—a randomized placebo-controlled double-blind clinical trial. Phytomedicine 1995; 2(1): 3–6
12. Mittman P. Randomized, double-blind study of freeze-dried Urtica dioica in the treatment of allergic rhinitis. Planta Med 1990; 56: 44–47
13. Melchart D, Linde K, Fischer P et al. Acupuncture for recurrent headaches: a systematic review of randomized controlled trials. Cephalalgia 1999; 19: 779–786

14. Walach H, Haeusler W, Lower T et al. Classical homeopathic treatment of chronic headaches. Cephalalgia 1997; 17: 119–126
15. Systematic review. spinal manipulation for headache. Compl Ther Med 1999; 7: 1442–1155
16. Gobel H, Fresenius J, Heinze A, Dworschak M, Soyka D. Effectiveness of Oleum menthae piperitae and paracetamol in therapy of headache of the tension type. Nervenarzt 1996; 67: 672–681
17. Engel J M, Rapoff M A, Pressman A R. Long-term follow-up of relaxation training for pediatric headache disorders. Headache 1992; 32: 152–156
18. Melis P M, Rooiman W, Spierings E L, Hoogduin C A. Treatment of chronic tension-type headache with hypnotherapy: a single-blind time controlled study. Headache 1991; 31: 686–689
19. Hesse J, Mogelvang B, Simonsen H. Acupuncture versus metoprolol in migraine prophylaxis: a randomised trial of trigger point inactivation. J Intern Med 1994; 235: 451–456
20. Melchart D, Thormaehlen J, Hager S, Liao J. Acupuncture versus sumatriptan for early treatment of acute migraine attacks—a randomized controlled trial. Forsch Komplementärmed Klass Naturheilkd 2000; 7: 53
21. Ernst E. Systematic review. Homeopathic prophylaxis of headaches and migraine? A systematic review. J Pain Symptom Manag 1999; 18: 353–357
22. Parker G B, Tupling H, Pryor D S. A controlled trial of cervical manipulation for migraine. Aust N Z J Med 1978; 8(6): 589–593
23. Egger J, Carter C M, Wilson J, Turner M W, Soothill J F. Is migraine food allergy? A double-blind controlled trial of oligoantigenic diet treatment. Lancet 1983; ii: 865–869
24. Mansfield L E, Vaughan T R, Waller S F, Haverly R W, Ting S. Food allergy and adult migraine: double-blind and mediator confirmation of an allergic etiology. Ann Allergy 1985; 55: 126–129
25. Systematic review. Feverfew for migraine. Cochrane Library 2000
26. Holroyd K A, Penzien D B. Meta-analysis. Pharmacological versus non-pharmacological prophylaxis of recurrent migraine headache: a meta-analytic review of clinical trials. Pain 1990; 42: 1–13

27. Neild V S, Marsden R A, Bailes J A, Bland J M. Egg and milk exclusion diets in atopic eczema. Br J Dermatol 1986; 114: 117–123

28. Morse P F, Horrobin D F, Manku M S et al. Meta-analysis of placebo-controlled studies of the efficacy of Epogam in the treatment of atopic eczema. Relationship between plasma essential fatty acid changes and clinical response. Br J Dermatol 1989; 121: 75–90

29. Armstrong N C, Ernst E. The treatment of eczema with Chinese herbs: a systematic review of randomised clinical trials. Br J Clin Pharmacol 1999; 48: 262–264

30. Sokel B, Christie D, Kent A, Lansdown R, Atherton D. A comparison of hypnotherapy and biofeedback in the treatment of childhood atopic eczema. Contemp Hypnosis 1993; 10: 145–154

31. Ferley J P, Zmirou D, d'Adhemar D, Balducci F. A controlled evaluation of a homeopathic preparation in the treatment of influenza-like syndromes. Br J Clin Pharmacol 1989; 27: 329–335

32. Galand M L, Hagmeyer K O. The role of zinc lozenges in treatment of the common cold. Ann Pharmacother 1998; 32: 63–69

33. Douglas R M, Chalker E B, Treacy B. Systematic review. Vitamin C for respiratory tract infection. Cochrane Library. 1997

34. Melchart D, Linde K, Fischer P, Kaesmayr J. Systematic review. Echinacea for preventing and treating the common cold. Cochrane Library. 1998

35. Chan J, Carr I, Mayberry J F. The role of acupuncture in the treatment of irritable bowel syndrome: a pilot study. Hepatogastroenterology 1997; 44: 1328–1330

36. Nanda R, James R, Smith H, Dudley CR, Jewell DP. Food intolerance and the irritable bowel syndrome. Gut 1989; 30(8): 1099–1104

37. Pittler M H, Ernst E. Peppermint oil for irritable bowel syndrome: a critical review and meta-analysis. Am J Gastroenterol 1998; 93: 1131–1135

38. Bensousson A, Talley N J, Hing M, Menzies R, Guo A, Ngu M. Treatment of irritable bowel syndrome with Chinese herbal medicine. A randomized controlled trial. JAMA 1998; 280: 1585–1589

39. Harvey R F, Gunary R M, Hinton R A, Barry R E. Individual and group hypnotherapy in treatment of refractory irritable bowel syndrome. Lancet 1989; i: 424–425

40. Riordan A M, Hunter J O, Cowan R E et al. Treatment of active Crohn's disease by exclusion diet: East Anglian multicentre controlled trial. Lancet 1993; 342: 1131–1134

41. Beluzzi A, Brignola C, Campieri M, Pera A, Boschi S, Miglioli M. Effect of an enteric-coated fish-oil preparation on relapses in Crohn's disease. N Engl J Med 1996; 334: 1557–1560

42. Marzyk P M. Biofeedback for gastrointestinal disorders: a review of the literature. Ann Intern Med 1985; 103: 240–244

43. Jin P. Efficacy of Tíai Chi, brisk walking, meditation and reading in reducing mental and emotional stress. J Psychosom Res 1992; 36(4): 361–370

44. Witteman J C M, Grobbee D E, Derkx F H M et al. Reduction of blood pressure with oral magnesium supplementation in women with mild to moderate hypertension. Am J Clin Nutr 1994; 60: 129–135

45. Margetts B M, Beilin L J, Armstrong B K, Vandongen R. A randomized control trial of a vegetarian diet in the treatment of mild hypertension. Clin Exp Pharmacol Physiol 1985; 12(3): 263–266

46. Auer W, Eiber A, Hertkorn E et al. Hypertension and hyperlipidaemia: garlic helps in mild cases. Br J Clin Pract 1990; suppl 69: 3–6

47. Eisenberg D M, Delbanco T L, Berkey C S et al. Cognitive behavioral techniques for hypertension: are they effective? Ann Intern Med 1993; 118(12): 964–972

48. Ballegaard S, Meyer C N, Trojaborg W. Acupuncture in angina pectoris: does acupuncture have a specific effect? Intern Med 1991; 229(4): 357–362

49. Lai J S, Lan C, Wong M K, Teng S H. Two-year trends in cardiorespiratory function among older Tai Chi Chuan practitioners and sedentary subjects. J Am Geriatr Soc 1995; 43(11): 1222–1227

50. Singh R B. Serum concentration of lipoprotein (a) decreases on treatment with hydrosoluble coenzyme Q10 in patients with coronary artery disease: discovery of a new role. Int J Cardiol 1999; 68: 23–29

51. Heber D, Yip I, Ashley J M, Elashoff D A, Elashoff R M, Go V L W. Cholesterol-lowering effects of a proprietary Chinese red-yeast-rice dietary supplement. Am J Clin Nutr 1999; 69: 231–236

52. Silagy C, Neil A. Garlic as a lipid lowering agent—a meta-analysis. J R Coll Phys (Lond) 1994; 28: 39–45

53. Salenius J-P, Harjo E, Jokela H, Reikkinen H, Silvasti M. Long term effects of guar gum on lipid metabolism after carotid endarterectomy. BMJ 1995; 310: 95–96

54. Ornish D, Brown S E, Scherwitz L W et al. Can lifestyle changes reverse coronary heart disease? The Lifestyle Heart Trial. Lancet 1990; 336: 129–133

55. Pittler M H, Ernst E. Gingko biloba extract for the intermittent treatment of claudication: a meta-analysis of randomized trials. Am J Med 2000; 108: 276–281

56. Ernst E, Pittler M H. Systematic review. Ginkgo biloba for dementia. A systematic review of double-blind, placebo controlled-trials. Clin Drug Invest 1999; 17: 301–308

57. Ernst E, White A R. Acupuncture for back pain, meta-analysis. Arch Intern Med 1998; 158: 2235–2241

58. Bonfort G. Spinal manipulation, current state of research and its indications. Neurol Clin North Am 1999; 17(1): 91–111

59. Ernst E, Chrubasik S. Phyto-antiinflammatories. A systematic review of randomized, placebo-controlled, double-blind trials. Rheum Dis Clin North Am 2000; 26: 13–27

60. Berman B M, Sing B B. Chronic low back pain: an outcome analysis of a mind–body intervention. Compl Ther Med 1997; 5: 29–35

61. Nespor K. Psychosomatics of back pain and the use of yoga. Int J Psychosom 1989; 36: 72–78

62. White A R, Ernst E. Systematic review. A systematic review of randomized controlled trials of acupuncture for neck pain. Rheumatology (Oxford) 1999; 38: 143–147

63. Aker P D, Gross A R et al. Systematic review. Conservative management of mechanical neck pain: systematic overview and meta-analysis. BMJ 1996; 313: 1291–1296

64. Berman B M, Singh B B, Lao L et al. A randomized trial of acupuncture as an adjunctive therapy in osteoarthritis of the knee. Rheumatology 1999; 38: 346–354

65. Long L, Ernst E. Homeopathic remedies for the treatment of osteoarthritis: a systematic review. British Homeopathic Journal 2001; 90: 37–43

66. Gottlieb M S. Conservative management of spinal osteoarthritis with glucosamine and chriropractic treatment. J Manip Physiol Ther 1997; 20: 400–414

67. Garfinkel M S, Schumacher H R, Husain A, Levy M, Reshetar R A. Evaluation of a yoga based regimen for treatment of osteoarthritis of the hands. J Rheumatol 1994; 21: 2341–2343

68. Meta-analysis. Glucosamine for osteoarthritis. Arthritis Rheum 1998; 41: S198

69. McAlindon T M, LaValley M P, Gulin J P, Felson D M. Glucosamine and chondroitin sulfate for treatment of osteoarthritis: a systematic quality assessment and metaanalysis. JAMA 2000; 283: 1469–1475

70. Maheu E, Mazieres B, Valat J P et al. Symptomatic efficacy of avocado/soybean unsaponifiables in the treatment of osteoarthritis of the knee and hip. Arthritis Rheum 1998; 41: 81–91

71. Ernst E. Phyto-anti-inflammatories: a systematic review of randomized, placebo-controlled, double-blind trials. Rheum Dis Clin: Compl Alt Ther Rheum Dis II 2000; 26: 13–27

72. Mills S M, Jacoby R K, Chacksfield M et al. Effect of a proprietary herbal medicine on the relief of chronic arthritic pain: a double-blind study. Br J Rheumatol 1996; 35: 874–878

73. DeLuze C, Bosia L, Zirbs A, Chantraine A, Vischer T L. Electroacupuncture in fibromyalgia: results of a controlled trial. BMJ 1992; 305: 1249–1252

74. Jonas W, Linde L, Ramirez G. Homeopathy and rheumatic disease. Rheum Dis Clin North Am 2000; 26: 117–123

75. Kjeldsen-Kragh J, Haugen M, Borchgrevink C F, Forre O. Vegetarian diet for patients with rheumatoid arthritis—status: two years after introduction of the diet. Clin Rheumatol 1994; 13(3): 475–482

76. Kjeldsen-Kragh J, Haugen M, Borchgrevink C F et al. Controlled trial of fasting and one-year vegetarian diet in rheumatoid arthritis. Lancet 1991; 338: 899–902

77. Fortin P R, Lew R A, Liang M H et al. Validation of a meta-analysis: the effects of fish oil in rheumatoid arthritus. J Clin Epidemiol 1995; 48: 1379–1390

78. Ernst E. Phyto-anti-inflammatories: a systematic review of randomized, placebo-controlled, double-blind trials. Rheum Dis Clin: Compl Alt Ther Rheum Dis II 2000; 26: 13–27

79. Ernst E. The efficacy of phytodolor for the treatment of musculoskeletal pain – a systematic review of randomized clinical trials. Natural Medicine Journal 1999; 2(5): 14–17

80. Lundgren S, Stenstrom C H. Muscle relaxation training and quality of life in rheumatoid arthritis. A randomized controlled clinical trial. Scand J Rheumatol 1999; 28: 47–53

81. Berman B M, Ezzo J, Hadhazy V, Swyers J P. Systematic review. Acupuncture for fibromyalgia. J Fam Pract 1999; 48: 213–218

82. Fisher P, Greenwood A, Huskisson E C et al. Effect of homeopathy on fibrositis (primary fibromyalgia). BMJ 1989; 299: 365–366

83. Brattberg G. Connective tissue massage in the treatment of fibromyalgia. Eur J Pain 1999; 3: 235–245

84. McCarthy D J, Csuka M, McCarthy G, Trotter D. Treatment of pain due to fibromyalgia with topical capsaicin: a pilot study. Semin Arthritis Rheum 1994; 23(suppl 3): 41–47

85. Haanen H C M, Hoenderdos H T W, van Romunde L K J et al. Controlled trial of hypnotherapy in the treatment of refractory fibromyalgia. J Rheumatol 1991; 18(1): 72–75

86. Kaplan K H, Goldenberg D L, Galvin-Nadeau M. The impact of a meditation-based stress reduction program on fibromyalgia. Gen Hosp Psychiatry 1993; 15: 284–289

87. Gowans S E, deHueck A, Voss S, Richardson M. A randomized, controlled trial of exercise for fibromyalgia syndrome. Arthritis Care Res 1998; 11: 196–209

88. Oleson T, Flocco W. Randomized controlled study of premenstrual symptoms treated with ear, hand, and foot reflexology. Obstet Gynecol 1993; 82: 906–911

89. Kleijnen J, Ter Riet G, Knipschild P. Vitamin B$_6$ in the treatment of premenstrual syndrome—a review. Br J Obstet Gynaecol 1990; 97: 847–852

90. Choi P Y L, Salmon P. Symptom changes across the menstrual cycle in competitive sportswomen, exercises and sedentary women. Br J Clin Psychol 1995; 34: 447–460

91. Helms J M. Acupuncture for the management of primary dysmenorrhea. Obstet Gynecol 1987; 69(1): 51–56

92. Kokjohn K, Schmid D M, Triano J J, Brennan P C. The effect of spinal manipulation on pain and prostaglandin levels in women with primary dysmenorrhea. J Manipul Physiol Ther 1992; 15: 279–285

93. Wyon Y, Lindgren R, Hammar M, Lundeberg T. Acupuncture against climacteric disorders? Lower number of symptoms after menopause. Lakartidningen 1994; 91: 2318–2322

94. Dalais F S, Rice G E, Wahlqvist M L et al. Effects of dietary phytoestrogens in postmenopausal women. Climacteric 1998; 1: 124–129.

95. Pittler M H, Ernst E. Ginkgo biloba extract for the treatment of intermittent claudication: a meta-analysis of randomized trials. Am J Med 2000; 108: 276–281

96. Boblitz N, Schrader E, Henneicke-von Zepelin H H, Wüstenberg P. Benefit of a fixed drug combination containing St John's wort and black cohosh for climacteric patients—results of a randomized clinical trial. Focus Alt Compl Ther 2000; 5: 85–86

97. Chow R, Harrison J E, Notarius C. Effect of two randomised exercise programmes on bone mass of healthy post-menopausal women. BMJ 1987; 295: 1441–1444

98. Wilt T J, Iskani A, Stark G, McDonald R, Lan J, Murlow C. Meta-analysis. Saw palmetto extracts for treatment of benign prostatic hyperplasia. JAMA 1998; 280: 1604–1609

99. Awdry R. Homeopathy may help ME. Int J Alt Compl Med 1996; 14: 12–16

100. Beatty C. Prescriptions used by medical herbalists in the treatment of chronic fatigue syndrome and depression. Eur J Herb Med 1999; 4: 35–37

101. Deale A, Chalder T, Everitt B, Marks I, Wessely S. Cognitive behavior therapy for chronic fatigue syndrome: a randomized controlled trial. Am J Psychiatry 1997; 154: 408–414

102. Field T, Grizzle N, Scafidi F, Schanberg S. Massage and relaxation therapies' effects on depressed adolescent mothers. Adolescence 1996; 31: 903–911

103. Cooke B, Ernst E. Aromatherapy for anxiety: a systematic review. Br J Gen Pract 2000; 50: 493–496

104. Pittler M H, Ernst E. The efficacy of kava extract for anxiety. A systematic review and metaanalysis. J Clin Psychopharmacol 2000; 20: 84–89

105. Eppley K R, Abrams A, Shear J. Differential effects of relaxation techniques on trait anxiety: A metaanalysis. J Clin Psychol 1989; 45(6): 957–974

106. Astin J A. Stress reduction through mindfulness meditation. Effects on psychological symptomatology, sense of control and spritual experiences. Psychother Psychosom 1997; 66: 97–106

107. Miyake Y, Nakagawa M, Asakura Y. Effects of odors on humans (I). Effects on sleep latency. Chemical Senses 1991; 16: 183

108. Hughes R J, Sack R L, Lewy A J. The role of melatonin and circadian phase in age-related sleep maintenance insomnia: assessment in a clinical trial of melatonin replacement. Sleep 1997; 21: 52–68

109. Stevinson C, Ernst E. Valerian for insomnia: a systematic review of randomized clinical trials. Sleep Med 2000; 1: 91–99

110. Stanton H E. Hypnotic relaxation and the reduction of sleep onset insomnia. Int J Psychosom 1989; 36: 64–68

111. Morin C M, Culber J P, Schwartz S M. Nonpharmacological interventions for insomnia: a meta-analysis of treatment efficacy. Am J Psychiatry 1994; 151: 1172–1180

112. Luo H, Jia Y, Zhan L. Electro-acupuncture vs amitriptyline in the treatment of depressive states. J Trad Chin Med 1985; 5: 3–8

113. Field T, Morrow C, Valdeon C, Larson S, Juhn C, Schanberg S. Massage reduces anxiety in child and adolescent psychiatric patients. J Am Acad Child Adolesc Psychiatry 1992; 31: 125–131

114. Janakiramaiah N, Gangadhar B N, Naga Venkatesha Murthy P J, Harish M G, Subbakrishna D K, Vedamurthachar A. Antidepressant efficacy of Sudarshan Kriya Yoga in melancholia: a randomized comparison with electroconvulsive therapy and imipramine. J Affect Dis 2000; 57: 255–259

115. Gaster B, Holroyd J. St John's wort for depression: a systematic review. Arch Intern Med 2000; 160: 152–156

116. Lawlor D A, Hopker S W. The effectiveness of exercise as an intervention in the management of depression: systematic review and meta-regression analysis of randomised controlled trials. BMJ 2001; 322: 763

117. White A R, Rampes H, Ernst E. Metaanalysis. Acupuncture for smoking cessation. Cochrane Library 1999

118. Vickers A J. Can acupuncture have specific effects on health—a systematic review of acupuncture trials. J Soc Med 1996; 89: 303–311

119. Corner J, Cawley N, Hildebrand S. An evaluation of the use of massage and essential oils on the wellbeing of cancer patients. Int J Palliative Nursing 1995; 1: 67–73

120. Ferrell-Torry A T, Glick O J. The use of therapeutic massage as a nursing intervention to modify anxiety and the perception of cancer pain. Cancer Nursing 1993; 16: 93–101

121. Ernst E. Can allium vegetables prevent cancer? Phytomedicine 1997; 4: 79–83

122. Spiegel D, Bloom J R, Kraemer H C. Effect of psychosocial treatment on survival of patients with metastatic breast cancer. Lancet 1989; ii: 888–891

123. Ter Riet G, Kleijnen J, Knipschild P. Acupuncture and chronic pain: a criteria-based meta-analysis. J Clin Epidemiol 1990; 43: 1191–1199

124. Kabat-Zinn J, Lipworth L, Burney R, Sellers W. Four year follow-up of a meditation-based program for the self-regulation of chronic pain: treatment outcomes and compliance. Clin J Pain 1986; 2: 159–173

KEY FURTHER READING

Acupuncture
Filshie J, White A 1997 Medical acupuncture. Churchill Livingstone, New York. This is a practical in-depth manual of medical acupuncture.
Kaptchuk T 1983 Chinese medicine: the web that has no weaver. Rider, London. A well-written voyage into the world view of TCM for the general reader.
Maciocia G 1989 The foundations of Chinese medicine. Churchill Livingstone, New York. For those who want in-depth reading about clinical practice.

Herbal medicine
Mills S, Bone K 2000 Principles and practice of phytotherapy. Churchill Livingstone, New York. An in-depth manual of herbal medicine which provides an accessible glimpse of its world view.
Newall C A, Anderson L A, Phillipson J D 1996 Herbal medicines: a guide for health-care professionals. Pharmaceutical Press, London. A simple, practical guide to basic herbal medicine.

Homeopathy
Leckridge B 1997 Homeopathy: a practical guide for the primary care team. Butterworth-Heinemann, London. A textbook for those wanting a structured approach for applying homeopathy.
Schiff M 1995 The memory of water. Thorsons, London. An interesting book which speculates on the biophysics of high dilutions.
Swayne J 1998 Homeopathic method: implications for clinical practice and medical science. Churchill Livingstone, Edinburgh. A thoughtful account for practitioners wanting to consider homeopathy in depth.
Royal London Homoeopathic Hospital Academic Unit 1999 The evidence base of complementary medicine. RLHH, Parkside Health Trust, London. Useful summary of the evidence for homeopathy and other therapies.

Manipulative therapies
Burn L 1998 A manual of medical manipulation. Petroc Press, Newbury. Provides a practical guide to basic techniques.
DiGiovanna E L, Schiowitz S, Dowling D 1996 An osteopathic approach to diagnosis and treatment. Lippincott Raven, Plymouth.

Gives insight into the osteopathic perspective and a detailed account of its application.
Ward R (ed) 1997 Foundations for osteopathic medicine. Williams & Wilkins, Baltimore

Hypnosis and relaxation
Karle H, Boys J 1996 Hypnotherapy: a practical handbook. Free Association Books, London. This book covers just what the title states.
Siegel B 1989 Love, medicine and miracles. Arrow, London. A touching and persuasive account of the effectiveness of the therapeutic relationship and the power of vizualization techniques.
Watkins A (ed) 1997 Mind–body medicine: a clinician's handbook of psychoneuroimmunology. Churchill Livingstone, New York. A collection of writing from mainstream clinicians exploring theory and practice of a wide range of approaches.

Massage and touch-based therapies
Vickers A 1998 Massage and aromatherapy: a guide for health professionals. Stanley Thornes, Cheltenham. A thorough exploration of techniques, practical issues and available research.

Naturopathy
Pizzorno J, Murray M 1999 Textbook of natural medicine, 2nd edn. Churchill Livingstone, Edinburgh. An impressive textbook to broaden conventional practitioners' appreciation of the potential of naturopathy.

Nutritional therapies
Brostoff J, Gamlin L 1992 Complete guide to food allergy and intolerance. Bloomsbury, London. Thorough and enlightening account of current thinking and practice.
Davies S, Stewart A 1987 Nutritional medicine. Pan, London. This is still the best introductory book.
Werbach M 1999 Nutritional influences on illness, 3rd edn. Third Line Press, Tarzana, CA. A compendium of lab-based and clinical trial evidence.

FURTHER READING

General
Dekker M, Schouten EG, Klootwijk P et al 1997. Heart rate variability from short electrocardiographic recordings predict mortality from all causes in middle age and elderly men. The Zutohen Study. American Journal of Epidemiology 145(10): 899–908
Engels G 1977 The need for a new medical model: the challenge for biomedicine. Science 4(286): 129–135
Ernst E, De Smet P A G M 1996 Adverse effects of complementary therapies. In: Dukes M N G (ed) Meyler's side effects. Elsevier, Amsterdam
Geschwind N, quoted in Locke S E, Hornig-Rohan M 1983 Mind and immunity. Institute for the Advancement of Health, New York
Greenwood D J, Levin M 1998 Introduction to action research: social research for social change. Sage, Thousand Oaks
Kaptchuk T J 1998 Powerful placebo: the dark side of the randomised controlled trial. Lancet 351: 1722–1725
McCraty R et al 1996 Music enhances the effect of positive emotional state on serum immunoglobulin A. Stress Medicine 12: 167–175
Mitchell A, Cormack M 1998 The therapeutic relationship in complementary care. Churchill Livingstone, New York
Oschman J L 2000 Energy medicine. Churchill Livingstone, New York
Pert C 1997 Molecules of emotion. Simon & Schuster, New York
Reason P, Bradbury H (eds) 2000 Handbook of action research: participative inquiry and practice. Sage, London and Thousand Oaks

Selye H 1982 History and present status of the stress concept. In: Goldberger L, Breznitz S (eds) Handbook of stress. Macmillan, New York, pp 7–20
Van Haselen R, Fisher P 1998 Evidence influencing British Health Authorities' decisions in purchasing complementary medicine. Journal of the American Medical Association 280: 1564
Vickers A 1998 Bibliometric analysis of randomised controlled trials in complementary medicine. Complementary Therapies in Medicine 6: 185–189
Vickers A, Cassileth B, Ernst E et al 1997 How should we research unconventional therapies? A panel report from the conference on Complementary and Alternative Medicine Research Methodology, National Institutes of Health. International Journal of Technology Assessment in Health Care 13(1): 111–121.

Websites
Bandolier Jan 2000: 71–72
Bandolier is an NHS site devoted to EBP: *www.jr2.ox.ac.uk/Bandolier/index.html* www.quackwatch.com is worth visiting if you are concerned about the benefits or otherwise of alternative therapies.

Acupuncture
Systematic reviews
Vickers A J 1996 Can acupuncture have specific effects on health? A systematic review of acupuncture antiemesis trials. Journal of the Royal Society of Medicine 89: 303–311.

White A R, Rampes H 1998 Acupuncture for smoking cessation. In: Cochrane Collaboration. The Cochrane Library. Issue 2. Update Software, Oxford

RCTs
Johansson K, Lindgren I, Widner H, Wiklund I, Johansson B B 1993 Can sensory stimulation improve the functional outcome in stroke patients? Neurology 43: 2189–2192
Kovacs F M, Abraira V, Pozo F et al 1997 Local and remote sustained trigger point therapy for exacerbations of chronic low back pain. A randomised, double blind, controlled, multicentre trial. Spine 22: 786–797
Pintov S, Lahat E, Alstein M, Vogel Z, Barg J 1997 Acupuncture and the opioid system: implications in management of migraine. Pediatric Neurology 17: 129–133
Vincent C A 1989 A controlled trial of the treatment of migraine by acupuncture. Clinical Journal of Pain; 5: 305–312
White A R, Eddleston C, Hardie R, Resch K L, Ernst E, 1996 A pilot study of acupuncture for tension headache, using a novel placebo. Acupuncture in Medicine 14: 11–15

Books
Ernst E, White A (eds) 1999 Acupuncture: scientific appraisal. Butterworth Heinemann, Oxford
Myers T 2001 Anatomy trains. Churchill Livingstone, Edinburgh

Papers
Al Sadi M, Newman B, Julious S A 1997 Acupuncture in the prevention of vomiting. Anaesthesia 52: 658–661
Andrzejowski J, Woodward D 1996 Semi-permanent acupuncture needles in the prevention of post-operative nausea and vomiting. Acupuncture in Medicine 14: 68–70
Ernst E 1995 The risks of acupuncture. International Journal of Risk and Safety in Medicine 6: 179–186
Ernst E, White A 1997 Acupuncture: safety first. British Medical Journal 314: 1362
Ernst E, White A R 1999 Indwelling needles carry greater risks than acupuncture techniques. British Medical Journal 318: 536
Helms J M 1987 Acupuncture for the management of primary dysmenorrhoea. Obstetrics and Gynaecology 69: 51–56
Hesse J, Mogelvang B, Simonsen H 1994 Acupuncture versus metoprolol in migraine prophylaxis: a randomised trial of trigger point inactivation. Journal of Internal Medicine 235(5): 451–456
Jin-Ling Tang, Si-Yan Zhan, Edzard E 1999 Review of RCTs of traditional Chinese medicine. Bmj.com
Kovacs F M, Abraira V, Pozo F et al 1997 Local and remote sustained trigger points therapy for exacerbations of chronic low back pain. A randomized, double-blind, controlled, multicenter trial. Spine 22: 786–797
McConaghy P, Bland D, Swales H 1996 Acupuncture in the management of postoperative nausea and vomiting in patients receiving morphine via a patient-controlled analgesia system. Acupuncture in Medicine 14: 2–5
Pintov S, Lahat E, Alstein M, Vogel Z, Barg J 1997 Acupuncture and the opioid system: implications in management of migraine. Pediatric Neurology 17: 129–133
Schwager K L, Baines D B, Meyer R J 1996 Acupuncture and postoperative vomiting in day-stay paediatric patients. Anaesthesia and Intensive Care 24: 674–677
Shen J, Wenger N, Glaspy J et al 1996 Adjunct antiemesis acupuncture in myeloablative chemotherapy. Forschung Komplementarmedizin 3: 325
Thomas M, Lundeberg T, Bjork G et al 1995 Pain and discomfort in primary dysmenorrhoea is reduced by pre-emptive acupuncture or low frequency TENS. European Journal of Physical and Medical Rehabilitation 4: 71–76
Vickers A J 1996 Can acupuncture have specific effects on health? A systematic literature review of acupuncture anti-emesis trials. Journal of the Royal Society of Medicine 89: 303–311
Vickers A, Zollman C 2000 ABC of complementary medicine: acupuncture. bmj.com

Website
Acupuncture Resource Research Centre website www.demon.co.uk/acupuncture/arrc.html

Herbalism
Systematic reviews
Cochrane Library 1999 Issue 3. Update Software, Oxford
Linde K, Ramirez G, Mulrow C D, Pauls A, Weidenhammer W 1996 St John's wort for depression: an overview and meta-analysis of randomised clinical trials. British Medical Journal 313: 253–258
Melchart D, Linde K, Fischer P, Kaesmayr J. Echinacea for preventing and treating the common cold. In: Cochrane Collaboration
Wilt T J, Ishani A, Stark G, MacDonald R, Lau J, Mulrow C 1998 Saw palmetto extracts for treatment of benign prostatic hyperplasia: a systematic review. Journal of the American Medical Association 280: 1604–1609

RCTs
Sheehan M P, Rustin M H, Atherton D J et al 1992 Efficacy of traditional Chinese herbal therapy in adult atopic dermatitis. Lancet 340: 13–17

Books
Mills S 1993 The essential book of herbal medicine. Arkana, London
For an in-depth listing of practically all the research into this subject readers are directed towards Botanical influences on illness by Melvyn Werbach and Michael Murray (Third Line Press, 4571 Viviana Drive, Tarzana, CA91356)

Papers
Bent S 1999 Commentary: Adulterants in herbal products: dangerous and deceitful. Western Journal of Medicine 170: 259–260
Ernst E, Pittler M H 1999 Ginkgo biloba for dementia: a systematic review of double-blind, placebo-controlled trials. Clinical Drug Investigation 17: 301–308
Ernst E, Rand J I, Barnes J, Stevinson C 1998 Adverse effect profile of the herbal antidepressant St John's Wort (Hypericum perforatum L). European Journal of Clinical Pharmacology 54: 589–594
Keane F M, Munn S E, du Vivier A W P, Higgins E M, Taylor N F 1999 Analysis of Chinese herbal creams prescribed for dermatological conditions. Western Journal of Medicine 170: 257–259
Linde K, Ramirez G, Mulrow C D, Pauls A, Weidenhammer W, Melchart D 1996 St John's Wort for depression—an overview and meta-analysis of randomised clinical trials. British Medical Journal 313: 253–258
Pittler M H, Ernst E 1998 Horse-chestnut seed extract for chronic venous insufficiency: a criteria-based systematic review. Archives of Dermatology 134: 1356–1360
Shaw D 1998 Risks or remedies? Safety aspects of herbal remedies in the UK. Journal of the Royal Society of Medicine 91: 294–296
Vickers A, Zollman C 2000 ABC of complementary medicine: herbal medicine bmj.com
Wagner P J, Jester D, LeClair B et al 1999 Taking the edge off: why patients choose St John's wort. Journal of Family Practice 48: 615–619

Sources of information on safety of herbal products
EXTRACT database. Centre for Complementary Health Studies, Exeter University, Exeter EX4 4RG. Tel: 01392 264496
PhytoNet Home Page www.exeter.ac.uk/phytonet/ (an information resource concerning development, manufacture, regulation, and surveillance of herbal medicines)
National Poisons Unit (contact details for poisons information centres available in the British National Formulary)

Homeopathy
Systematic reviews
Kleijnen J, Knipschild P, ter Riet G 1991 Clinical trials of homeopathy. British Medical Journal 302: 316–323
Linde K, Clausius N, Ramirez G et al 1997 Are the clinical effects of homeopathy placebo effects? A meta-analysis of placebo-controlled trials. Lancet 350: 834–843

RCTs
Papp R, Schuback G, Beck E et al 1998 Oscillococcinum in patients with influenza-like syndromes: a placebo controlled double blind evaluation. British Homeopathic Journal 87: 69–76
Reilly D, Taylor M A, Beattie N G et al 1994 Is evidence for homeopathy reproducible? Lancet 344: 1601–1606

Laboratory studies
Belon P, Cumps J, Ennis M et al 1999 Inhibition of human basophil degranulation by successive histamine dilutions: results of a European multi-centre trial. Inflammation Research 48(suppl 1): S17–S18
Linde K, Jonas W B, Melchart D, Worku F, Wagner H, Eitel F 1994 Critical review and meta-analysis of serial agitated dilutions in experimental toxicology. Human Experimental Toxicology 13: 481–492

Books
Downey P 1997 Homeopathy: a practical guide for the primary care team. Butterworth-Heinemann, London

Papers
Barnes J, Resch K-L, Ernst E 1997 Homeopathy for postoperative ileus? Journal of Clinical Gastroenterology 66: 207–220
Dantas F, Rampes H 1999 Do homeopathic medicines provoke adverse effects? Conference proceedings: Improving the success of homeopathy 2. Royal London Homeopathic Hospital, London, pp 70–74
Ernst E 1995 The safety of homeopathy. British Homeopathic Journal 84: 193–194
Ernst E, Fugh-Berman A 1999 Complementary/alternative medicine—a critical review of acupuncture, homeopathy and chiropractic. NHS conference on PCGs and complementary medicine, 2 September 1999
Reilly D T, Taylor M A, McSharry C et al 1986 Is homeopathy a placebo response? Controlled trial of homeopathic potency, with pollen in hayfever as model. Lancet ii: 881–886
Vickers A, Zollman C 1999 ABC of complementary medicine: homeopathy. British Medical Journal 319: 1115–1118/bmj.com

Manipulative therapies
Systematic reviews
Koes B W, Assendelft W J, van der Heijen G J M G, Bouter L M, Knipschild P G 1991 Spinal manipulation and mobilisation for back and neck pain: a blinded review. British Medical Journal 303: 1298–303
Koes B W, Assendelft W J, van der Heijen G J M G, Bouter L M 1996 Spinal manipulation for low back pain. An updated systematic review of randomised clinical trials. Spine 21: 2860–2871

RCTs
Balon J, Aker P D, Crowther E R et al 1998 A comparison of active and simulated chiropractic manipulation as adjunctive treatment for childhood asthma. New England Journal of Medicine 339: 1013–1020
Boline P D, Kassak K, Bronfort G et al 1995 Spinal manipulation vs. amitriptyline for the treatment of chronic tension-type headaches: a randomised clinical trial. Journal of Manipulative and Physiological Therapeutics 18(3): 148–154
Koes B W, Bouter L M, van Mameren H et al 1992 Randomised clinical trial of manipulative therapy and physiotherapy for persistent back and neck complaints: results of one year follow up. British Medical Journal 304: 601–605
Meade T W, Dyer S, Browne W, Townsend J, Frank A O 1990 Low back pain of mechanical origin: randomised comparison of chiropractic and hospital outpatient treatment. British Medical Journal 300: 1431–1437
Meade T W, Dyer S, Browne W, Frank A O 1995 Randomised comparison of chiropractic and hospital outpatient management for low back pain: results from extended follow up. British Medical Journal 311: 349–351

Books
Hurwitz E L, Aker P D, Adams A H et al 1996 Manipulation and mobilization of the cervical spine. A systematic review of the literature. Spine 21: 1746–1759
Kaptchuk T J, Eisenberg D M 1998 Chiropractic: origins, controversies and contributions. Archives of Internal Medicine 158: 2215–2224
RLHH 1999 The evidence base of complementary medicine, 2nd edn. RLHH, Parkside Health Trust, London

Papers
Anon 1998 New England Journal of Medicine 339: 1013–1019
Assendelft W J J, Koes B W, Knipschild P G, Bouter L M 1995 The relationship between methodological quality and conclusions in reviews of spinal manipulation. Journal of the American Medical Association 274: 1942–1948
Assendelft W J, Bouter S M, Knipschild P G 1996 Complications of spinal manipulation: a comprehensive review of the literature. Journal of Family Practice 42: 475–480
Assendelft W J J, Koes B W, van der Heijden G J M G, Bouter L M 1996 The effectiveness of chiropractic for treatment of low back pain: an update and attempt at statistical pooling. Journal of Manipulative and Physiological Therapeutics 19: 499–507
Boesler D, Warner M, Alpers A et al 1993 Efficacy of high-velocity low-amplitude manipulative technique in subjects with low-back pain during menstrual cramping. Journal of the American Osteopathic Association 93(2): 203–208, 213–144
Ernst E 1994 Cervical manipulation: is it really safe? International Journal of Risk and Safety in Medicine 6: 145–149
Gottlieb S 2000 Chiropractic treatment is of limited benefit. Bmj.com
Hurwitz E L, Aker P D, Adams A H, Meeker W C, Shekelle P G 1996 Manipulation and mobilization of the cervical spine. A systematic review of literature. Spine. 21: 1746–1759
Koes B W, Assendelft W J, Van der Heijden G J, Bouter L M 1996 Spinal manipulation for low back pain. An updated systematic review of randomized clinical trials. Spine 21: 2860–2871
Kokjohn K, Schmid D M, Triano J J et al 1992 The effect of spinal manipulation on pain and prostaglandin levels in women with primary dysmenorrhea. Journal of Manipulative and Physiological Therapeutics 15(5): 279–285
Parker G B, Tupling H, Pryor D S 1978 A controlled trial of cervical manipulation of migraine. Australian and New Zealand Journal of Medicine 8(6): 589–593
Vickers A, Zollman C 2000 ABC of complementary medicine: manipulative therapies. bmj.com
Waddell G, Feder G, McIntosh A, Lewis M, Hutchinson A 1996 Clinical guidelines for the management of acute low back pain: low back pain evidence review. Royal College of General Practitioners, London

Exercise systems
Kirsteins A E, Dietz F, Hwang S M 1991 Evaluating the safety and potential use of a weight-bearing exercise, tai chi chuan, for rheumatoid arthritis patients. American Journal of Physical Medicine and Rehabilitation 70(3): 136–141
Lai L S, Lan C, Wong M K, Teng S H 1995 Two-year trends in cardiovascular function among older tai chi chuan practitioners and sedentary subjects. Journal of the American Geriatrics Society 43(11): 1222–1227
Nagarathna R, Nagendra H R 1985 Yoga for bronchial asthma: a controlled study. British Medical Journal 291: 1077–1079
Sing Lee 2000 Chinese hypnosis can cause qigong induced mental disorders. British Medical Journal 320: 803

Healing
Benor D 1993 Healing research, vol I. Research in healing. Helix, Munich/Oxford
McCraty R, Atkinson M, Tiller W A et al 1995 The effects of emotion on short term powerspectrum analysis of heart rate variability. American Journal of Cardiology 76(14): 1089–1093
Russek L G, Schwartz G 1996 Energy cardiology—a dynamic energy systems approach for integrating conventional and alternative medicine. Advances—the journal of mind body health 12: 4–24

Hypnosis and relaxation
Systematic reviews
Carroll D, Seers K 1998 Relaxation for the relief of chronic pain: a systematic review. Journal of Advanced Nursing 27: 476–487
Eisenberg D M, Delbanco T L, Berkey C S et al 1993 Cognitive behavioral techniques for hypertension: are they effective? Annals of Internal Medicine 118: 964–972
Kirsch I, Montgomery G, Sapirstein G 1995 Hypnosis as an adjunct to cognitive-behavioral psychotherapy: a meta-analysis. Journal of Consulting and Clinical Psychology 63: 214–220

RCTs
Ewer T C, Stewart D E 1986 Improvement in bronchial hyper-responsiveness in patients with moderate asthma after treatment with a hypnotic technique: a randomised controlled trial. British Medical Journal (clinical research edn) 293(6555): 1129–1132
Harvey R F, Hinton R A, Gunary R M, Barry R E 1989 Individual and group hypnotherapy in treatment of refractory irritable bowel syndrome. Lancet i: 424–425
Syrjala K L, Donaldson G W, Davis M W, Kippes M E, Carr J E 1995 Relaxation and imagery and cognitive–behavioural training reduce pain during cancer treatment: a controlled clinical trial. Pain 63: 189–198

Books
Waxman D 1988 Medical–dental hypnosis. Baillière Tindall, London

Papers
Anon 1968 Hypnosis for asthma—a controlled trial. A report to the Research Committee of the British Tuberculosis Association. British Medical Journal 4(623):71–76
Dahlgren L A, Kurtz R M, Strube M J et al 1995 Differential effects of hypnotic suggestion on multiple dimensions of pain. Journal of Pain and Symptom Management 10(6):464–467
Horton-Hausknecht J R 1995 The effects of clinical hypnosis and relaxation techniques on the functioning of the immune system: new directions for Psychoneuroimmunology research and practice. Forschende Komplementärmed 2: 196–202
NIH Technology Assessment Panel on Integration of Behavioral and Relaxation 1996 Approaches into the treatment of chronic pain and insomnia. Integration of behavioral and relaxation approaches into the treatment of chronic pain and insomnia. Journal of the American Medical Association 276: 313–318
Stanton H E 1984 A comparison of the effects of an hypnotic procedure and music on anxiety level. Australian Journal of Clinical and Experimental Hypnosis 12(2): 127–132
Stanton H E 1992 Using hypnotic success imagery to reduce test anxiety. Australian Journal of Clinical and Experimental Hypnosis 20(1): 31–37
Vickers A, Zollman C 1999 ABC of complementary medicine: hypnosis and relaxation therapies. British Medical Journal 319: 1346–1349/bmj.com
Whorwell P J, Prior A, Faragher E B 1984 Controlled trial of hypnotherapy in the treatment of severe refractory irritable-bowel syndrome. Lancet 2(8414): 1232–1234
Whorwell P J, Prior A, Colgan S M 1987 Hypnotherapy in severe irritable bowel syndrome: further experience. Gut 28(4): 423–425

Massage and touch-based therapies
Systematic reviews
Vickers A, Ohlsson A, Lacy J B, Horsley A 1998 Massage therapy for premature and/or low birth-weight infants to improve weight gain and/or to decrease hospital length of stay. In: Cochrane Collaboration. Cochrane Library. Issue 3. Update Software, Oxford

RCTs
Field T, Morrow C, Valdeon C, Larson S, Kuhn C, Schanberg S 1992 Massage reduces anxiety in child and adolescent psychiatric patients. Journal of the American Academy of Child Adolescent Psychiatry 31: 125–131
Stevensen C 1994 The psychophysiological effects of aromatherapy massage following cardiac surgery. Complementary Therapies in Medicine 2: 27–35

Wilkinson S 1995 Aromatherapy and massage in palliative care. International Journal of Palliative Nursing 1: 21–30

Books
Lett A 2000 Reflex zone therapy for health professionals. Churchill Livingstone, New York
Price S, Price L 1999 Aromatherapy for health professionals. Churchill Livingstone, New York

Papers
Corner J, Cawley N, Hildebrand S 1995 An evaluation of the use of massage and essential oils on the wellbeing of cancer patients. International Journal of Palliative Nursing 1(2): 67–73
Dunn C, Sleep J, Collett D 1995 Sensing an improvement: an experimental study to evaluate the use of aromatherapy, massage and periods of rest in an intensive care unit. Journal of Advanced Nursing 21(1):34–40
Ernst E 1996 Acupuncture for nausea: a best evidence analysis. European Journal of Physical Medicine and Rehabilitation 6(1): 28–29
Fan C F, Tanhui E, Joshi S, Trivedi S, Hong Y, Shevde K 1997 Acupressure treatment for prevention of postpoperative nausea and vomiting. Anesthesia and Analgesia 84: 821–825
Ho C M, Hseu S S, Tsi S K, Lee Ty 1996 Effect of P-6 acupressure on prevention of nausea and vomiting after epidural morphine for post-cesarean section pain relief. Acta Anaesthesiologica Scandinavica 40: 372–375
O'Brien B, Relyea M J, Taerum T 1996 Efficacy of P6 acupressure in the treatment of nausea and vomiting during pregnancy. American Journal of Obstetrics and Gynecology 174: 708–715
Stein D J, Birnbach D J, Danzer B I, Kuroda M M, Grunebaum A, Thys D M 1997 Acupressure versus intravenous metoclopramide to prevent nausea and vomiting during spinal anesthesia for cesarean section. Anesthesia and Analgesia 84: 342–345
Stevensen C 1994 The psycho-physiological effects of aromatherapy massage following cardiac surgery. Complementary Therapies in Medicine 2(1): 27–35
Vickers A, Zollman C 2000 ABC of complementary medicine: massage therapies. bmj.com
Waldman C S, Tseng P, Meulman P et al 1993 Aromatherapy in the intensive care unit. Care of the Critically Ill 9(4): 170–174
Wilkinson S 1995 Aromatherapy and massage in palliative care. International Journal of Palliative Nursing 1(1): 21–30

Naturopathy and nutritional therapies
Systematic reviews
Budeiri D, Li Wan Po A, Dornan J C 1996 Is evening primrose oil of value in the treatment of premenstrual syndrome? Controlled Clinical Trials 17: 60–68
Douglas R M, Chalker E B, Treacy B 1998 Vitamin C for the common cold. In: Cochrane Collaboration. Cochrane Library. Issue 2. Update Software, Oxford
Fortin P R, Lew R A, Liang M H et al 1995 Validation of a meta-analysis: the effects of fish oil in rheumatoid arthritis. Journal of Clinical Epidemiology 48: 1379–1390
Wyatt K M, Dimmock P W, Jones P W, O'Brien P M S 1999 Efficacy of vitamin B-6 in the treatment of premenstrual syndrome: systematic review. British Medical Journal 318: 1375–1381

RCT
Schmidt M H, Mocks P, Lay B et al 1997 Does oligoantigenic diet influence hyperactive/conduct-disordered children: a controlled trial. European Journal of Child Adolescent Psychiatry 6: 88–95

Books
Anthony H, Birtwhistle S, Eaton K, Maberly J 1997 Environmental medicine in clinical practice. BSAENM, Southampton
Murray M, Pizzorno J 1999 Encyclopaedia of natural medicine. 2nd edn. Little, Brown, London
Quinn P 1998 Healing with nutritional therapy. Gill & Macmillan, New York

Vickers A, Zollman C 1999 Unconventional approaches to nutritional medicine. ABC of complementary medicine. bmj.com

Papers
Astarita C, Scala G, Sproviero S, Franzese A 1996 A double-blind placebo-controlled trial of enzyme potentiated desensitisation in the treatment of pollenosis. Journal of Investigative Allergy and Clinical Immunology 6: 248–255
Auer W, Eiber A, Hertkom E et al 1990 Hypertension and hyperlipidaemia: garlic helps in mild cases. British Journal of Clinical Practice suppl 69: 3–6
Beluzzi A, Brignola C, Campieri M, Pera A, Boschi S, Miglioli M, 1996 Effect of an enteric-coated fish-oil preparation on relapses in Crohn's disease. New England Journal of Medicine 334: 1557–1560
Broughton K S, Johnson C S, Pace B K, Liebman M, Kleppinger K M 1997 Reduced asthma symptoms with n-3 fatty acid ingestion are related to 5-series leukotriene production. American Journal of Clinical Nutrition 65: 1011–1017
Budeiri D, Li Wan Po A, Dornan J C 1996 Is evening primrose oil of value in the treatment of premenstrual syndrome? Controlled Clinical Trials 17: 60–68
Douglas R M, Chalker E B, Treacy B 1998 Vitamin C for the common cold. In: Cochrane Collaboration. Cochrane Library. Issue 2. Update Software, Oxford
Ernst E, Pecho E, Wirz P, Saradeth T 1990 Regular sauna bathing and the incidence of common colds. Annals of Medicine 22: 225–227
Fortin P R, Lew R A, Liang M H et al 1995 Validation of a meta-analysis: the effects of fish oil in rheumatoid arthritis. Journal of Clinical Epidemiology 48: 1379–1390
Hederos C A, Berg A 1996 Epogam evening primrose oil treatment in atopic dermatitis and asthma. Archives of Disease in Childhood 75: 494–497
Hodge L, Salome C M, Hughes J M et al 1998 Effect of dietary intake of omega-3 and omega-6 fatty acids on severity of asthma in children. European Respiratory Journal 11: 361–365
Jenkins M, Vickers A 1998 Unreliability of 19E/1994 antibody testing as a diagnostic tool in food tolerance. Clinical and Experimental Allergy 28: 1526–1529
Knipschild P 1988 Looking for gall bladder disease in the patient's iris. British Medical Journal 297(6663): 1578–1581
Lewith G T, Vincent C A 1997 The clinical evaluation of acupuncture. In: Filshie J, White A (eds) Medical acupuncture. Churchill Livingstone, New York, pp 216–218
Loeschke K, Ueberschaer B, Pietsch A et al 1996 n-3 fatty acids only delay relapse of ulcerative colitis in remission. Digestive Diseases and Sciences 41: 2087–2094
Machura E, Brus R, Kalacinnski W, Lacheta M 1996 The effect of dietary fish oil supplementation on the clinical course of asthma in children. Pediatria Polska 71: 97–102
Schmidt M H, Mocks P, Lay B et al 1997 Does oligoantigenic diet influence hyperactive/conduct-disordered children: a controlled trial. European Child Adolescent Psychiatry 6: 88–95
Sethi T J, Kemeny D M, Tobin S, Lessof M H, Lambourn E, Bradley A 1987 How reliable are commercial allergy tests? Lancet i: 92–94
Shaw D, Leon C, Kolev S, Murray V 1997 Traditional remedies and food supplements—a 5 year toxicological study (1991–1995). Drug Safety 17: 342–356
Vickers A, Zollman C 2000 ABC of complementary medicine: unconventional approaches to nutritional medicine. bmj.com
Witteman J M C, Grobbee D E, Derxx F H M et al 1994 Reduction of blood pressure with oral magnesium supplementation in women with mild to moderate hypertension. American Journal of Clinical Nutrition 60: 129–135

Research evidence summaries
Ernst E 1996 Complementary medicine: an objective appraisal. Butterworth Heinemann, London
Ernst E 2001 The desktop guide to complementary and alternative medicine—an evidence-based approach. Mosby, Edinburgh
Fugh-Berman A 1996 Complementary therapies: what works? Williams and Wilkins, Baltimore

Lewith G, Kenyon J, Lewis P 1996 Complementary therapies: an integrated approach. Oxford GP series. Oxford University Press, Oxford
Royal London Homoeopathic Hospital Academic Unit 1999 The evidence base of complementary medicine. RLHH, Parkside Health Trust, London

Placebo response
Chaput de Saintonge D M, Herxheimer A 1994 Harnessing placebo effects in health care. Lancet 344: 995–998
Dixon M, Sweeney K 2000 The human effect in medicine—theory, research and practice. Radcliffe Medical, Oxford
Harrington A (ed.) 1997 The placebo effect. An interdisciplinary exploration. Harrard University Press, Cambridge, MA
Kleijnen J, de Craen A J M, van Everdingen J, Krol L 1994 Placebo effect in double-blind clinical trials: a review of interactions with medications. Lancet 344: 1347–1349
Peters D 2001 Understanding the placebo effect in complementary medicine. Churchill Livingstone, New York, in press
Rees I, Weil A 2001 Integrated medicine. British Medical Journal 322: 119–120

Safety
General
Angell M, Kassirer J P 1998 Alternative medicine—the risks of untested and unregulated remedies. New England Journal of Medicine 339: 839–841
Ernst E, Fugh-Berman A 1999 Complementary/alternative medicine—a critical review of acupuncture, homeopathy and chiropractic. NHS conference on PCGs and complementary medicine, 2 September 1999
Royal London Homoeopathic Hospital 1999 The safety of complementary medicine. In: The evidence base of complementary medicine, 2nd edn. RLHH, Parkside Health Trust, London

Acupuncture
Ernst E, White A R 1997 Life threatening adverse events after acupuncture? A systematic review. Pain 71: 123–126
Ernst E, White A R 2000 Acupuncture may be associated with serious adverse events. British Medical Journal 320: 513
Norheim A J 1996 Adverse effects of acupuncture: a study of the literature for the years 1981–1994. Journal of Alternative and Complementary Medicine 2(2): 291–297
Norheim A J, Fønnebø V 1995 Adverse effects of acupuncture. Lancet 345: 1576
Norheim A J, Fønnebø V 1996 Acupuncture adverse effects are more than occasional case reports: results from questionnaires among 1135 randomly selected doctors and 197 acupuncturists. Complementary Therapies in Medicine 4(1): 8–13
Onizuka T, Oishi K, Ikeda T et al 1998 A fatal case of streptococcal toxic shock-like syndrome probably caused by acupuncture. Kansenshogaku Zassi 72: 776–780
Rampes H 1997 Adverse reactions to acupuncture. In: Filshie J, White A (eds) Medical acupuncture. Churchill Livingstone, New York, pp 375–387
Rampes H, James R 1995 Complications of acupuncture. Acupuncture in Medicine 13: 26–33
Yamashita H, Tsukayama H, Tanno Y, Nishijo K 1998 Adverse events related to acupuncture (letter). Journal of the American Medical Association 280: 1563–1564

Herbal medicine
Bayly G G, Braithwaite R, Sheehan M P 1995 Lead poisoning from Asian traditional remedies in the West Midlands—a report of a series of 5 cases. Human Experimental Toxicology 14: 24–28
Gottlieb S 2000 Chinese herb may cause cancer. New York bmj.com
Janetzky K, Morreale A P 1997 Probable interactions between warfarin and ginseng. American Journal of Health System Pharmacology 54: 692–693
Keane F M, Munn S E, du Vivier A W P, Taylor N F, Higgins E M 1999 Analysis of Chinese herbal creams prescribed for dermatological conditions. British Medical Journal 318: 563–564

Lord G M, Tagore R, Cook T, Gower P, Pusey C D 1999 Nephropathy caused by Chinese herbs in the UK. Lancet 354: 481–482

McIntyre M 2000 A review of the benefits, adverse effects, drug interactions, and safety of St John's wort (*Hypericum perforatum*): the implications with regard to the regulation of herbal medicines. Journal of Alternative and Complementary Medicine (2): 115–124

Miller L G 1998 Herbal medicinals: selected clinical considerations focusing on known or potential drug–herb interactions. Archives of Internal Medicine 158: 2200–2211

Shaw D 1998 Risk or remedies? Safety aspects of herbal remedies in the UK. Journal of the Royal Society of Medicine 91: 294–296

Shaw D, Leon C, Kolev S, Murray V 1997 Traditional remedies and food supplements—a five year toxicological study (1991–1995). Drug Safety 17: 342–356

Homeopathy

Dantas F, Rampes H 1999 Do homeopathic medicines provoke adverse effects? Conference proceedings: Improving the success of homeopathy 2. Royal Homeopathic Hospital, London, pp 70–74

Ernst E 1996 Direct risks associated with complementary therapies. In: Ernst E (ed.) Complementary medicine: an objective appraisal. Butterworth Heinemann, Oxford, pp 112–125

Kerr H D, Yarborough G W 1988 Pancreatitis following ingestion of a homeopathic preparation. New England Journal of Medicine 314: 1642–1643

Manipulative therapies

Dabbs V, Lauretti W J 1995 A risk assessment of cervical manipulation vs NSAIDs for the treatment of neck pain. Journal of Manipulative and Physiological Therapeutics 18: 530–536

Ernst E, Assendelft W J J 1998 Chiropractic for low back pain: we don't know whether it does more good than harm. British Medical Journal 317: 160

Leboeuf-Yde C, Hennius B, Rudberg E, Leufvenmark P, Thunman M 1997 Side effects of chiropractic treatment: a prospective study. Journal of Manipulative and Physiological Therapeutics 20(8): 511–515

Senstad O, Leboeuf-Yde C, Borchgevink F 1996 Side-effects of chiropractic spinal manipulation: types, frequency, discomfort and course. Scandinavian Journal of Primary Health Care 14: 50–53

Senstad O, Leboeuf-Yde C, Borchgrevink C 1997 Frequency and characteristics of side effects of spinal manipulative therapy. Spine 22: 435–441

Chapter 2 REFLECTIVE LEARNING CYCLE AUDIT

1. **What did you need to know?** *(clarify learning objectives)*

2. **What did you notice?** *(key points)*

3. **What have you learned?** *(learning evaluation)*

4. **How will you apply it to practice?** *(clinical relevance)*

5. **What do I need to do next?** *(reflective educational audit)*

6. **Proceed to next area of interest / section you have identified**.

CT service implementation

3

Designing an integrated service

INTRODUCTION

The provision of CTs in a mainstream primary care service is beset by a number of practical difficulties. Different units have tried to address them in a variety of ways. Consequently, there are various models for provision of CTs, so the best option for any particular practice needs careful consideration. CTs will survive in the mainstream only if they improve the effectiveness, efficiency or quality of care. So whatever the approach chosen, it should encourage evidence-based practice by including ways of collecting and managing data about referrals, encounters and outcomes. Only then can claims of clinical effectiveness and cost-efficiency be supported.

The NHS Executive has defined clinical effectiveness as 'the extent to which a specific clinical intervention when deployed for a particular patient or population does what it is intended to—that is . . . to secure the greatest possible health gain from the available resources'.[1] Obviously cost effectiveness has become a crucial issue in the purchasing and evaluation of every kind of health technology in the NHS. The above statement implies that resources will be targeted to prioritize need and it intimates that real-world health gain will become an important consideration. These are key issues for those concerned to develop an effective role for CAM in the mainstream. What, for example, might CTs contribute to the care of national priority conditions: heart disease, cancer, mental health and diabetes? In what sorts of common health problems might certain CTs usefully augment conventional approaches to treatment? Where in fact can we expect CAM to add value and how? Such questions about effectiveness and efficiency are important whether the cost of CTs is to be met by the state, an individual or employer or a medical insurer. A growing concern for consumer protection and clinical quality assurance will inevitably influence the way all future health care—CTs included—is organized in both the public and private sector.

These are important messages for complementary therapists in both NHS and independent practice. How we as practitioner-researchers respond will determine whether CT services survive in our health centres and in the NHS as a whole. Given the limitations on time and funding, CT provision in the NHS will have to develop rationally. And, since it will inevitably be rationed, we will have to find ways of using CTs efficiently and be able to demonstrate that this is so.

The NHS is an increasingly multidisciplinary service, and problems around communication come with the primary care team territory. Yet there is never enough time for reflection. Increasingly, healthcare professions need to optimize their collaboration. At Marylebone Health Centre, where a range of CTs has been available since the late 1980s, we rely on part-time complementary practitioners for CT service delivery. However, before the Smith Project (see p. 286) began, the service as a whole had never developed clear intake or exclusion criteria, nor clarified the outcomes expected. Therefore in order to focus and evaluate our CT service we decided to develop clear guidelines for treating some common illnesses.

Bringing about a CT service in the mainstream calls for a major piece of practice development. Consensus and teamwork are likely to be the keys. Its management will require efficient (that word again!) data collection, monitoring and a built-in capacity for closing learning loops. An organization that can complete learning loops is capable of quality assurance. Clinical governance is quality assurance in practice, and must in the case of CT service development be supported by both practitioner and patient education about complementary treatment. The appropriate integration of CTs is such a challenging piece of practice development that the processes and structures needed for clinical governance have to be considered at the outset. Once they are in place and working well, this system will ensure the best use of CTs by monitoring their appropriateness and effectiveness on a daily basis.

However, this kind of clinical audit will not provide evidence about which aspect of a therapy has produced a clinical benefit, nor whether improvement is due to natural remission; RCTs would be required for this (see Ch. 2, p. 37). GPs as well as patients may have unrealistic expectations of CTs or simply misunderstand their nature and relevance. They therefore need information about their appropriateness, about what a particular treatment entails, and about how well the complementary practitioner has been trained. It is valuable to have a range of user-friendly literature and self-help information available for patients; background material for GPs, clarifying the role and potential of CTs, is essential too. All these and other issues of practical importance that must be considered at the design stage are dealt with in this chapter.

Box 3.1 summarizes the structures, processes and outcomes required for the development of the CT field.

KEY ISSUES AND QUESTIONS FOR PRACTICE DEVELOPMENT AND CLINICAL GOVERNANCE

There are many issues and questions that arise when a practice is considering complementary medicine as an option within primary care. These can be grouped into three broad categories.

Needs

- Which conditions are poorly managed conventionally?
- In which conditions might conventional management be effectively improved by CTs?
- How prevalent are these conditions amongst your patient population?

Box 3.1 Structures, processes and outcomes required for the further development of the CT field

Structures
- Mainstream practitioners need appropriate referral guidelines based on need and evidence
- The public and the public sector need well-educated, professionally regulated therapists
- The capacity for research and the creation of large outcome data sets require the development of competent networks of practitioners and researchers
- Organizations involved must be capable of collaboration and reflective practice
- Reflective practice of CTs requires the development of systems for data collection and consistent methods for reporting outcomes

Processes

As an academic field the development of 'CT studies' will depend on:

- The further development of an interprofessional ethos
- Appropriate interdisciplinary referral activity and reflection
- Ways of improving access to CTs that optimize the relevance and effectiveness of CTs
- Practical approaches to evaluation that reflect everyday practice
- Evaluation of processes and outcomes relevant to patients' (and students') needs
- Continual clinical learning cycles to improve the delivery and relevance of CT services
- Appropriate action on reflection in order to optimize professional and practice development

Outcomes
- The developing CT field needs to build a consensus. What are our objectives in CT education, research, service delivery?
- Can we identify and agree appropriate outcomes for these areas of work?
- In developing service delivery models, for instance, are our outcomes individual or population based?; short or long term?; to cure, contain or maintain?; and what part can CTs play in health creation?
- In developing a consensus on these issues, how can soundings be taken from all the stakeholders?

• Is a comprehensive service feasible? Or might it be best to start with some simple changes?

Service innovation

• Are there potentially useful CTs to which patients need access?
• What primary interventions could feasibly be introduced (e.g. GP prescribing and self-care approaches, use of information leaflets, etc.)?
• What criteria should be set for recommending CTs?
• How should referral and communication processes be set up?

Quality assurance

• Can the practice provide appropriate knowledge, skills and evaluation of a new service?
• Should the service be provided by skilled doctors or professional CPs?
• If new team members are introduced how can effective teamwork be developed?
• How should data be gathered, analysed and evaluated?
• How should clinical audit be established?

The questions relating to needs (i.e. 'why integrate?') were addressed in Chapter 1, and the evidence for the usefulness of various CTs in particular conditions was examined in the last chapter. Assuming, then, that a practice team wishes to try offering CTs to its patients, the next set of questions revolves around: 'how best to do this?' and 'how will we judge whether the CT service is worthwhile?'

Before proceeding to the purely practical question of how to set up the CT service, a number of wider, but pertinent, issues should first be considered.[2] The first of these relates to the people involved and the 'cultural divide' that can open up between them. Particularly in the less-established CTs, complementary practitioners may adhere to very different understandings of the nature of health and illness, and therefore the type of healthcare management needed. This can produce tensions between people working at the conventional–complementary medicine boundaries. The problems arising from different models and the need for a common language have been addressed in Chapter 2. Attitudes, assumptions and unconscious prejudices can be an obstacle to team working. Some GPs may feel, for instance, that certain fringe CTs are simply not credible; obviously the issue of what they find acceptable needs to be addressed openly before implementation.

CPs without a medical or nursing background may not be accustomed to team working in a clinical setting let alone the distinctive structure, organization and procedures of the NHS. The potential for interprofessional misunderstanding in primary care team has been widely written about; differences exist and have to be recognized and acknowledged. The question of CP autonomy, and how working within the NHS will affect their clinical accountability, professional status and working practices, should be thought about at an early stage. The different options for employment of CPs have medicolegal implications, and both doctors and CPs need to be aware of these. Funding will largely determine the way CTs are made available and will influence how delivery is organized. At present there is wide variation in access within the NHS and any movement towards equity is likely to depend ultimately on whether pilot projects can demonstrate not only effectiveness and quality, but also cost effectiveness. Resources will always be limited, so wherever a pilot project is planned, integrative teams would be well advised to agree early on about how they select patients appropriately, how many treatments can be offered and how outcomes are to be evaluated. Inappropriate referrals can swamp a service and undermine its effectiveness, so referring doctors must understand intake guidelines and be persuaded they are important. Therefore the final challenge to integration is knowledge, for most primary care practitioners do not have a good understanding of what CTs involve in practice and so will be on a steep learning curve. Practitioner and practice development should be integrated into service design process from the outset, because they are essential components.

The Marylebone principles for developing CT services in the NHS (Box 3.2) can be adapted to suit particular practices. Reasons to integrate CTs into the primary care team are listed in Table 5.1.[5]

Box 3.2   Principles for developing CT services in the NHS

• CT service provision in the NHS must be fully integrated.
• The principles of clinical governance apply to CTs.
• Education for practitioners and patients is a key component.
• The service should be audited against agreed criteria and standards.[3]
• An integrative project should ideally be able to rely on funding for a period long enough to ensure the continuity and stability that a complex development requires.
• Maxwell's criteria for service quality apply when commissioning CTs (see Box 3.3, p. 78):[4]
— acceptability
— appropriateness
— accessibility
— effectiveness
— efficiency
— equity.

MODELS OF INTEGRATION AND DELIVERY

A primary care-driven health service[6] has opened up opportunities for primary care organizations to commission an extended range of services to patients in primary care settings.[7] Teams planning integrative projects must realistically assess CTs' strengths and limitations for themselves. At MHC we consider there is adequate evidence to justify their targeted implementation for certain common health problems.[8]

In 1987 Richard Tonkin described his vision of an NHS that embraces CAM as follows.[9]

The long-term benefits that can be expected from successful integration of properly trained and registered complementary therapists with conventional scientific practitioners are far reaching. First it would relieve the severely restrictive and indeed often crippling overload with which both the GP and hospital services are faced today. Secondly, it should effect substantial economies in the management of the majority of patients suffering from non-life threatening undifferentiated illness, for whom neither expensive high technology services nor costly and potentially toxic agents are necessarily appropriate.

Tonkin's vision will have to be supported by research and development resources through well-organized initiatives that can determine the problems and benefits of implementing CAM. This suggests the need for pilot units where the capacity to collaborate and reflect can develop. If the NHS is to provide greater access to CTs, then cooperation between CPs and doctors must be properly evaluated.

Approaches to CT provision[10]

Different ways of providing CTs have been tried out in and around the NHS over the past 10 years.[10] Once a practice team has agreed that aspects of CT are relevant to meeting identified needs, it is worth considering three different approaches to CT service delivery.

- *The bolt-on approach.* This approach aims to offer a broader and more responsive range of provision, in which CTs are 'added' to conventional medicine to address its clinical shortcomings. However, critics of this approach warn of the dangers of reducing CTs to sets of techniques, and of using them as a kind of superficial first aid, in ways that are unholistic.
- *Integrative-settings approach.* This approach entails certain minimum characteristics: multiprofessional working between conventional and complementary practitioners, patient-informed choice, and a commitment to service development based on reflective practice. It requires an ethos in which conventional and complementary therapists learn about (and question) one another's perspectives and practices. In units committed to this approach, coworkers should expect to explore the

problems of interprofessional learning and related issues around power and authority. The aim of integrative units is to effect change through collaboration with conventional practice in order to develop more effective and acceptable mainstream health care.

- *The transforming approach.* This approach takes the integration agenda rather further. Transformative aims are often expressed in terms of counteracting a biomedical tendency to fragment, mechanize or dehumanize people. Relevant objectives might include the 'rehumanizing' of health care through a renewed focus on care and healing, and a wish to empower patients and to encourage health creation. Transformative settings might, for example, be motivated by issues of community development, health promotion and participatory democracy. Some transformative settings tend to be explicitly countercultural and values driven—either spiritually or politically. It is not unusual for this type of practice to have a spiritual emphasis and to have concerns about the meaning of illness, whether to the individual, the family or the community the practice serves.

Examples of collaborative practice

The following pilot projects already in existence illustrate the different options.*

Glastonbury Health Centre

This health centre provides acupuncture, osteopathy, massage and herbalism, financed by a practice-based charity. Patients pay a small amount towards the cost of each treatment. Patients are referred by their general practitioner; guidelines for the service are used which are evidence based as much as possible. General principles used in drawing up guidelines are:

- CAM should only be treating conditions that it can reliably and effectively manage
- this should be substantiated where possible by clinical data
- the service is limited, so referrals need to be prioritized and treatments targeted as appropriately as possible.

The practice provides a total of 6 hours of osteopathy, 3 hours of herbal medicine, 3 hours of massage treatment and 3.5 hours of acupuncture per week for approximately 4500 patients. A long-term aim is to fund the services

---

* The following section is reproduced, with minor amendments and additions, with permission from the information booklet: Complementary medicine: information pack for primary care groups, June 2000 (available as a pdf document on the DoH, FIM, NHS Alliance and National Association for Primary Care websites).

Box 3.3 Defining a 'quality' integrated therapy service

APPROPRIATENESS
ACCESSIBILITY
ACCEPTABILITY
EQUITY
EFFECTIVENESS
EFFICIENCY

APPROPRIATENESS

	with collaboration	without collaboration
process	1. Complementary practitioners and GP have agreed to target patient groups – e.g. high utilizers and then GP and complementary practitioners work together to identify and share management.	1. The GP refers patients to the complementary practitioner and expects 'magic' to occur for a range of problem areas without discussion of the aims of the service.

APPROPRIATENESS

Structure	Process	Outcome
Are the providers of complementary therapies appropriately trained, supervised and supported?	Do team appropriately allocate complementary practitioner treatments to meet patient needs?	Do GPs successfully identify patients appropriate for complementary therapy treatment?

ACCEPTABILITY

Structure	Process	Outcome
Do the complementary services available reflect local health care needs?	Are patients satisfied with the procedures of intake into the complementary therapy service?	Are patients satisfied with the results of complementary therapy service?

EFFECTIVENESS

Structure	Process	Outcome
Do intake procedures make maximal use of resources?	Are complementary practitioners establishing and maintaining 'allied' relationships within the field of complementary therapy?	Are the results of complementary therapy considered clinically effective?

EFFICIENCY

Structure	Process	Outcome
Are resources allocated to monitoring and reducing non-attendance rates?	Are complementary therapies given to optimally balance treatment with need?	Is the allocation of complementary therapy treatments and their uptake considered to be cost effective?

APPROPRIATENESS

	with collaboration	without collaboration
structure	1. The complementary practitioners are supervised managerially in the practice. 2. The complementary practitioner has training funding to develop services. 3. The complementary therapist is appointed with the necessary skills in place to deliver the proposed service. 4. The practice has a clear idea of what they want and make sure they get it.	1 The complementary practioner has no contact and no identifiable manager. 2. The practice accepts no responsibility for professional development. 3. The complementary practitioner is appointed with no job description and is inadequately trained to deliver the planned service. 4. The GPs don't know what the complementary practitioner is doing except that they ask for a review once a year.

APPROPRIATENESS

	with collaboration	without collaboration
outcome	1. GPs correctly identify patients for complementary therapy using agreed protocols and guidelines. 2. Complementary practitioners are able to assess patients' suitability for complementary therapy and refer back those that are unsuitable and measure outcome.	1. Complementary practitioner expected to accept all patients referred and feels that they must cope – who else will otherwise? 2. GPs expect all patients referred to be seen and looked after by the complementary practitioner. No review of service requested.

ACCESSIBILITY

Structure	Process	Outcome
Are the complementary therapy services suitably located and available to all who might be in need of them?	Are waiting times for complementary therapies within the guidelines of the practice's Patient's Charter?	Do complementary practitioners enhance accessibility through detailed patient feedback to GPs?

EQUITY

Structure	Process	Outcome
Are minority groups catered for in terms of resources?	Are procedures applicable to all minority groups?	Are treatment outcomes equitable with other complementary therapy services?

Reproduced with permission from: Foundation for Integrated Medicine 1997 Integrated healthcare: a way forward for the next five years? FIM, London, p. 39

to the whole of the PCG, focusing on certain conditions to ensure greater clinical and cost effectiveness. (This project is discussed in detail in Ch. 4, p. 138.)

St Margaret's Surgery, Wiltshire

This practice serving approximately 3000 patients provides a homeopathy medical service within a primary care setting. This service was started in 1993 and was originally funded via fundholder savings. All members of the primary care team are able to refer patients on to the homeopath for treatment subject to GP approval. Nine hours of homeopathy are provided per week. A wide range of complaints were selected for homeopathic treatment as those thought to be the most common and successfully treated in clinical practice. It is possible that continuation of this service will be based on it forming a pilot study of homeopathic treatments on behalf of the PCG, with the interventions used based on evidence of effectiveness.

South Norfolk Primary Care Group

This PCG has set up an acupuncture service covering the whole PCG population of 107 000, first providing the service on a trial basis for 5 months before taking a decision about further provision. There are four local BMAS-accredited GPs working from four locations within the PCG. Guidelines have been agreed for referral, and only GPs may refer patients. A budget of £13 000 was set aside to cover the service in order to treat about 150 patients during the trial period.

Somerset Coast Primary Care Group

A group of three fundholding practices had developed guidelines for referral for patients with back pain (based on existing RCGP guidelines) or neck problems, to a chiropractic service. This service has been in operation for over 3 years. The PCG agreed to fund this service until March 2000. From April 2000 a pilot study was set up to run across the PCG, all referral for back, shoulder and knee problems being triaged by an interface doctor and referred to either:

- physiotherapy, orthopaedic services, pain clinic, (covering one-half of the PCG) or to
- chiropractic, physiotherapy, orthopaedic services, pain clinic (covering the other half).

Southampton Centre for the Study of Complementary Medicine

A unique contract arrangement for CT provision within the NHS has been set up between this centre and the Dorset Health Authority. It is composed of two parts. First, an integrated medicine unit is operated by the centre for one day each month in a GP practice in Dorset. Patients with any of six identified conditions (i.e. CFS, IBS, migraine, child behavioural problems, eczema or non-specific allergy) may be referred to this unit from other local clinics. Secondly, patients with the above conditions (although there is some flexibility here) may travel for treatment to the centre in Southampton. This part allows an initial six appointments to be made on the basis of a referral letter from the GP; a letter of progress is also sent to the referring GP. Subsequent appointments may also be arranged if the GP seeks permission in writing from the health authority.

Table 3.1 lists some other NHS institutions and practices that have used CTs, and the therapies offered.

A recent research study examined 10 existing schemes of CT provision in primary care throughout England. The different models of collaborative practice chosen by each are summarized in Table 3.2.[10]

Table 3.1 Examples of collaborative practice[11]

Integrative model	Therapies involved
Hospital-based	
Warwick Hospital	Acupuncture/maternity
Queen Mary's, Sidcup, Kent	Reflexology/maternity
Freedom Fields, Plymouth	Acupuncture/maternity
Radcliffe, Oxford	Aromatherapy/maternity
Hinchinbrook, Hertfordshire	Aromatherapy/maternity
Norfolk and Norwich Hospital	Aromatherapy/maternity
Community clinics	
Lewisham Hospital Complementary Therapy Centre	Acupuncture, homeopathy, osteopathy/outpatients
Tower Hamlets	Acupuncture/mental health
Liverpool Centre for Health	Various/family health clinic
Hoxton Health Group	Various/community—aged
GP—multiple practices	
Huddersfield and Dewsbury	Various
Wigan and Bolton	Acupuncture, chiropractic, osteopathy, musculoskeletal, medicine
GP—individual practices	
Wells Park, London	Acupuncture, osteopathy, health promotion
Leyton Green, London	Osteopathy
Stockwell Group Practice, London	Osteopathy
St Margaret's Surgery, Bradford on Avon	Homeopathy
College Surgery, Cullompton	Healing
St Albans	Healing
GP—multidisciplinary centres	
Glastonbury Complementary Health Service	Various
Marylebone Health Centre	Various
Phoenix Surgery, Cirencester	Acupuncture, osteopathy
Warwick House Medical Centre, Taunton	Various

Table 3.2 Existing types of CT provision and therapies offered

'Character' of provision	Funding (1997–1998)	Provider type	Therapies offered
A side-by-side service	Charitable trust	Sessional complementary practitioners in-house	Acupuncture, osteopathy
A focused interest	Fundholding	Service provided by GPs, by sessional complementary practitioners in-house, and by referrals to a local independent complementary therapy clinic	Herbalism, homeopathy, chiropractic, acupuncture
A one-stop shop	Fundholding	Sessional complementary practitioners in-house	Homeopathy, acupuncture, osteopathy
A parallel existence	Health authority	Sessional complementary practitioners in-house	Acupuncture, osteopathy
A team with a 'boss'	Fundholding	Sessional complementary practitioners in-house	Osteopathy, acupuncture and Chinese herbs, massage
'Muddling along'	Fundholding	Sessional complementary practitioners in-house	Osteopathy, traditional and medical acupuncture, reflexology
An instant service	Fundholding	Complementary practitioners in an adjacent complementary health centre	Osteopathy, chiropractic. Privately: massage, aromatherapy, colonic irrigation, homeopathy, acupuncture, Alexander technique, reflexology, hypnotherapy
Reluctantly private	Fee for service	Sessional complementary practitioners in-house	Acupuncture, Alexander technique, herbalism, homeopathy, osteopathy, massage, reflexology, aromatherapy
A new health care model	Community Trust	Independent centre accepting local GP referrals. Service provided by complementary practitioners on a sessional basis	Acupuncture, homeopathy, osteopathy, massage, hypnotherapy.
A personality-led service	Registered charity	Independent centre accepting funded and non-funded referrals from local GPs	Healing, acupuncture

Delivery options

Some doctors offer complementary treatment themselves—most commonly acupuncture or homeopathy—either in their own general medical appointment times or by organizing separate clinics. In other centres nurses, physiotherapists or non-medically qualified practitioners (NMQPs) provide the service. In a third type of provision doctors send their patients to a practitioner's own premises. Finally, family doctors may be able to refer patients to units where doctors, nurses or physiotherapists (but less commonly NMQPs) work on hospital wards, or in outpatient departments attached to a hospital. Each option will have different resource implications for the primary care practice concerned.

In some of the examples given in Table 3.2, CP practitioners provided services in the same location—for example, in a designated part of the practice or hospital. However, there are as yet few UK examples of services available on one location that provide an integrated model of care accessible to all who need it.

PEOPLE ISSUES

Working together: some questions to consider

Complementary or polarizing?

It is relatively easy for doctors to introduce CTs using a 'bolt-on model', beginning by incorporating into their own work certain techniques gleaned from CAM. However, the full mainstream potential of CAM is unlikely to be realized unless practitioners collaborate. The opportunity for experienced mainstream and complementary practitioners to explore one another's thoughts and methods while sharing patient management is irreplaceable. CPs, for their part, have much to learn about the challenges primary care teams face: the diversity, depth and difficulty of the case mix, coping with chronic as well as catastrophic disease, and dealing with levels of despair and deprivation they are unlikely to have witnessed in private practice. Yet working relationships between mainstream and complementary practitioners are potentially difficult because of fundamental differences between their clinical concepts; holistic diagnosis and treatment may be the mutual aim, but without a good enough common language and compatible attitudes, practitioners will retreat into a struggle for dominance when their viewpoints seem irreconcilable. This is in a sense the territory, for professionals under pressure often revert to tribal allegiances and reject outsiders. In order for the current truce between complementary and conventional health care to hold, so that the two cultures can explore their potential to complement one another, two urgent challenges will have to be faced: the *educational* challenge of joint learning, and the *organizational* challenges of managing innovative approaches to clinical cooperation and evaluation.

If you are a GP contemplating adding CTs to your practice you probably have specific ideas of the needs that you might want them to meet. These might include, for instance, working with patients where:

- conventional treatment has little to offer
- the patient cannot adhere to the proposed conventional treatment
- the patient finds the conventional treatment of choice inappropriate or unacceptable
- biomedical treatment has been relatively ineffective
- the patient shows a strong preference for CT
- the patient has had previous positive experience with CTs.

Complementary practitioners

Complementary practitioners may want to work in the public sector to bring CTs to people who could never afford to pay for treatment themselves. Another aim is to treat patients with the kinds of chronic illness rarely seen in private practice. CPs recognize that working in general practice will give them opportunities to develop their skills. There is ample scope to achieve this without compromising the needs of the practice. These include:

- the opportunity to specialize (e.g. rheumatology)
- the opportunity to work multiprofessionally
- the opportunity to develop new clinical skills
- access to resources and expertise—e.g. audit and evaluation
- opportunities to work with students from other disciplines
- opportunities to share skills with others
- opportunities to embed CTs into mainstream health care
- opportunities to shape local healthcare policies.

Are CPs 'specialists'?

GPs are used to referring to specialists within the biomedical system: specialities categorized by the organ system or age group involved. Here the relationship between the consultant and the accepted protocol is clear enough, the practitioners concerned speak the same clinical language, have a common basic training and share a set of expectations about patient behaviour and presentation and what might be expected of treatment. Referring patients to CPs who work in ways outside doctors' current experience is different from this. CPs tend to be regarded as specialists brought in to treat a specific type of problem and meet specific needs—for instance, to hold a migraine clinic or a pain clinic. Such problems are often complex, chronic and relatively intractable and it would be unrealistic to expect CPs to effect rapid change within a short time-frame. CPs are not 'magical specialists'. Far from being specialist at all, many practitioners of 'complete' systems like homeopathy or acupuncture see themselves as generalists dealing with people rather than diseases (in much the same way as a GP might) and practising a comprehensive system of medicine based on internally coherent approaches to diagnosis and treatment. Such systems claim an existence that is historically and intellectually independent of biomedicine. There is a potential mismatch of perception between 'specialist' and 'generalist' practitionership that can cause problems if it is not recognized and explored. This may not become obvious until a problem over expectations about treatment occurs.

Case selection

The efficient use of CP services requires appropriate case selection, and this will be one of the keys to successful CP/GP cooperation. Specific disease-based clinics, though they provide strict intake criteria, restrict CPs' generalist role. On the other hand, too open-ended an intake will result in overload, often with chronic and 'thick-notes' patients,[12] who are difficult to discharge even when progress is slow. When good channels of communication are established, working practices supporting two-way referral of patients can be agreed and evaluated and, in working collaboratively together, CPs and mainstream health workers can achieve a better understanding of one another's approaches. Proof of efficacy and cost–benefit alone will not determine whether CAM becomes more widely available within the NHS. Managing the interface between complementary and conventional practitioners will be equally influential.

Are certain patients suitable for CT?

These questions become further complicated because GPs will reasonably want to refer patients with whom they are having difficulty, including frequent attenders, patients labelled as 'somatizing' and those with a long history of multiple symptom presentation. As one GP put it, 'Why would a GP want to refer someone they could adequately treat themselves?'. CPs also know that their work is under scrutiny and there will be pressure to show success even in cases where biomedicine has consistently failed.

In private practice CPs have ongoing relationships with people who seek them out and treatment is often as much about health maintenance as it is about treating disease. The reality of the GP's task, although in theory not much different to this, is to see people as they choose to present with their ailments and not to treat on an on-going basis once the presenting problem is resolved. CPs when working for the first time within the public sector may therefore need to change the way they practise. With experience it becomes clear which patients the CP will be able to help the most within the confines of a limited service. We suspect the following groups of patients should be considered as more likely to respond well to a CT:

- those patients with newly diagnosed problems whose general health is good
- those patients where the CP can make a clear diagnosis of the problem from within their discipline and where this diagnosis does not imply an overly complex and deep-seated underlying problem
- patients with a positive expectation and who are well motivated towards the CT in question
- patients with conventional diagnoses that are known to respond quickly to treatment
- patients who are motivated to support themselves through self-help measures
- patients where the conventional treatment they are receiving does not inhibit their response to treatment by a CT.

CPs, especially those practising systems of medicine that have a comprehensive diagnostic system that allows for everything to be diagnosed, will need to learn to say 'no' to referrals they believe are inappropriate. In this respect an initial assessment consultation is crucial to running a CT service. Prospective patients need to know that the first session with the CP is purely for the assessment of whether they will be suitable to receive treatment.

Loss of CP autonomy

CPs new to the public sector will want to work to the best of their ability and will be aware that this may mean working in very different ways to those of working privately. They will not know, however, what this means in practical terms. Their main concern will be to be able to treat in a way that gives maximum benefit to patients.

Anxieties will arise if they are expected to work in a restricted way using their therapy, for example, only to address the superficial symptoms of an illness and not to work with what they would see as the deeper level of disease. This stems from fear that the therapy in its entirety will be rejected by doctors and concern about how to describe their therapy and what it can do in a way that would be acceptable and understandable. Doctors and other members of the primary healthcare team may have particular views about the scope of specific CTs and what they can treat, sometimes without realizing so.

Deciding on the number of treatments

A CP will sometimes find it frustrating to have to work within a framework where the number of treatments available is capped. Perhaps it might be possible to achieve more if only more treatment sessions were available; yet resources are limited. However, a lot can in fact be achieved in six to eight treatments and CPs have found they become more rigorous and focused in their treatments to make the most of what is possible. Engaging patients in activities that support their health and working with their motivation to get well become more important elements of the consultation when the service is limited. However, service delivery criteria may need to be flexible to be able to provide additional maintenance sessions to patients who have improved.

One of the strengths of having CPs who practise 'complete' systems within a team is that they come with an alternative understanding of how signs and symptoms might be patterned. These 'alternative syndromes' can sometimes help practitioners or patients make sense of a configuration of symptoms that fit no recognizable pattern within biomedicine. For example, the referral 'treat this person's knee pain' might appear simple from the doctor's point of view but for the acupuncture practitioner the simple knee pain may be related to long-standing 'Kidney Qi deficiency', which is associated with other symptoms such as sore back, tiredness and frequent urination—symptoms the patient may not have even mentioned to the doctor. Can the acupuncturist treat the knee pain without addressing the underlying complaint? Not comfortably. Does the practitioner need to go back to the doctor for permission to treat what is seen as the underlying cause? How does the CP obtain informed consent from the patient where the emphasis of the 'best possible treatment' may not be centred wholly on the referral problem? What happens if the CP considers the simple knee pain to be a symptom of a more complex problem that can be treated but would take longer than the number of treatments allocated?

GPs who are new to working with CPs may find it confusing that the problem referred to the CP may not always be the primary focus of the treatment that the CP provides, but is treated simply as an indication of an imbalance that becomes the main focus of treatment. In this circumstance, GPs need to remain open about the possibility that other complaints the patient has may also improve with treatment or that the referral problem does not improve but the patient is more able to cope with it because of other health changes—for example, being less anxious or less tired.

A lot of learning and adaptation of the use of CTs occurs for both GPs and CPs, and our experience and those of others working together within the health service shows that it takes about a year for CPs and biomedics to work together completely productively. It must also be remembered that GPs refer to a specific practitioner as well as the therapy, and this underlying relationship between practitioners is worth developing.

Skilled doctors or imported CPs?

Though their training imbues them with the assumptions and values of conventional, biotechnical medicine, doctors nevertheless participate in 'unorthodox' subcultures if they find them relevant. Health professionals seek out new approaches for many reasons, and innovation may be acceptable to them even without efficacy having been demonstrated by formal research.[13] CTs are increasingly popular in the UK and Europe and with the growing recognition of non-medical CPs' potential contribution, a new spirit of 'pluralism' now prevails.[14] In the UK, several significant trends are at work: high-quality research implies their potential effectiveness; more GPs want to learn about and use CT knowledge and skills;[15] CP education and professionalization continue to improve; highly trained non-medical CPs are entering the field and progress towards proper professional regulation has brought their inclusion into the NHS a step nearer.[16] Those responsible for undergraduate and postgraduate medical education are increasingly aware of CAM, and the undergraduate curriculum is beginning to include some teaching about it.[17] Co-operation with CPs will become more widespread if doctors feel more secure about complementary practitioners' levels of training and in addition all these developments are likely to encourage more doctors to use CT methods themselves.

Integrating new professions into primary care teams

When integration works CPs will stay because they enjoy seeing patients and feel their contribution is valued. GPs then benefit from having colleagues they know and trust to help them cope with the practice caseload. The very least that is required to ensure CPs are properly integrated into the practice, are structures and processes for referral and a system for feedback between practitioners. GPs also need an understanding of CT therapies and their scope. Lack of time for joint meetings can be problematic but informal conversations after clinics or over lunch can also be effective ways to develop good team relationships which will be essential if doctors and CPs are to work together effectively.

Primary care teams already include personnel with a range of medical, nursing and social work skills who work together; often not without interprofessional difficulties. It has been proposed that the wider integration of CPs into the NHS could solve some of the problems posed by some painful, chronic and functional disorder, undifferentiated disease[18] and some patients with problems mediated by stress[19]—conditions that occupy a good deal of primary care time. Yet, in one study[20] the use of alternative treatment outside general practice did not lead to an equivalent reduction in demand on GPs' time. This study identified problems around continuity of care, clinical responsibility and GPs' inability to be sure of CPs' professional accreditation. These concerns reflect how CAM and conventional medicine have been seen as two separate cultures. Their different languages and myths, the 'illicit' traffic of patients between them, poor communication across the 'borders' and the beliefs that have grown up about other cultures being 'foreign' all serve to confirm this picture. Practitioners who intend to work across this CP/GP boundary will need to learn how to avoid the pitfalls: problems of power, resource allocation, differing clinical models, communication and the logistics of the referral process.[21,22] Professions have an interest in retaining their frames of orientation for as Erich Fromm[23] points out, our capacity to act as professionals depends upon them and, in the last analysis, our sense of professional identity. If other professionals express ideas that disturb our own frame of reference it can seem very threatening. Yet integration does indeed challenge everyone involved to confront their own interdisciplinary issues, and when primary care teams include CPs, the many factors influencing cooperation—autonomy and resources, knowledge, language, communication and referral—have be addressed. Our group tackles them in twice-monthly 'case and process' meetings that incorporate elements of the 'Balint group'.[24] We have found this case-based supervision model of learning helps pave the way for better interprofessional working and learning between CPs and doctors. We suggest that an integrative team should aim to build into their project ample opportunity to look at the personal as well as the clinical interface between practitioners and provide the chance to reflect on one another's values and attitudes.

Skills

Some CT systems and techniques can appear quite unrelated to scientific medicine. Because of this doctors and nurses may learn most effectively about CT models and methods through practical, problem-oriented approaches. The MHC project has entailed learning from CPs directly, through joint casework allowing team members to experience how CPs think and work. This approach to learning about CTs has meant putting some basic CT skills into the hands of our mainstream colleagues. But are there truly certain aspects of CT diagnostic and treatment modalities that can be separated from their system of origin, and used as techniques? We would certainly argue, for instance, that GPs and nurses can achieve a primary care level of competence needed to recommend simple exercise regimens, low-potency homeopathy, basic nutritional interventions and relaxation techniques. And after relatively brief training doctors could also use simple manipulation techniques and trigger-point needling. In fact it is unlikely that these non-conventional techniques (NCTs), which are widely practised by many doctors in other parts of the EU,[9] will remain the exclusive preserve of fully initiated CPs. The essential ingredient in such an integrative team approach is the common aim of enhancing the capacity for health and for recovery. Reilly has pointed out that such an approach should not fragment the total care of the patient and should increase the team's sense of delivering more integrated care.[25]

A pluralistic healthcare system might mean doctors, nurses and physiotherapists in primary care making daily use of simple CAM techniques, while working alongside highly trained CPs—as they do at MHC. This would be a way to increase access to basic CTs, as part of primary care yet in the context of a broad appreciation of CAM systems and a deeper kind of expertise. In which case the question is not about either skilling doctors (and other mainstream health workers) or of collaborating with CPs, because in this scenario collaboration in a multidisciplinary group actually depends on the sharing of skills and models. And, if common ground can be achieved and effectiveness demonstrated, then eventually career structures and even consultant roles for some CPs might feasibly be developed within the NHS.

If doctors are to appreciate fully the contribution that trained specialist CPs can make to primary care, they need to be more aware of the extent of training that these practitioners receive. Although CPs (other than osteopaths and chiropractors) can legally practise without any training whatsoever, most have completed some further education in their chosen discipline. Until recently, most complementary practitioners trained in small, privately funded colleges and then worked independently and in relative isolation. Though many still train and practice this way, several universities now offer accredited undergraduate and postgraduate degrees in the main complementary therapies, as well as shorter diploma courses. The requirements for accreditation for individual disciplines are detailed later in this chapter, but there is a drive towards standardization and implementation of high standards taking place in many therapies and several organizations now hold registers of accredited practitioners. Doctors can therefore feel reassured that, to an increasing degree, they are collaborating with well trained and properly regulated practitioners. CPs willing to develop collaborative work with doctors need for their part to be sure that their would-be coworkers understand that integrating CTs means more than just bolting them on. CPs are not simply firing new 'magic bullets' and their therapies cannot be understood in isolation from their human impact on healing processes.

FUNDING AND RESOURCE ISSUES

In the UK, funding may be obtained from a number of sources including the following:

- the NHS via PCO-commissioned project funding, e.g. waiting list initiatives, primary care development initiatives
- the NHS via an acute or community trust, e.g. pain clinics, physiotherapy services
- the NHS via targeted research-funding initiatives
- individual practitioners may be paid through private individual income or private medical insurance schemes
- charitable sector funded projects.

Public sector funding for CTs in the UK

By far the most common form of NHS access will be where GPs or practice nurses with some CAM training—most often acupuncture, homeopathy or hypnosis—provide it directly to their patients. Other less typical examples are where CT services are provided by CPs 'attached' or 'semidetached' and either paid for privately by patients, charitably funded or funded by development or research funds.[10] It requires no special funding arrangements for complementary medicine to be provided by conventional NHS healthcare professionals as part of everyday clinical care. But equally, there are therefore no direct financial incentives for GPs to do so since they cannot claim item of service payments for complementary treatments they give to their own NHS patients.

However, since 1991, health authorities have been permitted to reimburse GPs who employ complementary therapists, although the staff budget is limited and a CP is therefore employed at the expense of another member of staff.[26] GP fundholders had additional control over staffing budgets and fundholding savings, which some used to purchase CTs. More recently primary care groups have greater power to allocate funds as they choose, but it remains to be seen whether complementary medicine will be identified as a priority by sufficiently large numbers of GPs for the creation of any new initiatives. Indeed, the change from general practice fundholding to primary care groups may mean that some established complementary services will be lost.

Health authorities have sometimes used money from research and development budgets, or for waiting list initiatives, to finance complementary medicine. Block service contracts or individual extracontractual referrals can be made with complementary medicine providers, but in practice financial constraints currently restrict this type of access.

Voluntary sector funding and health insurance

Funds from the voluntary sector or charities may also be sought. The CT service at the Marylebone Health Centre in London was initially funded by a research grant from the Waites Foundation, a charitable trust. Then for a time a mix of health authority initiative funds plus fundraising and donations by the local patients were essential to its ongoing financial viability. More recently, the Smith's charity research project subsidized the cost of providing CTs. Currently, the CPs are paid out of PCG funds through a primary care pilot scheme. The service has always survived one step away from the brink! In many other units, charities such as the London Lighthouse for people living with HIV subsidize complementary medicine for people who could not otherwise afford treatment. Some occupational health services provide CTs for employees and most private medical insurance schemes fund CT, from a small number of approved providers.

Resource allocation

GPs are being exhorted to save money and become more efficient. They are urged to do this by prescribing more economically and referring to hospitals more appropriately. In addition, they are asked to promote health and prevent disease. Would wider availability of CAM within the NHS be cost beneficial? The fee-paying public generally turn to CPs with the kind of painful and stress-related conditions that many doctors do not feel particularly skilled at managing, and surveys suggest that CPs' clients are pleased with the outcome.[27] The Department of Health

(DoH) has recognized this growing patient demand for CTs and GPs' wish to access them within the NHS. The DoH's policy towards CAM has in fact encouraged a clinical pluralism the medical and political establishments would have found unthinkable in the 1980s, even though in most parts of the UK very little new funding was made available to help bring it about. Although surveys show that most people support increased provision of complementary medicine on the NHS, this does not mean that patients would necessarily prefer complementary to conventional care. When planning services, it is essential to try to distinguish between patients' desires and defined patients' needs that can be met by complementary medicine. The trend towards evaluating the cost effectiveness of health care and to restrict access to what can be evidence based is here to stay. Conventional clinicians and decision makers want persuasive evidence that complementary medicine can deliver safe, cost-effective solutions to problems that are expensive or difficult to manage with conventional treatment. Unfortunately, such evidence is both scarce and equivocal. Only a moderate number of randomized trials and very few reliable economic analyses of complementary medicine have been conducted. (The economic evaluation of CTs is dealt with in detail in Ch. 4.)

LEGAL CONSIDERATIONS

The medicolegal implications of use of or referral to complementary treatment differ according to the qualifications of the person providing the CT. Some general guidelines are as follows.

Doctors who use CTs

The Medical Act of 1858 allowed qualified doctors to administer unconventional medical treatments if they so wished, so long as they adhered to professional standards of care. In law the 'Bolam test' is used to establish whether these standards have been met.[28] It specifies that 'a doctor is not guilty of negligence if he or she has acted in accordance with a practice accepted as proper by a responsible body of medical men skilled in that particular art as long as it is subject to logical analysis'. This means that doctors can justify their use of complementary treatments if they have undertaken training in that complementary discipline and their use of the treatment is considered acceptable by a number (not necessarily a majority) of other medically qualified CPs.

Referral to medically qualified practitioners

The legal situation here is the same as if the GP had asked another qualified doctor to provide any other specialist medical service. That is, the second doctor assumes legal responsibility for the complementary treatment. The responsibility of the GP is simply to ensure that the decision to make the referral was appropriate.

Referral to state-regulated CPs

Legally this situation is similar to delegating care to a physiotherapist or other member of a state-regulated profession allied to medicine.

Referral to NMQPs

This is the situation that tends to concern doctors most. However, provided that certain guidelines are followed the risk in terms of possible legal action is very low. To date, there have been no substantiated claims sustained against doctors who have delegated to complementary practitioners.

When considering whether to delegate, doctors need to bear in mind the following points to ensure their delegation to a non-medically qualified complementary practitioner is acceptable from a legal viewpoint.*

1. As above, the initial decision to delegate to this CT must be appropriate:
   — in essence, it must pass the Bolam test
   — evidence-based decisions are most persuasive
   — commonly accepted but unproved indications are also acceptable.
2. Doctors must take reasonable steps to ascertain that practitioners are appropriately qualified and insured:
   — it is usually sufficient for delegating doctors to ensure that practitioners are a member of the main professional regulatory body responsible for that particular discipline
   — the main bodies require members to be fully indemnified.
3. Doctors must retain 'overall clinical responsibility'— that is, ensure appropriate and adequate follow-up, reassessment, etc.
4. Doctors should not issue repeat 'complementary' prescriptions without having or obtaining sufficient information to ensure safe prescribing.

To clarify the legal situation for both GPs and CPs, in 1996 the Scottish Office of the DoH set out a list of key elements of a suggested model contract for a non-medically qualified complementary practitioner providing services in the NHS.[29] Many of these elements, listed

in Box 3.4, come under the broad heading of clinical governance.

Obtaining lists of the main professional registers

Patients expect to be protected from unqualified CPs and inappropriate treatments. NHS provision of CTs will help drive the further development of higher standards of regulation, record keeping, effective channels of interdisciplinary communication, and strategic research effort. There is no overarching professional body for CAM and various professional bodies maintain registers of members. The addresses of the main organizations involved are given in the remainder of this chapter or in Appendix II (p. 319).

ISSUES OF LEARNING AND COMMUNICATION

Wherever there are plans to integrate CTs into primary care, some provision for education will have to be made. Currently the education of neither GPs nor CPs prepares them for this kind of collaboration. Those planning a primary care CT service should therefore consider what the various stakeholders need to know in order to devise and use the resource effectively. This means exploring the needs of practitioners, other members of the practice involved (e.g. administration and reception) and thirdly members of the community who hope to make use of the service.

Doctors' knowledge of CTs

Few doctors have more than a layman's understanding of alternative medical systems like homeopathy or TCM. Yet with so slim a grasp of CPs' frames of reference, and knowledge base or skills, GPs now influence CAM's availability in the NHS. Therefore, as CTs become available in the NHS and public and professional attitudes to health care change, mainstream health workers will need to become more familiar with CT models and methods. The future of collaboration within the NHS will depend on GPs developing a broad understanding of the implications and potential of CTs.

Some doctors do have an in-depth knowledge of 'mainstream' alternatives—manipulation, homeopathy or hypnotherapy, for instance—but the great majority of GPs have none.[30,31] And it has been observed that most GPs' limited knowledge of CTs comes from the types of brief programme designed to equip them with a limited number of simple but effective CAM techniques. However, the BMA's 1993 report New Approaches to Good Practice[32] recognized that these brief courses do not produce the level of competence of fully trained CPs, implying that doctors ought not to represent themselves

---

* From Zollman C, Vickers A 1999 ABC of complementary medicine. Complementary medicine in conventional practice. British Medical Journal 319:901–904

Box 3.4 Suggested key constituents of a model contract for a NMQP providing services in the NHS*

Qualifications
Practitioners should be in receipt of a recognized qualification from a training establishment that is accredited by a suitable regulatory body.

Registration
Practitioners must be registered with a recognized professional body that requires its members to abide by codes of conduct, ethics and discipline.

Insurance
Practitioners must have adequate professional indemnity insurance cover that applies to the period of their employment.

Consent to treatment
Patients must be fully informed about the nature of the therapy and its effects, including any side-effects, and have realistic expectations of its benefits. The informed consent of the patient or, in the case of young children, of the parent or guardian, must be gained and documented.

Medical responsibility
Practitioners should be aware that patients referred to them for treatment remain the overall responsibility of the referring clinician. CAM practitioners should not advise discontinuing existing orthodox treatments without the agreement of the referring clinician.

Documentation
A written record should be kept by practitioners of the consultation and each episode of treatment. All written (and oral information) should be treated as confidential and take account of the needs of the Data Protection Act and Caldicott review.

Refusal to treat
Practitioners have a duty not to treat a patient if they consider the treatment unsafe or unsuitable.

Education and training
Practitioners should take responsibility for keeping abreast of development in the practice of their therapy.

Quality standards
Practitioners, in conjunction with other health care professionals, should assist with the development of local standards and guidelines for practice.

Audit
Practitioners should undertake clinical audit and should report results to the employing or commissioning practice/PCG. They should be responsible for monitoring the outcome of therapy; opinions of patients should be actively sought and included in any evaluation.

Research
Practitioners should be expected to agree to take part in research trials to support the evaluation and development of treatment programmes.

Health and safety
Practitioners should comply with the requirements of Health and Safety legislation and adhere to good practice in the protection of staff, patients and the public.

Control of infection
Practitioners should adhere to regulations governing infection control and follow the procedure for reporting outbreaks of infection.

* Reproduced with permission from Complementary medicine information pack for primary care groups June 2000; Adapted from the Scottish Department of Health 1996 Complementary Medicine and the National Health Service.

as homeopaths or acupuncturists on the basis of such brief training.

The following section contains an overview of the main complementary therapies in terms of their integration potential, the practicalities of diagnosis and treatment, organizational structure, regulation and training. (The theories and research basis of these therapies were dealt with in Chapter 2.)

INFORMATION FOR DOCTORS ON SPECIFIC CT TECHNIQUES, TRAINING AND ORGANIZATION*

Acupuncture

The existing degree of integration of acupuncture into general health care is an indication of its easy acceptability by patients and practitioners alike, and its clinical value.

The consultation

The initial consultation and treatment can take up to an hour and a half, as TCM practitioners take a thorough multisystem history of patients' complaints, including their emotional state, which forms part of the aetiology of disease, to be able to make a diagnosis. There is also palpation of acupoints to see which are tender or painful. In addition, traditional acupuncturists use other observations they believe to be relevant to diagnosis, including the shape, colour and coating of the tongue, face colour, and 'character' of the pulse.

Traditional diagnosis is framed in terms of imbalances of Qi and other substances/principles recognized by the TCM system (Yin and Yang, Blood, etc.). These imbalances can have a wide range of causes, both external (such as the weather) and internal (such as poor diet, excesses of emotions).

Acupuncturists will use a combination of techniques to rebalance the body systems. They will insert very fine solid, usually stainless steel, needles (now almost universally disposable) into the acupoints; different needle techniques can be used to stimulate or sedate as appropriate. Typically, up to ten points are selected, and - inserted needles may be left for up to 30 minutes—although in some systems they are removed more quickly.

* Acknowledgement is made to the following as sources of the information on therapies summarized in this section: Zollman C, Vickers A ABC of complementary medicine (published as articles in the British Medical Journal and now available in book form from BMJ Publishing); and tables contained in Complementary medicine: information pack for primary care groups, June 2000, available as a pdf document on the DoH, FIM, NHS Alliance and National Association for Primary Care websites.

Some systems such as Japanese acupuncture entail quite shallow insertion but others go deeper, and some practitioners may even pass a small electrical current between needles, particularly when treating chronic pain. Although many patients do not feel when a needle has been inserted, some acupuncturists stimulate the points further by twirling the needles manually; this produces a sense of heaviness, soreness, or numbness at the point of needling (called 'Deqi', and pronounced derki). This is traditionally taken as a sign that the Qi is moving along the meridian.

Some practitioners use alternatives to needles, some ancient (such as magnets and pressure) and others very recent (such as electrical point stimulators and lasers). Some use points on the ear (auricular acupuncture). They may also use cupping over areas where they diagnose 'Qi stagnation', or if a Cold condition is diagnosed they may warm points by moxibustion (using a burning stick of the herb mugwort, *Artemisia vulgaris*). Practitioners also often give dietary and other lifestyle advice based on TCM principles. Some acupuncturists also prescribe Chinese herbal medicine.

Patients with chronic problems are generally advised to have 6–12 sessions over a 3-month period, after which it is usual to have occasional 'top-up' treatments to maintain the improvement.

Training

In the UK professional acupuncturists must train for up to 3–4 years full or part time at a privately funded college (there are several accredited colleges in the UK). It is now possible to study for a BSc in Acupuncture or in TCM at several universities. All accredited courses include conventional anatomy, physiology, pathology and diagnosis, and research and audit skills, as well as extensive clinical practice. Some courses include supervised practice in China.

Medical acupuncturists and other health care professionals (e.g. physiotherapists) generally train for shorter periods in specific acupuncture techniques. Generally, each discipline runs courses appropriate to its members. About 2000 GPs, physiotherapists, osteopaths, chiropractors, as well as specialists such as rheumatologists, practise acupuncture, generally as an adjunctive treatment—for instance, in pain clinics or in their general practice to treat acute of chronic pain. Acupuncturists who are NMQPs most often work in private practice, treating a wider range of conditions.

The narrow aspect of acupuncture usually studied by conventional practitioners roughly corresponds to the treatment a TCM practitioner would use to treat pain superficially, and would not take into account (or aim to treat) what TCM would regard as the causes of the condition. This is not to deny that using acupuncture in this way may be of great value and should be encouraged. However the potential added value of using TCM in its entirety would be lost to mainstream practice if this incomplete form of acupuncture were to become the dominant version in the West. Needless to say, traditionally trained acupuncturists and conventional medical practitioners who have taken the shorter acupuncture courses available to them almost inevitably end up on opposite sides of the fence over this issue, not least because they will have studied completely different theories explaining its mode of action: the doctors' neurophysiological, the NMPQs' version based on principles rooted in Taoist understanding.

Regulation

NMQP acupuncturists have a single regulatory body, the British Acupuncture Council (BAcC), with about 2100 members, which is ultimately aiming to achieve statutory regulation. It admits only those practitioners who have

Organization	Number of members	Educational requirements	Comments
The British Acupuncture Council (BAcC) 63 Jeddo Road, London W12 9HQ Tel: 020 8735 0399	2100	1200 hours	The BAcC has led the way in establishing standards of education. They work with relevant training colleges to set and audit standards of education and training
Acupuncture Association of Chartered Physiotherapists 18 Woodlands Close, Dibden Purlieu, Southampton SO45 4JG Tel: 02380 845901	1600	80 hours	Members are statutorily registered
The British Medical Acupuncture Society Newton House, Newton Lane, Whitley, Warrington Cheshire WA4 4JA Tel: 01925 730727	1680	100 hours	Members are statutorily registered medical practitioners

undergone a training that is independently accredited by the British Acupuncture Accreditation Board. Doctors who have completed the appropriate training are awarded a Certificate of Basic Competence or a Diploma of Medical Acupuncture by the British Medical Acupuncture Society. Physiotherapists have their own regulatory body, the Acupuncture Association of Chartered Physiotherapists (AACP).

Organizations

Organizations concerned with regulation and training in acupuncture are shown in the box at the bottom of p. 87 (see Appendix II, p. 319, for overseas addresses).

Herbal medicine

Herbal medicine offers a rational, relatively safe, highly researched approach whose rationale Western-trained physicians are likely to find easy to understand. That said there has been little integration of herbal medicine into the public health system. This lack of take-up may be related to concerns over the safety of herbal preparations and their possible interaction with prescription drugs and the cost to patients of the herbal remedies, which can be quite high.

Herbalists tend to concentrate on treating chronic conditions such as asthma, depression, eczema, RA, migraine, PMS, menopausal symptoms, CFS and IBS, rather than acute mental or musculoskeletal disorders. Some may be trained in the use of non-European herbal systems (e.g. Chinese herbalism, ayurveda). A small number of doctors also practise herbalism and there is great scope for GPs to direct some simple herbal remedies towards the relief of symptoms (e.g. St John's Wort for mild depression, peppermint for IBS, or valerian for sleep disturbance) and to suggest over-the-counter (OTC) herbal remedies as self-help advice to patients.

The consultation

The primary objective of a practitioner of herbal (phytotherapy or botanical) medicine is a balancing of dysfunctional organs and systems with the objective of restoring proper regulatory function. This might include general modulation of circulation, digestive function, eliminative functions, immune function, or more specifically liver or kidney functions. Hence a detailed medical interview gathers appropriate details of the patient's system functions, taking into account the personal characteristics of the individual and the perceived causes of disease or dysfunction. In addition to the herbal prescription, practitioners may advise on improvements in diet and other lifestyle factors such as exercise and emotional issues.

Herbal remedies and formulations are prescribed to suit the needs of the individual and not given purely to alleviate the symptoms of illness. Remedies are commonly prescribed in the form of tinctures or teas but can also take the form of pills, capsules and ointments. Herbal formulae may utilize the whole plant or part of the plant (leaf, root, flower, etc.). For the medical herbalist this is important as herbalists believe that, by using the entire plant or part of plant, safety is ensured as the various constituents are thought to work synergistically. An example is given of meadowsweet (*Filipendula ulmaria*), which is used as a digestive medicine. This plant contains salicylic acid (the basis of aspirin), which can cause mucous membrane irritation and bleeding. Because the plant also contains tannin and mucilaginous substances this tendency is neutralized, and the total effect is beneficial and the risk of irritation reduced. This effect is known as 'buffering'. Often different herbs are combined together in formulation to maximize the synergistic and buffering effects.

Follow-up appointments occur after 2–4 weeks. Progress is reviewed and changes made to drugs, doses, or regimen as necessary.

Organization	Number of members	Educational requirements for membership	Comments
National Institute of Medical Herbalists 56 Longbrook Street, Exeter EX4 4AH Tel: 01392 426022	340	4 years full time to 2 years part time	Associated with BSc university courses
Register of Chinese Herbal Medicine PO Box 400, Wembley, Middlesex HA9 9NZ Tel: 07000 790332	383		Associated with university diploma courses

Training

There is substantial variation in the content and standard of training. The most highly trained practitioners are members of the National Institute of Medical Herbalists (NIMH), and will have completed the equivalent of 4 years' full-time training, with at least 500 hours of supervised clinical practice and training in nutrition, pharmacology, pharmacognosy, botany, pathology, biochemistry, physiology, clinical diagnosis and communication skills, and research skills. Some courses lead to BSc degrees in herbal medicine. Courses in herbal medicine for doctors range from 2-day introductions to 2-year programmes leading to a diploma in herbal medicine.

In the UK, training in Chinese herbalism was originally incorporated into acupuncture training courses. However, it is now possible to study the subject on its own; there are accredited courses both at acupuncture colleges and at universities, which lead to membership of the Register of Chinese Herbal Medicine (RCHM); some of these include study in China.

Regulation

The NIMH is the main registering and regulating body for Western herbal practitioners; it accepts as members only graduates of its approved courses.

The Register of Chinese Herbal Medicine accepts graduates from a number of UK colleges.

Organizations

Organizations concerned with regulation and training in herbal medicine are shown in the box at the bottom of p. 88 (see Appendix II, p. 319, for overseas addresses).

Homeopathy

Homeopathy is probably the form of alternative and complementary health care most widely integrated into mainstream medicine in Europe. There are thousands of doctors using homeopathic methods of treatment, most notably in France and Germany. In the UK, homeopathy has been part of the NHS since its inception. Homeopathy is recognized as a postgraduate speciality with about 1000 doctors practising some form of homeopathy alongside conventional treatment. Several homeopathic hospitals remain active within the NHS, of which the two largest, in Glasgow and London, have inpatient units. Normal NHS conditions apply: patients receive services free at the point of care, the hospitals being reimbursed through block contracts. There are also at least 1500 professional non-medically qualified practitioners.

Homeopaths often treat chronic recurrent conditions such as common skin problems, headache, rheumatoid arthritis, IBS, asthma, fibromyalgia, and ill-defined complex conditions. Opinions about what can be effectively treated by homeopathy vary widely, medically trained practitioners generally being more conservative than non-medical ones. Many GPs have received only a basic training and generally restrict their prescriptions to a limited number of remedies for specific acute conditions.

Homeopathy is a very popular way of treating children. Many naturopaths and nutritional counsellors also use homeopathy in their work. In the USA and Germany homeopathy forms a major part of the training (as does herbalism) of state-boarded naturopathic practitioners (Heilpraktikers in German). Homeopathy has also been integrated into ayurvedic practice in India where it is used on a national scale.

The consultation

The selection of remedies in classical homeopathy is based only partly on the symptoms presented. It also takes account of constitutional characteristics and emotional responses of the individual. Therefore the homeopathic case history is necessarily extremely detailed and initial consultations can take over an hour. For example this would include eliciting details of:

- a person's likes and dislikes (sweet or salty foods, hot or cold weather),
- personality traits (ambitious, perfectionist, reactions to stress, etc.)
- colouring (pale, florid, dark haired, etc.)
- susceptibilities (joint pains, headaches, respiratory complaints, etc.)
- sensitivities (cold, heat), nature (quick tempered, calm, introverted, fearful, etc.).

A complete 'symptom picture' of the patient emerges from the history-taking based on these physical, emotional, intellectual and habitual characteristics as well as the presenting symptoms. Remedies are chosen on the basis of this symptom picture in its entirety, the most suitable remedy being the one whose characteristics most closely match those of the patient's symptoms. Patients and their symptom picture commonly do not exactly dovetail with a single remedy picture but their 'case' will be highly correlated with a few potential remedies.

Some examples of remedy pictures include the following.

Chamomilla—used in treating teething problems in children

- excitable, impatient, irritable

- likes to be carried
- screaming with pain
- sensitivity to pain
- stubbornness
- likes cold drinks
- heat—better for being uncovered.

Belladonna—used in treating inflammation

- onset of complaint is sudden
- shooting throbbing pain
- worse for being moved or touched
- better for lying down
- glands swollen and sensitive
- shining eyes
- tearful during fever
- sensitive to light and noise.

Remedies are commonly derived from plant, mineral or animal sources. For instance, the plant remedies include *Belladonna*, *Arnica*, *Chamomile* and *Ignatia*; mineral remedies include *Mercury* and *Sulphur*; animal remedies include *Sepia* (squid ink), *Lachesis* (snake venom) and *Cantharis vesticatoria* (Spanish fly).

Remedies are prepared in a liquid or solid form. In solid form the remedy will usually have been added to lactose tablets, powder or granules. The remedies are produced by a process of serial dilution and succussion (vigorous agitation). The greater the dilution and process of succussion the higher is the potency. The potency of the remedy is denoted by an 'X' to indicate a decimal dilution (1 : 10) or a 'C' to represent a centesimal dilution (1 : 100).

Follow-up appointments take place between 2 and 6 weeks after the initial remedy has been given. Follow-up appointments may take about 30–45 minutes. A review of progress is undertaken and any alterations, either with the remedy needed or with the potency, are made. If the patient is doing well the practitioner may not repeat the remedy but simply monitor changes; if symptoms have recurred the treatment may be repeated at the same or a higher potency. The development of an ongoing therapeutic relationship with the patient is important for the homeopath in order for the practitioner to make accurate adjustments to treatment.

'Classical homeopathy' is practised by medical as well as non-medically qualified practitioners. It aims to find the single closest-matched remedy for an individual patient at each consultation. 'Complex homeopathy' uses medicines made from a combination of low-potency remedies (which are less specific than higher-dilution or high-potency remedies). They are prescribed for particular conditions or diatheses but without the in-depth individualizing history that characterizes classical

homeopathy. Many homeopaths also recommend changes to diet and lifestyle; some advise against vaccination.

Common acute remedies include:

- *Belladonna* to treat scarlet fever (belladonna poisoning symptoms closely resemble the symptoms of scarlet fever)
- *Apis*, in its 6C potency, a remedy made from bees (including their sting), to treat inflammation accompanied by stinging sensations, such as nettle rash, bites and stings
- Grass pollen, in the 6C potency, for hay fever.

Complex and some single, low-potency remedies are often used to self-treat conditions such as the common cold, cuts, bruising and sprains. An estimated 10–20% of the UK population have bought homeopathic products over the counter at pharmacies, healthfood stores and even supermarkets.

Training

About 2500 homeopaths are practising in the UK, including over 1500 NMQPs and 1000 UK doctors. The Faculty of Homeopathy has various training courses for doctors, including a basic 40-hour course, and an examination leading to a primary care health care certificate, and intermediate and advanced study. The Faculty admits as members (MFHom) only those who have completed at least 150–180 hours of study.

The Homeopathic Hospitals in London and Glasgow have been offering postgraduate medical training for some years, and it is claimed that 20% of all Scottish GPs have now undertaken at least a basic training.

NMQP homeopathic training ranges from 3 years part time to 3 years full time; there are also university degrees in homeopathy.

Regulation

A register of medically qualified homeopaths is maintained by the Faculty of Homoeopathy; this body was incorporated by an Act of Parliament in 1950 to train and examine doctors in homeopathy. NMQP homeopaths may join the register of the Society of Homoeopaths.

Organizations

Organizations concerned with regulation and training in homeopathy include the following (see Appendix II, p. 319, for overseas addresses):

Organization	Number of members	Educational requirements for membership	Comments
Society of Homoeopaths (SOH) 2 Artizan Road, Northampton NN1 4HU Tel: 01604 621400	1400	3 years full-time to 3 years part-time	The SOH and UKHMA have cooperated on producing agreed National Occupational Standards for homeopathy
Faculty of Homoeopathy (FH) 15 Clerkenwell Close, London EC1R 0AA Tel: 020 7566 7810	660	150–180 hours	Members are statutorily registered

Osteopathy and chiropractic

With the establishment of a state registration procedure through the General Osteopathic Council and General Chiropractic Council the process of integration of osteopathy and chiropractic into mainstream health care has taken a great step forward. Many GP practices and hospitals are currently employing practitioners.

The professions are also widely and well established in Australia, New Zealand, South Africa and Canada and are gaining ground in Europe (with schools in France, Scandinavia and Spain). In the USA these independent professions are well recognized, there are over 130 osteopathic hospitals offering all the specialist services of a medical hospital, but in addition in some of these hospitals osteopathic manipulation is utilized as part of the general health care provision for patients, alongside their normal medical care.

The consultation

Despite focusing their therapeutic methods on the musculoskeletal system, both osteopathy and chiropractic aim to take a holistic approach. They take into account emotions, nutritional status, inherited factors and past medical history, as well as the more obvious postural and occupational factors affecting the muscles, joints and bones. A typical consultation lasts around 30 minutes; apart from normal medical diagnostic methods, diagnosis would be by physical examination and observation in which the feel and behaviour of muscles and joints are compared with what is known to be normal. In particular the following assessments would routinely be made:

1. *changes in symmetry in the body*—different strength or length of muscles when one side is compared with the other or one shoulder being higher than the other

2. *restrictions or changes in quality and range of joint movement*—compared with what is considered normal or with the same joint on the other side
3. *muscular coordination*—muscles being used by the body when they are not meant to be used, because of excessive tightness in some or weakness in others
4. *changes in the texture of soft tissues possibly because of overuse*—e.g. repetitive movements
5. *misuse*—inappropriate bending or loading in leisure (e.g. gardening) or work settings
6. *abuse*—injury caused by falls, car accidents or other sudden events
7. *disuse*—insufficient exercise or function.

If a problem is suspected to be arising from a more serious, underlying disease—arthritis, for example—blood tests, conventional radiographs or scans would be used to diagnose this accurately. Many chiropractors use radiographs to assist diagnosis, whereas osteopaths use them generally only for the purposes of excluding serious pathology.

Osteopaths and chiropractors aim to optimize the movement and support function. They do this using, in the main, manual methods to mobilize mechanical restrictions, especially around the spine and diaphragm. Treatment aims to relieve the associated discomfort of tight muscles and joints caused by injury, overuse, inappropriate use, postural habit or persistent stress and strain. Postural and respiratory re-education would also aim to prevent reoccurrence. Treatment considers the whole of the biomechanical function and not just the part. For instance someone regularly wearing high heels where the entire body's centre of gravity alters may eventually experience pain and stiffness in back muscles and joints. Overuse and patterns of misuse lead to changes of soft tissue and ultimately joint structure, such as fibrosis and early arthritic change. Chronic tension in muscles and stresses on joints lead not only to problems such as back pain but to energy being wasted, resulting in fatigue. Osteopathic and chiropractic techniques can help relieve such problems.

An osteopath is likely to commence any treatment by releasing and relaxing muscles and stretching stiff joint structures. Osteopathic soft tissue methods aim at mobilizing and normalizing restrictions and restoring normal pain-free function, whereas chiropractors take the view that although attention to soft tissues may be important the reflexive influence of active joint manipulation, via the nervous system is a better way of treating a problem, and many use a very wide range of manipulative techniques. McTimoney chiropractors use a gentle technique, known as the 'toggle' technique, that employs less direct mechanical pressure and movement than high-velocity thrusts. In a branch of osteopathy called cranial osteopathy (and the related discipline called craniosacral therapy) that is popular for treating problems in infants (colic, frequent crying, etc.), practitioners gently and rhythmically massage the bones of the skull, with the aim of correcting disturbances of the neuromuscular system.

A treatment course for back pain might consist of six sessions initially and then more at weekly intervals.

Training

In the UK, training of chiropractors and osteopaths, and subsequent entry into their respective professional organizations, is predominantly via full-time degree courses (BSc Hons). There are at least four major British osteopathic schools, all associated with universities, and two chiropractic colleges (also with university-validated degree programmes). Most McTimoney practitioners train part time for 4 years.

Training for doctors in aspects of manipulation, most notably soft tissue techniques, is readily available in the UK, as are fast-track training opportunities in osteopathy (1 year) by the London College of Osteopathic Medicine, where credit is given for prior medical studies. Several organizations run training courses for other conventional health care practitioners. The Manipulative Association of Chartered Physiotherapists runs and accredits postgraduate training in manipulation for physiotherapists. The British Institute of Musculoskeletal Medicine runs part-time courses for medically qualified practitioners.

Organization	Number of members	Comments
General Osteopathic Council Osteopathy House, 176 Tower Bridge Road, London SE1 3LU Tel: 020 7357 6655	2900	
General Chiropractic Council (GCC) 344–354 Gray's Inn Road, London WC1X 8BP Tel: 020 7713 5155	770+360	With the formation of the GCC the constituent Professions of Chiropractic will cease to have a formal role in registration
McTimoney Chiropractic Association 21 High Street, Eynsham, Oxon OX8 1HE Tel: 01865 880974	360	The title 'McTimoney practitioner' is being considered by practitioners who do not want to be statutorily registered
Craniosacral Therapy Association of the UK 27 Old Gloucester Street, London WC1N 3XX Tel: 07000 784735	290	Recent moves to integrate the craniosacral disciplines are underway

In the USA osteopaths have equivalent status to doctors (and in many states the same scope of practice).

Regulation

In the UK osteopaths and chiropractors are now regulated by legal statute. Two acts of parliament passed in the mid 1990s established the General Osteopathic Council and a General Chiropractic Council, which have similar powers to the GMC (i.e. they can remove practitioners from their register after disciplinary hearings).

Organizations

Organizations concerned with regulation and training in manipulative therapies are shown in the box at the bottom of this page (see Appendix II, p. 319, for overseas addresses).

Exercise systems

Exercise systems such as tai chi, qigong and yoga can be practised for general relaxation and health maintenance as well as medical conditions, and a small number of general practices offer regular classes.

Tai chi is a system of exercises originating from China; its 'solo form' is continuous sequence of slow and graceful movements performed in a state of relaxed concentration and with breath control. It is of low to moderate intensity and said to improve strength, balance and a state of inner calm. Although it is actually a type of 'internal' martial art that aims to utilize the internal flow of Qi, many people practise tai chi simply for health promotion on a daily basis.

Qigong (pronounced 'chi kung') is a related Chinese exercise system, which is more specifically orientated towards health maintenance. There are a variety of different exercise sets for specific medical conditions, as well as other exercises practised to maintain general health and keep the Qi of the body's organ systems in balance. The exercises are a combination of physical movements, visualization and mental focusing, and breathing exercises.

Yoga practice involves mainly static postures, breathing exercises and meditation aimed at improving mental and physical functioning.

Training

Yoga and tai chi can take years to master completely. Training in tai chi and qigong is traditionally handed down individually. There is now a university diploma course in qigong tuina for Western medical practitioners or qualified shiatsu or TCM practitioners.

Many yoga centres run courses to train yoga teachers. The Yoga Biomedical Trust also trains yoga therapists, who see patients individually and work on specific health problems.

Regulation

There is currently no official system of regulation of tai chi and qigong. The Chinese tradition is to pass on knowledge of this system from an individual teacher to personally selected students. In recent years, the UK Tai Chi Union has attempted to set some common standards by administering a test for membership. However, at present many teachers, particularly those of Chinese nationality, do not recognize its authority as a regulating body.

Some schools of yoga, such as the Iyengar school, have a well-established training system, and regulate the standards of their own teachers. Once again, there is as yet no nationally recognized national organization acting as a regulating body: however, the British Wheel of Yoga and the Yoga Biomedical Trust keep lists of trained members.

Organizations

Organizations concerned with training in exercise systems include the following (see Appendix II, p. 319, for overseas addresses).

Tai Chi Union
131 Tunstall Rd, Knypersley, Stoke-on-Trent ST8 7AA

British Wheel of Yoga
1 Hamilton Place, Boston Road, Sleaford, Lancs NG34 7ES
Tel: 01529 306851

Yoga Biomedical Trust
PO Box 140, Cambridge CB4 3SY

Healing

Some healers have specific diagnostic and treatment methods—for instance, qigong healers work by stimulating Qi via the TCM system of meridians and acupoints; others work completely intuitively and spontaneously.

The consultation

Healing is sometimes called the 'laying on of hands'. Generally the patient simply sits quietly in a chair while the practitioner moves his or her hands over the patient's body and at a slight distance away from it. Abnormal sensations of heat, cold, etc. in the palms reveal abnormalities in the 'biomagnetic field' or 'vital energy field' of the patient's body-mind, and the practitioner subse-

quently concentrates on these areas when beginning the treatment.

The exact method of treatment varies. Some healers will lay their hands directly on the person's body; others may keep their hands slightly away from the body. Different hand positions and movements may be used—open palms, one or two fingers pointed at a particular acupoint or meridian, and so on. Some healing organizations also make much use of distance healing or prayer, given often by groups.

Training

Training in this area is extremely variable. Members of organizations recognized by the Confederation of Healing Organizations (CHO) must complete 1–2 years' part-time training. The National Federation of Spiritual Healers (NFSH) and the College of Healing also run training courses. Reiki, a Japanese system, has a hierarchical structure of awards of 'Reiki master' of different levels, beginning with weekend trainings for the first level.

Regulation

Although there is little regulation in this area, the CHO is an umbrella organization. In addition, the members of the Doctor–Healer Network are statutorily registered medical practitioners.

Organizations

Organizations concerned with regulation and training in healing include the following.

Organization	Number of members	Educational requirements for membership	Comments
Confederation of Healing Organisations (CHO) The Red and White House, 113 High Street, Berkhampstead, Herts HP4 2DJ	11 000	1–2 years part-time	An umbrella body representing the interests of the majority of healing organizations.

Hypnosis and relaxation

Some GPs and other medical specialists such as dentists use hypnosis regularly. In addition there are practitioners trained in clinical hypnosis who practise independently.

Relaxation techniques are often used in public medicine as an adjunct; they may, for instance, be integrated into CBT programmes in pain clinics, or into occupational therapy in psychiatric units. Some nurses use relaxation techniques, for example, in preparation for surgery. A small number of general practices offer regular classes in relaxation.

The consultation

In hypnosis, there is usually a long initial consultation, followed by a course of shorter appointments. A patient may also be given a posthypnotic suggestion; this enables them to undergo self-hypnosis in between treatments or after the course is completed. Some practitioners (e.g. midwives) work with groups of people.

Practitioners of relaxation techniques do not make diagnoses, although they may use a medical practitioner's diagnosis as described by the patient to tailor their prescribed programme. They will prescribe techniques that generally need to be practised daily.

Relaxation techniques use various methods to encourage the removal of unconscious muscle tension in the body, by encouraging the patient to become aware of and release tension, for instance by breathing out. Visualization and imagery techniques, in contrast, are more like hypnosis—that is, a relaxed state is induced and then suggestions for visualization are given.

Typically, a relaxation technique may be learnt over a course of classes, and participants are also encouraged to practise by themselves between classes.

Training

Although there is no standard training in hypnosis for NMQP practitioners, the British Medical Hypnotherapy Examination Board (BMHEB) awards a certificate, a diploma (DHyp) and a postgraduate diploma (PDCHyp) in clinical hypnosis. The British Society of Medical and Dental Hypnosis runs courses for doctors and dentists. A Medical Diploma in Clinical Hypnosis (MDCH) may be taken by medical or dental graduates; there is also a Medical Course in Clinical Hypnosis validated by the Royal College of Psychiatrists for Continuing Professional Development (CPD) units. If hypnosis is used for psychotherapeutic or psychoanalytical purposes the practitioner must also be appropriately qualified in clinical psychology, counselling or psychotherapy, and be a member of the British Psychological Society, the British Association of Counselling and Psychotherapy or the United Kingdom Council of Psychotherapy.

Training in teaching relaxation techniques is provided by various means, from short courses to lengthy apprenticeships.

Regulation

In this area the lack of regulation is a serious issue. There is a large number of hypnotherapy registers but no single regulating body. Hypnotherapists who are also conventionally qualified as doctors, dentists, nurses or psychologists are regulated by the appropriate regulatory bodies. Some organizations registering NMQP hypnotherapists are member associations of the British Complementary Medicine Association.

For relaxation therapies the situation is even more unsatisfactory, but, given the relatively benign nature of many relaxation techniques, this variation in standards presents usually more of a problem of ensuring effective treatment and good professional conduct rather than one of avoiding adverse effects.

Organizations

Organizations concerned with regulation and training in hypnosis and relaxation are shown in the box below (see Appendix II, p. 319, for overseas addresses).

Organization	Number of members	Educational requirements for membership	Comments
UK Confederation of Hypnotherapy Organisations (UKCHO) Suite 401, 302 Regent Street, London W1R 6HH Tel: 0800 952 0560 Website:www. ukcho.co.uk	2000	Not less than 450 hours (120 hours being one to one tuition)	An umbrella body, the aim of which is to implement national standards and be a central information source
British Society of Medical and Dental Hypnosis 23 Broadfields Heights, 53/58 Broadfields Avenue, Edgware, Middx HA8 8PF Tel: 020 8905 4342 or 17 Keppel View Road, Kimberworth S61 2AP Tel: 07000 560309	331		Members are statutorily registered

Massage and touch-based therapies

Although, as with many CTs, massage is usually practised in private medicine, there is considerable potential to integrate it into the mainstream. In conventional health settings, it is used mainly in hospices and in units for learning disability and mental disorders, where it is often practised by nurses or unpaid practitioner volunteers. However, a few professional massage practitioners are being employed in NHS hospitals (e.g. in drug rehabilitation and in oncology units) and general practices. Tens of thousands of massage therapists practice in the UK. It is estimated that there are over 50 000 licensed therapists in the USA, where the largest professional body, the American Massage Therapy Association, has about 30 000 members.

Many associated forms of bodywork, deriving from different traditions, are now being offered to patients alongside standard European (Swedish) massage. These include:

- *acupressure/tuina*—a Chinese system using vigorous and penetrating techniques: deep pressure on acupoints and squeezing, pushing and kneading massage, to balance the flow of Qi through the meridians
- *Alexander technique*—education and hands-on postural correction
- *aromatherapy*—massage using highly aromatic plant oils
- *bioenergetics*—massage to aid the psychotherapeutic process
- *feldenkreis*—movements performed by the practitioner on the patient's body to improve posture, movement and function
- *reflexology*—a system that uses pressure, mainly on the feet or hands, to affect distant areas of the body
- *rolfing*—a Western form of deep-pressure massage
- *shiatsu*—a modified form of acupressure using slow and sustained static pressure to balance the flow of Qi through the meridians, systematized as part of traditional Japanese medicine
- *structural integration*—treatments that use deep-pressure massage to improve function of the muscular system
- *tragerwork*—an open-ended system of psychophysical integration in which the client's trunk and limbs are moved in a gentle, rhythmic way, but avoiding undue pressure and effort, to encourage free, light and flexible movements
- *zero balancing*—a therapy using finger pressure and gentle traction on the bones and joints underlying soft tissue.

The consultation

A standard therapeutic treatment involves taking a case history followed by a full body massage. Case history taking can be relatively short compared with other CTs, and systems such as reflexology also use a preliminary palpation to gain diagnostic information. Treatments usually last from 30 minutes to an hour, though they can be adapted to the time-frames of public sector care by focusing on one part of the body: for example head, neck and shoulders, or any area of increased muscle tension. Patients usually have to undress to their underwear.

A variety of strokes are used for treatment, depending on the patient's condition and the part of the body being treated. Some systems employ deep pressure, which can cause painful sensations, but these are usually short lived.

The patient generally lies on a specially designed massage couch. In the UK practitioners will often use oils to help their hands move over the patient's body; elsewhere in Europe, soap or talcum powder may be used. Adverse effects are rare. In aromatherapy, oils derived from plants ('essential oils') are added to a base massage oil. Although often used purely for their smell, the oils are claimed to have a wide range of medicinal properties, including effects on wound healing, infection, blood circulation, and digestion. However, many massage practitioners use essential oils without claiming to be practising aromatherapy.

In reflexology, practitioners use a moving-pressure technique, rather than massage strokes, concentrating on areas of the foot or hand ('reflex zones') that are believed to correspond to the organs or structures of the body in which there is imbalance, damage or disease.

Training

UK standards of training vary widely, from weekend courses in basic massage to 3-year full-time university BSc degree courses and 2-year MSc courses in therapeutic bodywork. The International Therapy Examinations Council (ITEC) qualification is a very basic qualification that includes anatomy and physiology, and is widely accepted. There are ITEC qualifications both in Western massage and in oriental systems such as tuina. There is also a university diploma course in qigong tuina.

If massage is to be incorporated widely into mainstream settings in the UK, NHS or private, training standards will certainly need to rise. The first specialized massage training courses in the UK are now developing and many nurses and some physiotherapists have chosen to augment their professional training by learning massage skills. The training of specialized groups within the profession (e.g. sports massage) is helping to form a core of well-trained professionals out of which a sound profession could emerge.

Training standards in the USA are more stringent than in the UK. The majority of therapists will have had at least 600 hours of direct contact training and this is gradually extending to around 1000 hours. In Canada, led by British Columbia standards, a 2200-hour training is required, soon to be extended to 3200 hours.

Regulation

The regulation of massage therapies is currently very unsatisfactory, as practitioners may be registered with one of many different organizations. However, umbrella organizations are attempting to unite these different bodies in massage and aromatherapy. Practitioners who are also conventional healthcare professionals are regulated by their own professional body; however, if integration into mainstream settings is to happen, these professions need to establish basic massage therapy competencies, standards (including compulsory continuing education), regulatory machinery and goals.

Standards in the USA and Canada are generally more than adequate in these terms, with state licensure and continuing education offering reassurance to those practitioners wishing to employ, or refer, to massage therapists.

Organizations

Organizations concerned with regulation and training in massage and touch-based therapies include the following (see Appendix II, p. 319, for other types of massage and pressure therapy and for overseas addresses).

Organization	Number of members	Educational requirements for membership	Comments
British Massage Therapy Council (BMTC) 17 Rymers Lane, Oxford OX4 3JU Tel: 01865 774123		100–1600 hours	Umbrella organization
British Association for Massage Therapy 36 Lodge Drive, Palmers Green, London N15 5JZ Tel: 020 8886 3120			Umbrella organization. Combines FSMT, LCSP, MTIGB, SMTO

Naturopathy

Many doctors would be surprised to realize that their everyday health promotion advice actually has its origins in naturopathic ideas. High-fibre–low-fat diets, the value of exercise, clean air and water and the importance of relaxation are basic to naturopathy. Long before their general acceptance by conventional medicine, these approaches were the core principles of naturopathic medicine. Integration with naturopathy is therefore well advanced in a general way! In integration terms, it remains for doctors to recognize the potential of more specific naturopathic methods, such as therapeutic fasting, orthomolecular nutrition, hydrotherapy and procedures involving homeopathy, herbal medicine and manipulation. Naturopathy can often be combined with mainstream methods, especially in care of chronic conditions, since its objectives are long term and its methods are seldom contraindicated

Naturopathy has much in common with ayurvedic medicine and therefore has a strong following in the Indian subcontinent.

The consultation

The initial consultation with a naturopath may last up to an hour. The practitioner will want to complete a comprehensive medical interview covering all aspects of physical and emotional well-being. A medical examination will generally form part of this procedure and radiography, blood, urine, and other tests may be ordered.

Naturopaths believe that their task is largely to remove obstacles to the body's natural self-healing process, as well as enhancing more efficient function, so the body can heal itself. The typical naturopathic client, whatever the conventional diagnosis, is generally feeling chronically and persistently under par—a condition attributed to an overload of 'toxins' that have accumulated because of poor diet, digestion, absorption or excretion. A naturopath may treat this by employing nutritional, herbal, homeopathic, manipulative, hydrotherapeutic and stress management approaches, as appropriate. Treatment of symptoms is avoided unless these are distressing, in which case attempts are made to modulate rather than suppress them. A great deal of naturopathic care entails teaching the patient prevention and self-help methods; dietary, exercise, hydrotherapy and relaxation all feature strongly.

Many naturopathic approaches entail altering habitual behaviour and trying out new regimens over often a long period of time. Temporary relapses known as 'healing crises' can occur as the detoxifying effects of treatment and recommendations begin to take effect. However, because naturopathy does not rely solely on one treatment modality it can provide some choice for patients, which helps those with long-term chronic problems to feel they have some control over and something to contribute to their healing process. Follow-up sessions will take between 20 and 40 minutes. The number of consultations will depend on the severity of the condition and the recuperative powers of the patient.

Training

In the UK there is only one 4-year full-time degree course (BSc Hons) in naturopathy; it includes anatomy, physiology, biochemistry and pathology as well as naturopathic and osteopathic principles and practice. A number of part-time courses are also available. The majority of naturopaths in the UK are also state-registered osteopaths.

In Germany, naturopathic-type care is state funded. In the USA 11 states (and several more where legislation is pending) license and reimburse the fees of naturopaths as family practitioners. Bastyr University, in Seattle, Washington, offers a full naturopathic medical training in close cooperation with the University of Washington Medical School. Modern American naturopathy includes in its 5 years of training nutrition, homeopathy, botanical medicine, TCM (including acupuncture), manipulative medicine (largely based on chiropractic and massage), psychotherapy and hydrotherapy. A high standard of training in naturopathy also exists in Australia, Canada, South Africa and Israel.

Regulation

The General Council and Register of Naturopaths registers and regulates the 300 or so naturopaths practising in the United Kingdom. Most of these are also trained osteopaths, and will therefore be subject to state regulation p. 93).

Organizations

Organizations concerned with regulation and training in naturopathy include the following (see Appendix II, p. 319, for overseas addresses):

Organization	Number of members
General Council and Register of Naturopaths 2 Goswell Road, Street, Somerset BA16 0JG Tel: 01458 840072	310

Nutritional therapy

The nutritional approach to healing fits readily into mainstream practice, as long as the measures have been well researched, which a great many have. As many people now purchase self-prescribed OTC vitamin and mineral supplements a nutritional approach to health care will be familiar and acceptable to a growing number of patients.

The consultation

The first consultation lasts about an hour and covers patients' current eating patterns, medical history, exercise habits, how much they smoke and drink and their emotional state as well as current symptoms and any medication they may be taking. A comprehensive evaluation is made of key indicators such as the status of skin, eyes, tongue, nails and reflexes. Clues will be looked for that suggest deficiencies, imbalances or toxicity by these means, as well as via the full case history and evaluation of the individual's dietary and lifestyle habits.

Exclusion dieting may be employed to determine allergenic foods. A range of standard testing procedures, including blood, stool, urine, sweat and hair analysis, may be used as well. However, some nutritional therapists also use less conventional assessment approaches for which at the present time there is less evidence. These methods include:

- *applied kinesiology, also called muscle testing.* The rationale for this is that substances to which the person is allergic or intolerant cause a detectable weakness in the person's muscle groups (usually tested in the arm)
- *hair testing.* This is analysis of strands of hair for, for example, vitamin or mineral deficiencies or toxic overload of heavy metals, etc.; the testing method is often unspecified, and can range from standard laboratory tests to dowsing
- *iridology.* This is based on the theory that the eye forms a 'map' of the body, hence changes within internal organ systems can be detected in different regions of the eye
- *vega testing.* This is testing of the 'state of balance' of the body's systems using a small meter applied to the end-points of various acupuncture meridians.

It has to be emphasized that there is almost no research-derived evidence for these methods. On the contrary, RCT studies of iridology, hair testing, kinesiology and vega testing suggest they do not provide reliable data about a person's diagnosis or food allergy (see Ch. 2).

Some practitioners use nutritional supplementation. Examples include:

- high-dose vitamin C for cancer
- zinc for the common cold
- high-dose vitamins for learning disability ('orthomolecular' therapy)
- evening primrose oil for atopic dermatitis and PMS
- vitamin B6 for morning sickness and PMS
- garlic for lowering cardiovascular risk
- multivitamins for improvement in general health.

Some nutritional therapists may utilize an approach based on the principles of naturopathy, recommend specific nutrients such as vitamins, minerals, plant-based supplements, etc. or advise on dietary changes, for example to help the patient cope with food intolerances. Food intolerances are not IgE-mediated immediate response type allergies and are said to be caused by gut mucosal hyperpermeability and to involve an IgG-mediated response to certain foods. Nutritionists and naturopaths attribute some chronic inflammatory disease to food intolerance.

A variety of specialized dietary protocols may be prescribed. These may include quite well-known dietary regimens such as vegan, vegetarian, raw food, food-combining (Hay diet) and high-fibre–low-fat healthy eating plans. Nutritional advice could also include more specialized recommendations such as following a macrobiotic diet, detoxification diet exclusion and rotation diet or oligoantigenic diet.

Training

Training courses range from short courses leading to a certificate in basic nutrition to full-time university BSc degree courses giving a qualification as a nutritional therapist.

Nutrition has long been a neglected aspect of the undergraduate medical curriculum, and many of today's doctors were never taught the scientific basis of nutritional therapy. However, it is making an increasingly important contribution to conventional clinical practice, creating a demand for training and education, and this deficiency is now being addressed by a joint intercollegiate committee including representatives of 11 medical royal colleges, so far resulting in a programme of 4-day intercollegiate courses. The intercollegiate committee believes that nutritional considerations must be part of the overall specialty training of doctors; ultimately, clinical nutrition may become recognized as a subspecialty with its own pathway of postgraduate training. There are also numerous other courses, some university based, in which MDs can readily familiarize themselves with current research, as well as computer programs (CD-ROMs, etc.) that can be used as instant sources of information.

SUMMARY

CAM: the UK training situation:

- UK complementary practitioners (other than osteopaths and chiropractors) are not regulated by the state
- most have completed some further education in their chosen discipline
- there is great variation in training CPs
- degree-level programmes began in the mid 1990s
- the University of Westminster School of Integrated Health has the UK's most comprehensive university degree programmes

CAM teaching in UK medical schools:

- developments toward integrated health care will depend on the availability of skilled doctors who can collaborate with CPs
- complementary medicine teaching in UK medical schools is expanding rapidly
- the number of schools providing dedicated CAM modules has risen by 50% to at least 15 out of 23 in the last 2 years
- in 1997,10 of 20 schools ran formal CM courses and a further four intended to do so by the academic year 1998/99

Regulation

The British Association of Nutritional Therapists registers practitioners who have completed one of its approved courses at selected training colleges.

Organizations

Organizations concerned with regulation and training in nutritional therapy include the following (see Appendix II, p. 319, for overseas addresses).

Organization	Number of membership
British Association of Nutritional Therapists BCM Bant, London WC1N 3XX Tel: 0870 606 1284	225

PRACTITIONER DEVELOPMENT
General practitioners

Although some knowledge of CAM is essential for appropriate referral and communication, as yet there are no broad programmes for doctors seeking a better understanding of the academic, scientific, political and clinical issues involved. A postgraduate foundation for collaboration between doctors and CPs is perhaps overdue. Such a programme would explore CTs' intellectual and cultural landscape and try to make some sense of an interface with conventional clinical science and practice. GPs also need to grasp certain key issues and controversies—clinical, political, conceptual and interprofessional—if they are to understand the current CT scene. It is useful for GPs to consider current projects where integration is under way, so that options for evaluating the process and outcome of innovative approaches is better understood. Such programmes can help clarify doctors' knowledge and attitudes, and reflect on the way our ideas about health and health care are changing. Perhaps, above all, such programmes will have to explore a common language for integrative joint working and be open to developing practitioners' capacity to care and communicate.

Components of continuing professional education and development

Continuing professional education and development may take many forms. These include ongoing lifelong learning, experiential learning, practice-based learning, participative and self-directed learning, reflective practice and portfolio-based learning.

The purpose of continuing medical education (CME) and continuing professional development (CPD) is to ensure improvement in clinical practice.[33] There is widespread consensus across disciplines (e.g. health and education) and continents on the importance of lifelong learning.[34] We learn as adults when we need to know something specific and we try to make sense of our experiences (experiential learning). The ideas and concepts generated by reflecting on an experience stimulate further experimentation and more learning. Kolb has described this experiential cycle of events.[35]

The reflective learning audit cycle

Development of a personal development plan may be broken down into the following stages:

1. *What* did I need to know?—needs assessment to clarify key learning objectives
2. How can I find out?
3. What did I *notice?*—key points
4. What did I *learn?*—learning evaluation
5. How will I *apply* this to practice?—clinical relevance
6. What do I need to do *next?*—reflective educational audit.

PRACTICE PROFESSIONAL DEVELOPMENT PLANNING

Practice professional development plans (PPDPs): 'are intended to ensure that continuing medical education, audit, research and effectiveness principles are applied more appropriately, to aid practices in identifying and achieving clear, focused, educational goals'.[36] They must respond to local as well as national community health priorities.[37] All practice members should be involved in the practice development process, which is an opportunity for team building, as well as ensuring that the team delivers high-quality service to patients.

In practice development planning the practice members tackle the following questions[37]:

• What things need to improve in our practice?
• How have they been identified? (discussions, surveys, audit, significant event analysis)
• Do these reflect priorities in the wider health care system? (although some problems, specific to practice, need to be mindful of external priorities)
• How are they to be addressed?
• How is successful outcome to be assessed?

Current policy emphasizes educational needs assessment at the level of the individual practitioner, practice, and locality[38] in order to deliver a high-quality service to patients. These needs can then be captured in personal learning plans;[39] practice development plans[36] and health improvement plans respectively. None can be viewed in isolation, but each is informed by the others in relation to the wider picture of health provision for a community[40]:

1. *individual practitioner*—education can be directed though formulating a personal learning plan about CTs
2. *practice*—education can be directed though formulating a practice development plan about how to include CTs
3. *community*—goals for health provision can be directed though formulating a locality development plan that explores the relevance of CTs to the local health improvement plan (in the NHS) or otherwise to identified local needs, organizational priorities or markets.

PATIENT INVOLVEMENT

There is an increasing use of OTC remedies by patients, both before and after consultation with a healthcare practitioner. This reflects the rise of self-care and patient autonomy on one hand (assisted by a proliferation of information sources, e.g. the internet) and rationing of public health care spending (often explicit in the field of prescribing but more covert in relation to practitioners' time and availability) on the other.

Patients will inform their self-selection of OTC remedies by advice, often initially sought from a pharmacist. Perhaps Balint's[24] 'doctor as drug' now has to be augmented by the notion of 'pharmacist as clinician', though some patients will find themselves redirected to their GP. A visit to the pharmacy, an information booth or a library, though it cannot replace the support of GP staff and other patients, can be an adequate background for self-care.

Knowledge about and availability of complementary and alternative medicines and dietary supplements will vary greatly from practitioner to practitioner, however, so reference to some kind of reliable database will become increasingly necessary (see Table 2.2, p. 59). Issues of safety and efficacy are paramount here; in particular, drug cross-reactions with active ingredients in 'natural' products need to be considered (see Ch. 2, p 50–51).

Patients also make their choice of remedy by reading relevant information. Too often, however, the readily accessible information is likely to be biased, simplistic or inaccurate; for instance, material is available from internet sites, but its content may be unreliable, biased or confusing. To ensure that patient self-care is well informed, at the MHC we developed a range of information leaflets and self-help instruction sheets (see p. 199).

DESIGN OF MATERIAL

Data collection

In designing the CT service process, the team will have to give proper thought to the means of recording information. Well-designed documentation will improve the interaction between the GP and the CP, yield important information on treatment preferences and effects, efficacy, etc. for evaluation, and so improve future decision making about treatment and service development. It can also help inform both the GP and the patient about available treatment options.

Design of documentation should encompass:

- essential data-entry forms
- patient record, treatment and referral forms (plus a guide to using the record system whether paper based or computerized)
- evaluation forms, e.g. questionnaires (plus clinician and patient guides for using them)
- GP information and self-help sheets as appropriate to the service.

The design of referral procedures and case notes needs to:

- reflect as accurately as possible what happens in practice
- communicate the most relevant information between the GP and the CP
- enable effective clinical encounters with patients
- be practical and feasible to use in a time-limited clinical session
- allow various kinds of reports to be produced easily.

The referral form

The referral form needs to:

- be quick and easy to use by all practitioners in a clinical setting
- be suitable in language and style for multiprofessional use
- include all essential information about a patient in a simple form
- have space for free text information to personalize the referral
- record the GP reason for referral
- include information on the 'complexity' of a case
- generate as much useful data for analysis as possible.

The ongoing patient record form

This has to:

- be easy to use
- allow free text entry about treatment
- act as an aide memoire for future care plan

- include a field for collecting feedback and comments back to GPs
- provide information on non-treatment factors impacting on outcome (life change, etc.)
- capture, summarize and allow easy tracking of outcome scores.

The information cards and leaflets

The GP cards need to be concise and clear, summarizing briefly the treatment choices, particularly salient research findings and any contraindications or safety pointers.

The patient self-care leaflets again should avoid over-wordiness, but clearly summarize the principles of particular therapies, what can be expected in and from a treatment, and include any well-established benefits of the therapy and ancillary information on, for instance lifestyle or nutrition.

Self-help leaflets

From the literature on patient education we knew that the following factors were important. First, repeating the educational message seems to produce the greatest persuasive effect. Secondly, educational messages should be tailored to fit the individual patient, addressing a patient's specific concerns, whereas 'canned' messages given to all patients are probably unwise and ineffective. Thirdly, use of multiple strong arguments in favour of an activity will have a greater persuasive impact than a single argument. Finally, any negative consequences should be addressed.

Bearing these factors in mind, we designed a variety of specific leaflets to give patients information about the different therapies available, about their condition and about other useful guidelines such as diets and exercise programmes. (Examples of these are given in Chapter 7.)

Questions we thought patients might want the leaflets to address included the following.

Why?
- Why am I being asked to do this?

How do I do it?
- How long does it take to do?
- How can I tell if I am doing it right?
- Where can I go if I need extra help?
- If I lapse how can I restart?

What will it be like?
- Will this procedure or suggestion hurt?
- Will it inconvenience me or my family/friends in any way?
- Is it difficult to learn?

Assessing progress
- How long will it be before I will notice any changes?
- How long will I have to do this (diet, exercise, taking supplements) for?

Costs
- Does it cost anything?
- How much will it cost me (on a weekly basis)?

Resources
- What will I need?
- Where might I be able to obtain the things suggested (general information)?

Design requirements
  These included:
- a simple attractive layout
- in clear simple language.

(Copies of forms developed at the MHC are included in Chapter 8.)

AN EXAMPLE OF SERVICE DESIGN: THE MARYLEBONE HEALTH CENTRE (MHC) PROJECT

In the mid 1980s at MHC the group formed under Patrick Pietroni to develop a multidisciplinary approach to inner city primary care. This included health education and counselling and, though it still does, it has usually been the CT aspect that attracted most attention. Patrick Pietroni, the lead GP, was able to raise grants to fund a small CT service and gradually a group of non-medically qualified complementary practitioners formed and began to work at MHC part-time—the first such group to work in NHS general practice.

Initially our research involved simply describing the kind of CTs used, the patients referred and what they and the doctors thought and felt about the therapies. Our published work confirmed our initial sense that including CTs was clinically useful, pleasing to patients and interesting to doctors.[41] Yet it proved unexpectedly difficult to define this sense or describe precisely what contributed to or undermined it. To help us understand more about the team dynamics—especially the problems of authority, communication and conflict inherent in multidisciplinary practice and interprofessional learning, two cooperative inquiries were organized.[21]

Still the outcomes in terms of cost–benefit or health gain were less easy to determine. For example although we knew the practice prescribed substantially less than the national average, there was no way of knowing whether this was because CTs were available, for we had no 'pre-CT' data to compare ours with. The opportunity to organize a CT back and neck pain clinic for a neigh-bouring practice—one with several years' records available—made up for this. We designed a study to see whether an osteopathy/acupuncture service would reduce referrals from this practice to hospital specialists (see Ch. 4, p. 121 for details of this study). This it did, substantially: an indication at last for cost-beneficial outcome from CT!

The study aimed to reflect the clinician's ordinary way of treating patients, and to work within the time constraints of ordinary NHS practice, while still entering the data needed. This had entailed entering clinical information on a laptop computer after the consultation. The analysis and reports generated were then discussed in monthly audit meetings with the GPs—over sandwiches—where referrals and treatment outcomes (derived from patient and GP questionnaires) could be continually updated. In this pilot study we were able to develop and test out the necessary elements of a learning cycle.

We next used what we had learned in the pilot to develop the CT service at MHC. The first step was to audit the range of approaches at MHC and take a close look at our own established CT team. The aim was to improve the extended primary care team's work and to develop the materials needed—from guidelines to patient leaflets. At MHC, as in most primary care units, there had been no stated intake and exclusion criteria for the CT service, nor had the expected outcomes been made explicit. In the 1990s as resources shrank the practice expanded and the imperative to use time effectively grew. Our research turned in the direction of outcomes and efficiency. So guidelines and clinical audit were the obvious way forward. In order to find answers, structured approaches had to be put in place for referral, collection of consultation data and assessment of treatment outcomes. We had to find ways of making every stage of the clinical work explicit: recording all activity and tracking clinical progress at each consultation. All this had to be achieved within the time and energy constraints of a busy general practice. And for the sake of efficiency and to avoid overloading the limited CT service we had to make patient self-help an easy option for GPs to choose.

Importing complementary therapies or complementary practitioners?

The majority of family practices where CTs became available over the last decade did not do so by expanding their primary care teams. Rather, in most cases it has tended to be doctors or nurses who were the providers. At MHC acupuncture, homeopathy, osteopathy, massage and, intermittently, naturopathy have been available for 12 years, and we rely on part-time CPs for CT service delivery. Primary care is an increasingly multidisciplinary venture, where problems around communication come with the territory; despite this our team mix is not just an historical accident: bringing in non-doctors was a deliberate attempt to enrich our ideas about health care. This is not to deny that difficulties are likely to increase as teams enlarge and intensify as new disciplines join the team. It makes time for meeting and discussion even more necessary, yet there is rarely enough time for reflection. So how, we wondered, could we make the best use of our time, make our communication more effective and ensure that CTs were used in appropriate, efficient and effective ways? To help us do this we chose an action research approach, based on the need to answer these questions, and devised ways of collecting the data needed in order to track referrals made and the outcomes of CPs, work. We took this step because having worked for over a decade as an extended primary care team we realized that the future of our work depended on adopting a more evidence-linked approach. The details of this design process are described in this section.

Our pragmatic method was a response to the sort of problems GPs face in family medicine when deciding how best to use CTs. We based our approach not only on an assessment of the available research evidence but on practitioners' experience as well. The aim has been to develop a system for evidence-based practice of CTs by making rationale choices about treatments and gather evidence about their use and their impact.

An action research approach to integration

Summary of the main action research cycles

The action research cycle is composed of six stages, as follows.

1. The practice review. The initial task is to agree on appropriate conditions and referral criteria and on the service aims: for instance, 'fix patients', 'maintain function', 'contain distress', 'improve coping', etc. At this stage a draft referral form has to be agreed. In order to achieve all this, the practice has to establish which needs are currently poorly met. This might be done through consensus, e.g. by circulating information and questionnaires. And if the practice has used CTs before then a retrospective analysis might clarify how and why and what happened. A review of internal costs (drug spend) and use of external resources (hospital specialist referrals) will highlight possible savings to be made. Patient meetings can provide user input. (This stage was discussed in detail in Chapter 1.)

2. Assessing resources. At this stage, it has to be decided which CTs are most likely to be relevant. Once again, this might involve team meetings, where the evidence available would be presented. This would include

summaries of experiential reports, well-designed studies such as RCTs, evidence reports and systematic reviews and expert opinion. (This stage was discussed in detail in Chapter 2.) The economic implications (e.g. potential savings, costs, external funds and possible subsidies, grants and targeted public sector sources) have to be decided. An assessment of the knowledge and skills required to implement the service is the next step. Are they available? How could they be developed? Is implementation feasible? How for instance might local CPs qualified and prepared to work in an integrated team be found?

3. Designing the service. Knowledge and skills of the existing team are reviewed. GPs' knowledge of CTs and skills in 'primary care CT' might need to be improved. Staff development sessions can be held. Consultation role play and question and answer sessions might be used to explore what is and is not understood about CTs, CPs and how they work. Documentation that helps ensure the smooth running of the service could include aide memoires of primary care advice, referral protocols (e.g. the maximum number of treatments a patient can have) and treatment guideline cards, etc. The best, or the most practical, options for service delivery have to be agreed and, if the team is to be expanded then this will involve new job descriptions and contracts.

Once agreement on CT options, referral pathways, resources available and outcomes expected has been reached, all staff need to understand how the GP/CP interface will work. Whether paper or computer systems are used, the team will need a user-friendly guide to data entry and use of the evaluation system chosen (e.g. use of MYMOP forms, etc.).

Patient information and self-care options can be addressed at this stage: leaflets informing patients about particular therapies and conditions, and self-help leaflets (on diets, exercise, etc.).

4. Delivering the service. Delivery could include the use of the primary care CT options perhaps as prereferral and self-care advice: OTC herbs, homeopathic remedies, nutritional supplements, diet, exercise, etc. All concerned have to be clear about the GP to CP pathway; what sort of referral is appropriate; how patients are informed about the referral process; what data has to be collected; and how to use referral, treatment and outcomes forms. Because this is almost certain to mean a steep learning curve—practitioners have to get used to new set ways of working together—developing the delivery process will require regular scheduled meetings and minutes, as well as easy aide memoires to manage the whole process. Our group meet mid week for 90 minutes at a sandwich lunch and keep a record of our discussions. (This stage will be discussed in detail in Chapter 4.)

5. Monitoring the service. We believe groups can only learn and lay claim to evidence-based CT practice if they are able to track and assess what has been happening in an extended service. We have developed a computer system to make data gathering and data processing easier and more effective. Our own audit meetings—held every 4–6 weeks to assess intake and outcomes—rely on structured reports to bring together referral data and clinical data We gather our data on screen using the practice's computer network. The same material could be captured with a paper-based system but we found that very labour intensive; even a computer-based approach still requires a staff member prepared to pull the report together. Our aim has been to circulate 6-weekly CP–GP reports and to include critical incident reports in preparation for audit meetings and to make them as effective as possible. (However, we have not always met this standard by any means!) Extended meetings are also held where we discuss clinical problems, difficult cases and team dynamics, and organize 'academic meetings' for more formal inter-professional learning through presentations or reading seminars. (See Ch. 4.)

6. Modifying the service. Finally, decisions can be taken on any actions needed to improve the service. Emerging questions can be discussed and possible solutions developed. (This stage will be discussed in detail in Ch. 4.) This is an ongoing process, the possible solutions in the form of service modifications (e.g. referral criteria) being themselves monitored and evaluated, and so on. So the action research process becomes a continuous cycle, as shown in Figure 3.1.

(A summary of our experience of CT service design at MHC, using this approach, appears in Chapter 5.)

How we integrated CPs into the primary care team

Box 3.5 summarizes our approach to the integration of CTs at the MHC.

The clinicians group (four GPs, a homeopath, three osteopaths, an acupuncturist and a massage therapist) had been meeting fortnightly since the late 1980s to review clinical problems. Several members of the group

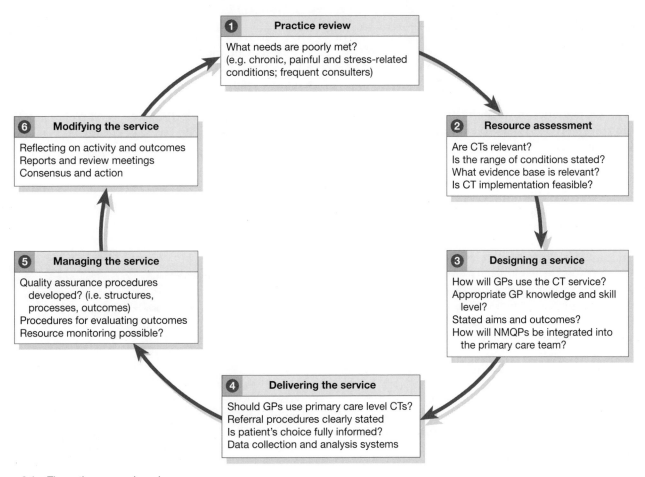

Figure 3.1   The action research cycle.

Box 3.5 How we approached the problem of integrating CTs into an NHS practice at MHC

We wanted to find out:

- what GPs and CPs thought a CT service could realistically achieve in an NHS setting
- whether guidelines for treating a range of agreed common conditions could include relevant aspects of certain complementary therapies
- whether an extended multidisciplinary primary care team could work together using these guidelines
- how to use a computer-based data collection system to manage the integration process
- whether outcomes of using the CT guidelines could be practically evaluated.

To do this we developed a series of action learning cycles:

- a series of meetings of the extended primary care team explored ways of developing a rational and quality-assured CT service
- this cycle defined core conditions, the practice's previous use of CTs, a relevant evidence base, agreed referral guidelines, initial methods for data collection and reporting structures and meetings that would be needed
- critical incidents were brought to fortnightly clinical discussion meetings
- a computer-based clinical database was developed (see screen examples and reports, pp. 000; 000) to record activity (referral and treatments) and outcomes
- we reflected on the CT service's development and the emerging problems of capturing data about intake and outcomes, through action research cycles.
- the process was supervised and evaluated through 6–8-weekly audit meetings
- methods were continually adapted as problems and new options emerged.

have worked together throughout that time. Two reflective inquiries had been held to explore the problems of collaboration.[21] In 1993 members of the group first developed a way of using rapid audit cycles as a way of making communication more effective and resource use more efficient. (See the N. W. Thames Study in Ch. 4, p. 127, for an example.) We eventually refined this approach in order to answer our MHC practice development questions (see list above). A grant from the Smith's charity funded a study to staff, organize and document the work entailed. The clinicians group met for 2 hours every 6–8 weeks to progress the development and discuss the emerging questions. In order to find answers, structured approaches had to be implemented for referral, collection of consultation data and assessment of treatment outcomes.

A number of key materials were used to gather the information needed:

- a GP referral form
- a clinical database used by CPs to record detail of clinical encounters
- a patient-centred evaluation (MYMOP) to track clinical change

- documented fortnightly 1-hour meetings of all clinicians
- CT activity reports reviewed at documented 6-weekly audit meetings.

(Examples of blank referral, treatment and MYMOP forms and computer screens, also report examples, are included in Chapters 4, 5, and 8.)

The process of implementing these approaches has entailed 3 years of participative action research during which the structures and linked processes were developed, adapted and gradually taken up by practitioners.

Design of the material

We began the project using a paper system and gradually moved to an entirely computerized approach. In the computer system all data, including patient case data, referral, treatment details, case records and other notes, was entered using a database based on a Filemaker Pro application (Fig. 3.2; see Chapter 8 for details of the computer system and Chapters 4 and 5 for screen shots of case records and treatment details.)

Leaflets and forms for doctors included the following:

- GP information leaflet—key points about the service and its evaluation
- GP referral form—completed at point of referral
- a 6–8-weekly report detailing all new referrals made by each GP
- follow-up form after discharge—completed at follow-up appointment with GP or next contact.

The in-house GP referral form is put into the patient notes when making a referral to the CP. It summarizes the problem, duration, aims and background information. It records the therapy requested, the category of problem

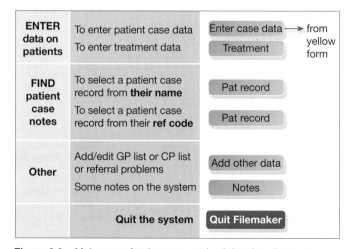

Figure 3.2 Main menu for the computerized data keeping system.

(i.e. one of the guideline conditions appropriate for CT referral) its duration and location, the aims of the referral, alternate options to CP referral the GP might consider and space for comments or background information. (Chapter 8 contains an example of a blank referral form.)

Leaflets and forms for CPs included the following:

- the completed referral form received from the GP
- CP case sheet
- CP treatment sheet
- MYMOP questionnaires
- guide to using MYMOP, which is given to patients.

During the pilot phase of the project we realized it would be essential to find ways of recording the treatment progress and outcomes. Some impression of effectiveness is clearly necessary and tracking encourages patient selection to improve so that effort can be targeted more effectively. The ability to do so will largely determine how efficiently CTs can be used. CPs nowadays use a database to record detail of clinical encounters, but the paper-based system though more difficult to analyse could still help structure a small CT service by providing a basis for tracking and feedback between practitioners.

The CP case sheet contains space to enter the referral problem, the referral aim, the presenting condition, the diagnosis, a decision on whether to treat, and record five problems and two activities as entered by the patient on the MYMOP questionnaire (see below), and whether the patient is a 'complex case'. (Chapter 8 contains an example of a blank case record sheet.) This information is recorded when a patient is first seen.

The treatment sheet is completed at each encounter and contains space to record the therapy used, details of the treatment given and any self-care advice. The patient's MYMOP problems, restricted activities and well-being score are all entered each time the patient is seen. We eventually added two additional fields on the treatment sheet where practitioners could add information about their impression and comments. We did this because we found that without this contextualizing information changes in MYMOP scores (or a lack of them) were sometimes impossible to interpret. (Chapters 4, 5, and 8 contain an example of various treatment screens and reports.) One example of a computer-generated report of the outcomes of a series of CT treatments using MYMOP scores is also given in Chapter 5.

The patient management system

The referral and data pathways

The dynamics of the CT service, including the pathways of GP to CP referral and the use of forms at each stage is summarized in a flow diagram. This is shown in Figure 3.3.

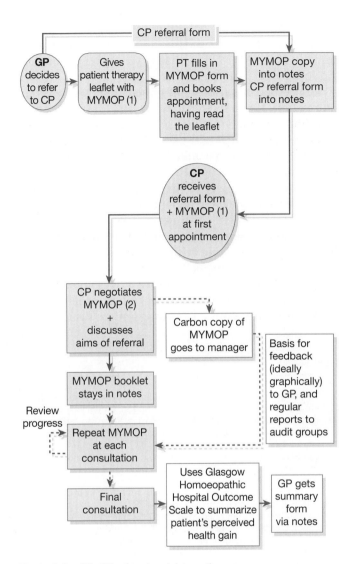

Figure 3.3 GP–CP referral and data pathways.

Informing patients

Our aim has been to put in place structures and processes to encourage evidence-based practice of CTs, to manage their delivery and evaluate their impact in practical ways. MYMOP asks patients to focus on a number of key symptoms or health problems whose improvement becomes the treatment objective. It asks them to gauge the subjective severity of these problems and the degree to which they interfere with aspects of daily life. In addition practitioners ask patients to estimate their 'level of well-being'. These are the sorts of question all practitioners ask and the only unusual aspect of MYMOP is that one links the questions to a figure between zero (no symptom, or no restriction in function or perfect well-being) and six (symptom, or restriction in function or well-being as bad as the patient could possibly imagine). We have found that in time this kind of systematic

106 DESIGNING AN INTEGRATED SERVICE

inquiry blends quite naturally into the consultation. However, at first one needs to inform the patient more formally about MYMOP perhaps even using the booklet and forms to explain the aim.

We also had to ensure that patients had the relevant information about their condition and the CT option, including information about what a particular CT consultation might entail and any side-effects. Patients also had to understand that initial consultations are always exploratory and that if CPs think they cannot help a patient then this will be explained and the patient referred back to the GP who will explore further options for treatment. Patients also needed to understand that they would be offered a maximum of six treatments and the importance of giving adequate notice of cancellation. By making all this explicit at the outset we hoped to improve the use of a scarce resource. It was intended that patients with inappropriate expectations, or suspicions, or with anxieties about CT treatment might decide not to

use the service—rather than fail to complete a programme of treatment or miss appointments without cancelling.

We therefore put in place a system for informing patients that would simultaneously fulfil the following aims:

1. outline possibilities for treatment
2. inform the patient about self-care options
3. explore patient preferences for treatment
4. provide an opportunity for the patient to discuss the therapies with the GP and the CP
5. provide written information on the therapies and on the evaluation process
6. inform patients about both what to expect from CT treatment and what it involves
7. inform patients about the MYMOP process
8. give information that improves efficiency of the service, e.g. days and times of CT clinics.

REFERENCES

1. Bonnet J 2000 Complementary medicine in primary care—what are the key issues? NHS Executive, London. January 2000
2. Patterson C 1999 Breaking the boundaries. Paper presented at NHS conference on CTs in primary care, University of Exeter, September 1999.
3. General Medical Services Committee 1996 Commissioning in a primary care led NHS: functions and principles. British Medical Association, London
4. Maxwell R 1992 Dimensions of quality revisited: from thought to action. Quality in Health Care 1: 171–177
5. Foundation for Integrated Medicine 1997 Integrated healthcare: a way forward for the next five years. FIM, London
6. Reith W 1996 Statement on a primary care led NHS. Royal College of General Practitioners, London
7. Pietroni C, Pietroni P (eds) 1996 Innovation in community care and primary health: the Marylebone experiment. Churchill Livingstone, New York
8. Chase D, Morrison S, Cohen J 2000 A complementary medicine project for the Marylebone primary care group; a millenium initiative. Marylebone PCG, London
9. Tonkin R D 1987 Role of research in the rapprochement between conventional medicine and complementary therapies: discussion paper. Journal of the Royal Society of Medicine 80:361–363
10. Luff D, Thomas K J 2000 Sustaining complementary therapy provision in primary care: lessons from existing services. Complementary Therapies in Medicine 8: 173–179
11. Peters D, Peacock W 1999 Integrating complementary therapies. Practice Nursing 9(14): 31–34
12. Gerard T J, Riddell J D 1988 Difficult patients: black holes and secrets. British Medical Journal 297: 530–532
13. Reilly D, Taylor M 1993 The evidence profile. In: Report of the RCCM Research Fellowship 1987–1990. Complementary Therapies in Medicine 1: 11–13
14. Fisher P, Ward A 1994 Complementary medicine in Europe. British Medical Journal 309: 107–110
15. Thomas K J, Carr J, Westlake L, Williams B T 1991 Use of non-orthodox and conventional health care in Great Britain. British Medical Journal 302: 207–210
16. Standen C 1993 The implications of the Osteopaths Act. Complementary Therapies in Medicine 1: 208–210
17. Reilly D, Taylor M 1993 Undergraduate medicine. In: Report of the RCCM Research Fellowship 1987–1990. Complementary Therapies in Medicine 1 (Suppl 1): 32–33
18. Lewith G 1988 Undifferentiated illness: some suggestions for approaching the polysymptomatic patient. Journal of the Royal Society of Medicine 81: 563–565
19. Patel C, Marmot M 1988 Can GPs use training in relaxation and management of stress to reduce mild hypertension? British Medical Journal 296: 21–24
20. Murray J, Sheperd S 1988 Alternative or additional medicine? A new dimension for doctors. Journal of the Royal College of General Practitioners 38: 511–514
21. Reason P, Chase H D, Desser A et al 1992 Towards a clinical framework for collaboration between general and complementary practitioners. Journal of the Royal Society of Medicine 85: 161–164
22. Reason P 1991 Power and conflict in multidisciplinary collaboration. Complementary Medicine Research 5: 144–150
23. Fromm E 1972 The anatomy of human destructiveness. Cape, London
24. Balint E, Courtenay M, Elder A et al 1993 The doctor, the patient and the group: Balint revisited. Routledge, London
25. Reilly D 2001 Enhancing human healing. British Medical Journal 322: 120–121
26. Hansard (HC) 1991: 585 Complementary therapies. (question put to Secretary of State for Health by Peter Rost). Written answer by Stephen Dorrell, 3 December 1991; press release by Department of Health, 3 December 1991
27. Fulder S 1988 Handbook of complementary medicine, 2nd edn. Oxford University Press, Oxford
28. Bolam v. Friern HMC [1957] 2 All ER 118
29. Scottish Office 1996 Complementary medicine and the National Health Service. An examination of acupuncture, homeopathy, chiropractic and osteopathy. Scottish Office Department of Health, London
30. Anderson E, Anderson P 1987 General practitioners and alternative medicine. Journal of the Royal College of General Practitioners 37: 52–55
31. Pietroni P 1992 Beyond the boundaries: the relationship between general practice and complementary medicine. British Medical Journal 305: 564–566

32. British Medical Association 1993 Complementary medicine: new approaches to good practice. Oxford University Press, Oxford
33. Calman C 1998 A review of Continuing Professional Development in General Practice. DOH, London
34. OECD 1996 Lifelong Learning for All. Background report. pp 25–85
35. Kolb D 1984 Experiential Learning: experiences as the source of learning and development. Englewood Cliffs, NJ: Prentice-Hall
36. Karim S 1999 Practice Professional Development plans: first steps. Update 9 September

37. Roland S, Baker R 1999 Clinical Governance, a practical guide for primary care teams. National Primary Care Research and Development Centre. University of Manchester
38. Wilson T 1998 Establishing educational needs in a new organisation. British Medial Journal Classified. Dec 19: 2–3
39. Gallen D. Personal Development Plan. Update London 2000
40. DoH 1999 Continuing professional development: quality in the new NHS. DoH, London
41. Pietroni C 1996 Innovations in primary care. Churchill Livingstone, New York

FURTHER READING

Key evaluation reports from NHS complementary medicine services:

Hills D, Welford R 1998 Complementary therapy in general practice: an evaluation of the Glastonbury Health Centre Complementary Medicine Service. Somerset Trust for Integrated Health Care, Glastonbury

Hotchkiss J 1995 Liverpool Centre for Health: the first year of a service offering complementary therapies on the NHS. Observatory report series no. 25. Liverpool Public Health Observatory, Liverpool

Richardson J 1995 Complementary therapy in the NHS: a service evaluation of the first year of an outpatient service in a local district general hospital. Report prepared by Health Services Research and Evaluation Unit. Lewisham Hospital NHS Trust, London

Scheurmier N, Breen A C 1998 A pilot study of the purchase of manipulation services for acute low back pain in the United Kingdom. Journal of Manipulative Physiology and Therapeutics 21: 14–18

Books

BMA 1993 Therapies and the medical profession. In: Complementary medicine: New approaches to good practice. Oxford University Press, Oxford, pp 37–59

BMA 1999 Referrals to complementary therapists: guidance for GPs. General Practitioners Committee, London

CISCOM: Research Council for Complementary Medicine database

Lewith G, Kenyon J, Lewis P 1996 Complementary therapies: an integrated approach. Oxford GP series. Oxford University Press, Oxford

Luff D, Thomas K 1999 Models of CT provision in primary care. Medical Care Research Unit, University of Sheffield

Mills S, Budd S 2000 Professional organisation of complementary and alternative medicine in the United Kingdom 2000. Centre for Complementary Health Studies. University of Exeter, Exeter

Royal London Homoeopathic Hospital Academic Unit 1999 The evidence base of complementary medicine. RLHH, London

Papers

Ernst E 1996 Regulating complementary medicine. Only 0.08% of funding for research in NHS goes to complementary medicine. British Medical Journal 313:882

Patterson C 1996 Measuring outcomes in primary care: a patient generated measure, MYMOP, compared to the SF36 health survey. British Medical Journal 312: 1016–1020

Peters D, Davies P, Pietroni P 1994 Musculo-skeletal clinic in general practice—a study of one year's referrals. British Journal of General Practice 44: 25–29

Peters D, Davies P Rapid audit cycles: an approach to introducing and evaluating a complementary therapy service into general practice, in press

Studdert D M, Eisenberg D M, Miller F H et al 1998 Medical malpractice implications of alternative medicine. Journal of the American Medical Association 280: 1610–1615

KEY INFORMATION SOURCES

General databases

CINAHL. Information on the CINAHL® database including journal coverage (currently 32 journals in the CAM field). Website: www.cinahl.com

CISCOM database. A specialist database of published research. Research Council for Complementary Medicine. Email: info@rccm.org.uk

Cochrane resources. The Cochrane Collaboration and the Cochrane Library include many published CAM trials and most systematic reviews. Website: www.cochrane.org

Medline. Includes most of the CT research published in peer reviewed journals on complementary medicine. Website: www.omni.ac.uk/medline/

TRIP. An amalgamation of 26 databases of hyperlinks from 'evidence based' sites around the world. Website: www.ceres.uwcm.ac.uk

Books and reports

Foundation for Integrated Medicine 1997 Integrated healthcare: a way forward for the next five years. Foundation for Integrated Medicine, London. Tel: 0207 633 1881; website: www.fimed.org

Mills S, Budd S 2000 Professional organisation of complementary and alternative medicine in the United Kingdom 2000. Centre for Complementary Health Studies. University of Exeter, Exeter Royal London Homeopathic Hospital Academic unit 1999 The evidence base of complementary medicine. RLHH, London

Zollman C, Vickers A 2000 ABC of complementary medicine. BMJ, London. The contents of this book are also available as articles on the bmj.com website

Journals and bulletins

Bandolier. Evidence-based medicine monthly reports, free within NHS. Pain Research, The Churchill, Headington, Oxford OX3 7LJ. Tel: 01865 226132; website: www.ebandolier.com

BMC Complementary and Alternative Medicine. Newly established online journal. Covers the evaluation of alternative and complementary health interventions. To receive updates on research, reviews and editorials published by BioMed Central, register at: http://www.biomedcentral.com/registration/

Complementary Therapies in Medicine. Aimed at GPs, nurses and allied health professionals; four issues per year. Journals Marketing Department, Harcourt Publishers Ltd, 32 Jamestown Road, London NW1 7BY. Tel: 020 8308 5790; website: www.harcourt-international.com/journals CompMed Bulletin. Evidence base of selected clinical topics; bimonthly. Church Farm Cottage, Weethley Hamlet, Evesham Rd, Alcester, Warwickshire B49 5NA. Tel: 01789 400295

Journal of Alternative and Complementary Medicine: Research on Paradigm, Practice and Policy. Reports on CAM treatments, case reports, and current concepts; six issues per year. Website: www.liebertpub.com

Websites
General
Alternative Medicine Foundation: www.amfoundation.org
Alternative medicine homepage: www.pitt.edu/-cbw/altm.html
British Medical Journal: www.bmj.com
Foundation for Integrated Medicine: www.fimed.org
Health A to Z. Conventional and complementary medicine site: www.healthatoz.com
Omni. A catalogue of sites covering health and medicine: omni.ac.uk
OneMedicine. A subscription site with information about CM and conventional treatments: www.onemedicine.com/alert/subscribe
Research Council for Complementary Medicine: www.rccm.org.uk

Search engines
MedHunt: www.hon.ch/MedHunt
Medical Matrix. Search on 'alternative medicine': www.medmatrix.org
Medical World Search. A very clever search engine, with multiple search words: www.mwsearch.com
PubMed. The US National Library of Medicine's search service, providing access to over 11 million citations in Medline, PreMedline and related databases: www.ncbi.nlm.nih.gov
SUMSearch. University of Texas search for evidence based information which splits results according to the source: sumsearch.uthscsa.edu

Academic
University of Exeter Centre for Complementary Health Studies: www.ex.ac.uk/chs
University of Exeter Department of Complementary Medicine: www.ex.ac.uk/pgms/comphome.htm
University of Maryland Complementary Medicine Program: www.compmed.ummc.umaryland.edu/
University of Maryland School of Medicine Cochrane Collaboration field on complementary medicine: www.compmed.ummc.umaryland.edu/compmed/cochrane/cochranefr.htm
University of Westminster. Degree programmes in CTs: www.westminster.ac.uk

For a sceptical view of complementary medicine
Quackwatch: www.quackwatch.com

US National Institutes of Health
Memorial Sloan-Kettering Cancer Center, New York, United States Integrative Medicine Service: www.mskcc.org/patients_n_public/patient_ care_services/outpatient_services_and_facilities/integrative_medicine_service/index.html

National Center for Complementary and Alternative Medicine: nccam.nih.gov

Websites on individual CTs
Acupuncture
Acupuncture Association of Chartered Physiotherapists: www.aacp.uk.com
Acupuncture.com. A broad TCM site: www.acupuncture.com
British Acupuncture Council: www.acupuncture.org.uk/
British Medical Acupuncture Society: www.medical-acupuncture.co.uk
International acupuncture associations: directory.google.com/Top/Health/Alternative/Acupuncture_and_Chinese_Medicine/Professional_Organizations/

Chiropractic
Cochrane Collaboration and the Cochrane Library: www.cochrane.org
General Chiropractic Council: www.gcc-uk.org
International chiropractic organizations: directory.google.com/Top/Health/Alternative/Chiropractic/Organizations_and_Associations/UK Chiropractic Website:www.chiropractic.org.uk

Herbal medicine
American Botanical Council: www.herbalgram.org/
Phytone: www.exeter.ac.uk/phytonet/

Homeopathy
Faculty of Homeopathy: www.trusthomeopathy.org
Homeopathic Trust: www.trusthomeopathy.org/
National Center for Homeopathy in the US: www.homeopathic.org/
Society of Homeopaths: www.homeopathy-soh.org

Hypnosis
British Society of Medical and Dental Hypnosis: www.bsmdh.org/
US Society for Clinical and Experimental Hypnosis: sunsite.utk.edu/ijceh/scehframe.htm

Massage
American Massage Therapy Association: www.amtamassage.org/
Aromatherapy Organisations Council: www.aromatherapy-uk.org

Osteopathy
General Osteopathic Council: www.osteopathy.org.uk
Osteopathic Information Service: www.osteopathy.org.uk/
US osteopathic medicine at the Student Doctor Network: osteopathic.com/

Chapter 3 REFLECTIVE LEARNING CYCLE AUDIT

1. **What did you need to know?** *(clarify learning objectives)*

2. **What did you notice?** *(key points)*

3. **What have you learned?** *(learning evaluation)*

4. **How will you apply it to practice?** *(clinical relevance)*

5. **What do I need to do next?** *(reflective educational audit)*

6. **Proceed to next area of interest / section you have identified**.

4

Delivering and evaluating the service

INTRODUCTION

Although an open access arrangement might be appropriate in a consumer-centred model of health care, UK convention makes GPs the gatekeepers to many NHS resources. In our centre GPs maintain this role for several reasons. First, any attempt to model a new kind of collaboration that could be applied elsewhere in the NHS would have been marginalized had we done otherwise. Secondly, in countries where GPs do not retain this role and patients freely refer themselves to specialists the overall cost of health care rises. Thirdly, without a generalist's overview the patient's care becomes fragmented. Finally, no matter how CTs are incorporated into the mainstream, the historical and positional power of doctors is likely to continue and this will have to be taken into account by CPs who enter the arena and by organizations that hope to encourage collaboration. To make the 'gatekeeper' task work in this situation any referral criteria and guidelines, while they should be based on the available range of evidence, also have to be established *collaboratively* and through *consensus*. Conflict and misunderstanding will be minimized if the primary team can achieve this.

Though teamwork is fraught with problems, it seems the only practical way to deliver integrated care on a large scale. The range of knowledge skills and attitudes needed goes so far beyond the purely biomedical that only multidisciplinary teams could provide the necessary depth and breadth. In the NHS, primary care teams already include medical, nursing and social work personnel, working together across the boundaries of their individual disciplines. How feasible is it then to bring CPs into these teams? Each therapy has different theories and therapeutics, which are in turn different from those of GPs. However, the similarities between their values, the challenges they face and their practical aims actually fit well into primary care. The overlap between their approaches is substantial—therapeutic methods notwithstanding. Primary care culture has a natural affinity with CAM; they are both, from their own perspective, 'holistic'. They are also committed to self-care, and both value and use the therapeutic relationship.

GPs and CPs, at their best, try to see how patients' conditions arise out of their individuality, the life they lead, their relationships and predicaments. Out of this psychosocial 'diagnosis' arise ideas for encouraging healthy adaptation, promoting recovery or limiting further organic, personal and social damage. Though counsellors, psychotherapists and behavioural therapists are the experts in this aspect of health and social care, GPs and CPs often have to suggest ways of changing diet or lifestyle or introducing stress management techniques. At the MHC we prepared a series of leaflets to help all practitioners to promote this primary care level of *psychosocial interventions*.

We also agreed that there is an appropriate level of CT prescribing that is absolutely appropriate for primary care: for instance, recommending simple homeopathic remedies, herbal medicines, or nutritional supplements. A 'practice formulary' approach linked to a series of common conditions is available for GP prescribing. We see this is as the primary care level of *biochemical interventions*.

Although most practitioners are familiar with both the prescribing and the advising roles, it is more unusual for a GP to suggest exercises and body-centred approaches. But we see this is as a primary care level of *biomechanical interventions*. Once again our emphasis has been on guidelines suggesting which interventions might be appropriate. We have encouraged GPs to try out this sort of self-help and invite patients to give feedback about this and the other GP primary CAM interventions using MYMOP forms and leaflets (see Ch. 8) to self-rate how the suggested interventions affect their condition.

The further integration of complementary therapy services—whether in general practice, community-based centres or in hospital settings—requires rigorous quality assurance. We have tried to develop the necessary structures (knowledge and skills, guidelines and data instruments), processes (feedback and learning loops) and outcomes (appropriate, sustainable primary care) for quality assurance of an NHS CT service, and to evaluate them through continuous learning cycles. Difficult, chronic and complex cases are commonly referred to CPs, so limits need to be set and, given the lack of experience in the area, unpredictable, potentially expensive and inappropriate patterns of referral to CT services can always be expected. Therefore, when developing CT services it is essential for coworkers to take into account local need, to optimize patient self-help, to explore stakeholder expectations, and to develop evidence-linked guidelines and the clinical audit processes needed to keep them on track. In this chapter we look at how the integrated provision of

CTs within primary care works out in practice. It is based largely on our experience at the MHC, but uses also the experience of other centres where the processes of service delivery and evaluation are being explored.

THE SERVICE DELIVERY PROCESS

The bullet-point lists in this section indicate the standards that we aim to reach at each stage of the delivery process. We offer them as examples for colleagues to consider when setting their own.

The consultation and referral procedure

The patient and the GP—the first consultation

The possibility of offering CT begins when patients present with a condition on the 'conditions suitable for referral' list. CT should be considered particularly where:

- conventional treatment appears to have been unsatisfactory
- there is a new diagnosis of a condition where, according to guidelines, CTs have something to contribute to treatment
- unacceptable side-effects of conventional treatment have been experienced
- patients have specifically asked about what else they can do to help themselves
- they show a particular interest in the potential part CTs might play in their treatment (and their problem lies within the boundaries of our guidelines).

The GP begins by consulting the guideline cards for guidance on appropriate self-care options in this particular condition. (Examples of guideline cards used at the MHC can be found in Ch. 6.) This would be followed by a discussion with the patient on the feasibility of trying options for self-help. If there is agreement the patient leaves the first consultation with the appropriate self-help leaflets.

Assisting the patient to make the most use of these leaflets is helped by:

- giving patients a lot of information at the time of the consultation
- making the giving of the leaflets a central part of the consultation
- where possible demonstrating any exercises suggested
- (usually) by arranging for a follow-up appointment—especially where the self-help suggested is complex.

Sending to classes

Many of the issues considered above in relation to the use of self-care materials obviously apply to recommending patients to self-care classes. Whilst some may not wish to have their symptoms 'demedicalized', there is the possibility to link lifestyle and health, and the challenge to make a difference through regular commitment rather than 'a quick fix'.

There are issues about ensuring the standard and usefulness of classes, and also the cost of provision has to be considered; in some areas, local authorities provide a wide range of options (e.g. yoga, tai chi or stress management). Linked with quality is also the challenge of maintaining provision.

The group situation may provide support from members who share similar symptoms but, conversely may produce social unease in some patients; indeed, some will not tolerate this type of setting. Appropriate selection of patients for particular classes or approaches is essential, and this demands particular GP knowledge.

It is vital that groups seek regular and detailed evaluation from members, and are professionally quality assured.

Follow-up (possibly split into two sessions)

The GP begins by asking about the patient's experience of using the self-care advice. If the patient has persevered with this advice and any conventional care but still needs some help, the GP discusses the possibility of CT with the patient and assesses which therapy might suit the person best, using the following procedure. The GP:

- checks the *guideline* card for that condition for guidance on CTs that might be appropriate
- considers any possible *contraindications* and *side-effects* for each therapy (see Box 4.1)
- outlines any CTs that might be *appropriate* for treatment

Box 4.1   CT contraindications and side-effects

Contraindications

Acupuncture:
- anyone who absolutely hates needles
- anyone on any form of steroid medication
- people taking anticoagulants will bruise very badly
- patients will also be asked not to drink alcohol on the day of treatment
- deep needling is contraindicated in patients with bleeding disorders or taking anticoagulant drugs
- although systemic infection is very uncommon, acupuncture should probably be avoided in patients with valvular heart defects

Herbalism:
- if patients are taking conventional drugs, herbal preparations should be used with extreme caution and only on the advice of a herbalist familiar with the pharmacology

Homeopathy:
- people with poor spoken English
- psychotic/borderline patients
- those who lack motivation

Naturopathy:
- lack of motivation to change diet/lifestyle
- poor locus of control

Osteopathy:
- reluctance to undress
- acute inflammatory disease (e.g. RA)

Exercise:
- sequential muscle relaxation and abdominal tensing in people with poorly controlled cardiovascular disease

Massage:
- patients diagnosed with somatization disorder
- patients who are psychotic
- doctor or practitioner experiences incomprehensible discomfort in the presence of the patient
- in patients with burns, deep-vein thrombosis, or serious or life-threatening illness such as cancer, or after myocardial infarction, techniques using brisk rubbing, deep pressure, kneading or other overstimulating techniques are inadvisable

(however, there is no evidence that gentle massage puts an undue strain on the heart, or increases metastatic spread in cancer cases, even though this is often cited as a contraindication, although it is obviously inadvisable to direct firm pressure over sites of active spread)
- since specific oils are thought to be abortive, emmenagogic or uterotonic and contraindicated in particular stages of pregnancy, aromatherapy should be used with great care in these circumstances

Nutritional therapy:
- high dosages of vitamin E are contraindicated in people with hypertension, rheumatic heart disease or ischaemic heart disease
- children, pregnant and lactating women, and patients with chronic illness should undertake major dietary changes only under professional supervision

Side-effects

Acupuncture:
- local bruising around site of needle
- tiredness after treatment, especially the first treatment—can feel light-headed
- indwelling 'press' needles, commonly used in treating addiction, should be used with care as they have been associated with infections such as perichondritis

Homeopathy:
- sometimes symptoms can get worse before they get better; steroid medication in certain circumstances

Naturopathy:
- healing crisis: feeling ill as healing/detoxifying processes take place

Osteopathy:
- stiff, sore reaction after treatment sometimes; rarely requires mild pain killers (fades after 24–48 hours); discuss if more than minor and transient

Massage:
- deep relaxation is an unfamiliar feeling for some people, and may occasionally be accompanied by uncomfortable thoughts and feelings—if so discuss it with the therapist or GP involved

- ascertains whether the patient is *interested* in trying CTs generally for this condition
- asks whether patient has a *preference* for any of the CTs indicated as being of potential benefit
- checks the patient's current *understanding* of the therapies, and if appropriate gives the patient one or more therapy leaflets (which includes information on the evaluation process and what to expect from treatment)
- checks that the patient has all the information necessary to make a *decision* whether to have CT treatment
- explains to the patient what coming for CT treatment would *entail*, and what to expect (for instance, the days that the patient would be expected to attend for treatment)
- explains the *evaluation* process, and if the patient is to proceed with this fills in the first MYMOP together with the patient
- informs the patient that the first consultation with the CP is always *exploratory*, and that if the CP feels that the therapy is unlikely to be helpful then the patient will be referred back to the GP.

The MYMOP process

At this point the patient may have already made the choice to opt for CT treatment. If so the GP explains the MYMOP form to the patient together with the guide to using it (copies of these can be found in Ch. 8). It is well worth spending time at this stage to discuss the MYMOP, as how it is introduced sets the tone for its use over the entire course of treatment. It is also worth emphasizing its value to both the practitioner and the patient, as well as its wider use as a means of evaluation to the practice and by extension to other patients. The GP may need to help the patient with the initial MYMOP—for instance in negotiating the problems to enter, and asking specifically for any questions or comments. It should be pointed out that:

- patients can pick whatever symptom is most important to them
- they don't have to use medical terms
- they will normally be asked to fill the form out before the session, but it can be used within the consultation for discussion
- it takes less than a minute to fill in once they understand the MYMOP
- they don't have to fill in everything (for instance, if they have only one problem)
- their confidentiality will be maintained throughout the CT referral process
- they will be able to use MYMOP to keep a record of their progress if they so wish

- there are no right or wrong answers and they are not being tested.

This initial MYMOP has three objectives. First, it helps generate the patient's appointment. Secondly, it gives the CP a clear idea of the patient's main concerns. Finally, it gives a measure of the severity of symptoms and sense of well-being at the time of referral, by the GP.

After the consultation, the patient takes the completed MYMOP form to the reception and makes an appointment with the CP. Only when the MYMOP form is filled in can an appointment be made. This part of the process was designed to engage the patient fully in the choice of coming for CT treatment and was intended to help minimize the rate of non-attendance.

Referral to a CT practitioner

Whenever a GP refers a patient to a colleague, there is some loss of therapeutic relationship. It may be possible to maintain an 'integrated care' pathway but this is often difficult. The possibility for the patient to 'split' the two practitioners into 'good' and 'bad' therapist is also created. Although the GP is likely to remain as 'key worker' it is essential that a relationship of trust exists between the two colleagues. This is no mean achievement, especially in an environment of restricted resources, and the interprofessional dynamics demand much attention.

Within a primary care setting, a referral to a CP may be either 'primary' or 'secondary'. Although clear criteria will have been agreed for patient referral, it will in some cases be strongly influenced by what the GP knows of the CP, rather than the therapy.

Reasons for referral will tend to have a local bias, depending on the skills, attitudes and knowledge in any one environment. Main categories include:

- assessment of condition
- treatment of symptoms
- relief for clinician
- patient support
- clarification of diagnosis
- patient request.

Experience has revealed that 'complex' or 'heartsink' patients figure highly in referred groups (see discussion in Ch. 5, p 166–170), and here clinicians need to be especially careful about specific reasons for referral.

At the MHC the GP–CP referral process is an attempt to make patient-led treatment available within the resources and structural limitations of public sector medicine. It accepts, however, that this movement towards patient-centred care may well demand a higher degree of commitment on the part of the patient, and that this should be understood at the beginning. It sometimes has had to be explained to patients that not every condition, nor every patient, will be suitable for referral to CT. At the MHC the CT referral process cannot be simply on demand, but, having said this, general principles for the referral process to CT have been developed; the process can be depicted in the form of a flow diagram. Figure 4.1 summarizes the sequence and aims of consultation and referral in the MHC project.

Consultation with the CP

At the initial consultation the CP has received the patient file (or has on-screen access to the patient notes and the GP referral form) containing the referral form and the patient's initial MYMOP. (The CP protocol is illustrated in Figure 3.3.)

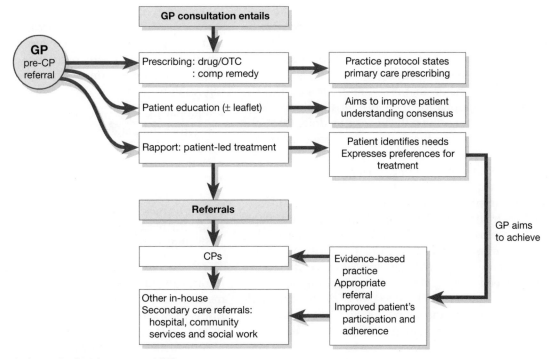

Figure 4.1A   The consultation and referral process at MHC.

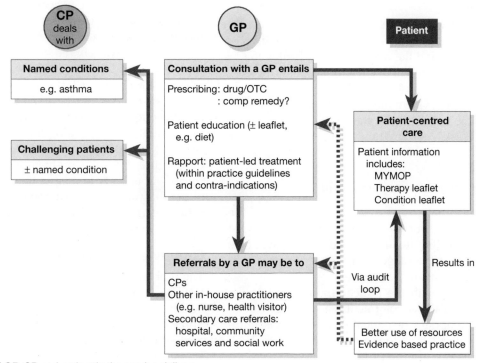

Figure 4.1B   The roles of GP, CP and patient in the service delivery.

The CP first checks that the patient understands the basic idea of the particular therapy chosen, also what the treatment will involve—and what is required of the patient during the course of treatment. Next, the CP assesses (through history taking and examination) the presenting problems and either decides the referral is appropriate or, if not, explains why the treatment approach will probably not be suitable. If the CP decides not to treat the patient the reasons are written in the notes (or on the screen) and placed in the GP's pigeonhole to alert the GP to the need for a brief CP–GP discussion. The patient is then asked to make an appointment with the GP to discuss other options.

Apart from a decision that it is inappropriate to treat, there are other reasons for the CP referring the patient back to, or contacting, the GP. This can be done through the patient notes, using the in-house pigeonholes, or on screen (or by in-house email or phone if contact is required quickly). For example, during the course of the initial (or subsequent) consultations a patient may develop signs or symptoms requiring immediate further investigation or treatment. These are known as 'red flag' criteria for medical opinion. They are listed in Box 4.2.[1]

If, however (as happens in the great majority of cases), the patient and the practitioner jointly agree that they want to proceed with treatment then, once it is clear that the patient has understood the MYMOP process, the CP answers any detailed questions on the therapy and the treatment planned. If the patient decides to proceed with CT treatment:

- then the CP completes the MYMOP with the patient
- treats the patient
- updates the MYMOP graph (if using a paper system) to show the symptoms of patient seen at the point when the GP referred the patient to the CP, plus the MYMOP scores at the initial CP appointment (they commonly differ)
- if using the paper system the MYMOP copy-form can be given to the patient at the start of the next session, when the CP asks 'has anything changed since we last met?'.

The course of complementary treatment

We provide an initial course of six appointments at the MHC. So, by session four, the CP should have a clear idea of the effects of the treatment and might want to approach the GP at this stage about future treatment or follow-up if this seems to be indicated.

The CP together with the patient should update the MYMOP graph at each appointment. The computer database, if used, can update the patient's MYMOP table automatically and will create various report formats (see Ch. 5). MYMOP graphs can also be produced between sessions 3 and 5 and given to patients. This allows them to see the

results, to check the validity of their experience against the graph, and to validate their participation.

Discharging the patient: closing the loop

When the previously agreed course of treatment is complete the CP needs to discharge the patient back to the referring GP by completing a discharge summary form. (Note: the computer database can produce a clinical summary of the treatment series and related MYMOPs that incorporates a discharge summary. It is possible to email this report directly on to the referring practitioner.)

The discharge summary should include the following information:

- whether the patient's problem(s) improved
- whether the patient persisted with the treatment
- the number of DNAs
- post-treatment arrangements/management plan
- outcomes of the treatment
- CP evaluation
- long-term self-care advice given to patients
- any further options for management or significant findings that need to be passed on.

The discharge summary should be attached to the patient file and an entry made in the 'comments' box on the treatment sheet. If CP feels the door should be left open (e.g. if it is long term/chronic) then this needs to be communicated in the discharge summary.

A distinction has to be made between the treatment of acute conditions, and more persistent problems where management must rely heavily on patients' committed use of self-care programmes. However, some patients do receive more than six treatments—and although this choice is not always based on clear criteria, whoever initiates further treatment (or, rarely, who declines to offer it)— whether the CP or the GP—will need to communicate the reason for the request. To avoid raising expectations, CPs also have to be very clear when discussing with patients the possibility of extending the treatment course. When a second course of treatment is given, the GP needs a report on progress. And if a problem has been helped by a CT course but is likely to relapse then the CP should communicate this (to both patient and GP) and make it clear that future referral by the GP (for more CT) might be an option. Here too expectations may have to be carefully managed.

Quality assurance (QA) for CT services

The problem of defining a 'quality service' is not peculiar to CTs. There are various ways of defining 'quality' in health care delivery: 'clinical effectiveness'; Maxwell's 'three As and three Es' (acceptability, appropriateness, accessibility, effectiveness, efficiency and equity);[2] or Donabedian's quality assurance (QA) model of structures, processes and outcomes. The notion of 'cost effectiveness'

Box 4.2 'Red flag' criteria for referring a patient for medical opinion

Pain:
— any pain that is persistent, particularly if severe, or in the head, abdomen, or central chest.
* pain in the eye or temples, with local tenderness, in the elderly, rheumatic patient
— pain on passing urine, in a man
— cystitis recurring more than three times in a woman
— absence of pain in ulcers, fissures, etc.
* sciatic pain, if associated with objective neurological deficit

Bleeding:
— blood in sputum, vomit, urine or stools
* vomit containing 'coffee grounds'
* black, tarry stools
— non-menstrual vaginal bleeding (intermenstrual, postmenopausal, or at any time in pregnancy)
* vaginal bleeding with pain, in pregnancy, or after 'missed one period'

Persistent:
— vomiting &/or diarrhoea
* vomiting &/or diarrhoea in infant
— thirst
— increase in passing urine
— cough
— unexplained loss of weight (1 lb/wk or more)

Sudden:
* breathlessness
* swelling of face, lips, tongue or throat
* blueness of the lips
* loss of consciousness
* loss of vision
* convulsions
— unexplained behavioural change

Difficulty:
— swallowing
— breathing

Change:
— in bowel habit
— in a skin lesion (size, shape, colour, bleeding, itching, pain)

In cases of fever:
* over 106°F (41.1°C)
* patient less than 4 months old
* level of consciousness affected
* fits or convulsions
* neck becomes stiff
* breathing becomes very rapid or laboured
* intuition says the patient is 'very sick'
— fever unresponsive and persists over 104°F (40°C)
— persists 24 hours in patient 4–24 months old

In cases of headache:
* level of consciousness affected
* any severe, unexplained headache
* if neck stiffness &/or high fever &/or photophobia
* following head injury, especially if drowsy or vomiting
— if continues without signs of improvement for some days, even if mild
— if any other neurological symptoms (e.g. disturbed speech, sensation or vision, dizziness, weakness, etc.)

Psychological:
— deep depression, with suicidal ideas
— hearing voices
— delusional beliefs

— incongruous behaviour

In cases of eye problems:
* any deterioration/loss of vision
* severe pain
* damage by foreign body or chemical
— thick green or yellow discharge
— pain persists
— photophobia esp. if circumcorneal redness or loss of light reaction
— if any skin rash or infection near eye

In cases of ear problems:
* drowsiness, lethargy, severe headache, neck stiffness
— if baby persistently pulls or rubs an ear
— severe pain
— if also has measles
— any discharge from ear
— mastoid becomes tender or red
— hearing significantly/persistently impaired

In cases with throat problems:
* if swelling causes difficulty breathing
* if severe pain causes dysphagia/drooling
* in measles, if bleeding from the mouth
— if unusual/very marked swelling around tonsil(s)
— persistent severe sore throat in small child
— if past history of rheumatic fever

In cases of cough:
* with severe dyspnoea
* if confused or drowsy
* if marked chest pain
* if wheezing stops, but dyspnoea continues
* if something solid has been inhaled
* if cyanosed
— if cough persists a week and pt is weak
— if breathing laboured or very rapid
— if wheezing occurs
— in measles, if cough persists 4+ days without improvement

In cases with abdominal problems:
* if significant signs of dehydration, esp. in baby, e.g.:
  sunken eyes
  sunken fontanelle in baby
  dryness of mouth or eyes
  loss of skin turgor
  oliguria, concentrated
* persistent vomiting
* blood or 'coffee grounds' in vomit
* stool bloody or tar-like, esp. in measles
* if following injury to abdomen or head
* if abdominal pain severe
* if child persistently vomiting, inconsolably screaming or lethargic
* if any suspicion of drugs or poisons having been taken
— swelling, pain or tenderness in groin, scrotum or inner/upper thigh
— constipation plus pain &/or vomiting for 24+ hours
— if diabetic
— if pregnant
— if jaundiced, or dark urine/pale stools
— urinary symptoms accompanied by low back/loin pain

Others:
— pallor
— unexplained swelling or lumps
* neck stiffness in a patient with a fever
— unexplained fever, particularly if persistent or recurrent.

Adapted from How to use homeopathy effectively by Dr Chris Hammond. Those marked (*) usually require urgent referral.

also needs to be unpacked: the concepts of healthcare need and health gain are complex, and particularly so in the area of CTs. Defining and developing an appropriate quality service is more difficult here because:

- there is a scarcity of high-quality studies (defined as RCTs) to guide service development
- there is a lack of good pragmatic evidence demonstrating CAM's cost effectiveness in 'real-world' situations
- there are special problems of QA in CT, concerned with practitioner skills, non-standardized treatments, working context and appropriate evaluation methods.

The current emphasis on evidence-based effectiveness as the key determinant for commissioning is problematic, and the reorganization of the NHS may pose threats to existing CT provision if the 'lack of evidence' argument prevails. Indeed, at the time of writing, access to CTs at primary care level has declined significantly as the new PCGs struggle to find their feet. As these organizations develop and stabilize, all primary care commissioning will require new tools and processes for decision making. Commissioning of all health care services will be targeted to meet identified local needs through the local health improvement plan (HImP). The 'care pathways' designed to meet these needs could, in theory at least, include aspects of CAM and they could to a degree be the basis for national standards of care. The delivery of the care pathways will be implemented through 'long-term service agreements'. As this process unfolds, the case supporting the role and relevance of CAM, particularly as a care option in national priority conditions (cancer, cardiovascular disease, diabetes and mental health), will need to be carefully explored. Practical steps towards the cost-effective use of CAM include: building on existing experience of good practice, piloting commissioning methods in selected primary care groups, developing patient-centred needs identification and patient-centred outcome measures, producing clinical guidelines based on best available evidence and consensus, and ring fencing funds for key units with the potential for research into this complex area of service delivery. The main opportunity will probably arise in primary care organizations (PCOs) where there is strong support at the highest level for this kind of innovation. It will depend on a few PCO Chairs and Chief Executives who have the enthusiasm and commitment required and their ability to gain the necessary support to include CAM options and to back their initiative with the necessary funds. In all probability, creative use of the PCO's primary care investment plan will be the key that unlocks the complex professional, practice and service development needed to move integration forward. Fortunately attempts to integrate CAM appropriately fit well into the programme of 'quality improvement', which is a central component of the government's NHS 'modernization'

project. Widely known as 'clinical governance', its components are already familiar to primary healthcare workers, and they will increasingly involve all clinical and administrative members of an integrated primary healthcare team as well as patients. They include:

- accountability (practitioner and practice)
- responsibility (individual and corporate)
- continuing professional development
- clinical audit
- teamwork and communication
- partnership with patients and carers
- management policies
- risk management
- performance monitoring.

Some of these processes, such as professional development, teamwork, communication and responsibility, were discussed in the last chapter. In the following sections we will look specifically at aspects of the clinical governance process dealing with audit, performance monitoring and economic evaluation.

Maxwell's six criteria for service quality form a basis around which integration processes in general practice can be structured. Different questions arise in connection with each of the criteria. Those concerned with acceptability, appropriateness and accessibility relate largely to issues of unmet needs, the evidence base and service design, discussed in the earlier chapters. Under the heading of effectiveness, efficiency and equity the following questions would occur:

- Does access to a range of CTs improve clinical outcomes in the patients and conditions treated?
- Does access to a range of CTs improve the practice's use of resources, to produce individual or population health gain?
- Is a range of CTs accessible to all those who might benefit?

To answer the first question, on delivering the service, appropriate research methods could include action research on structures put in place and processes of referral and treatment, asking what patients say about the process, and reflection on reports of clinical activity. Monitoring of service outcomes could include analysis of resource use—for instance, GP time, prescribing costs, referrals out, plus epidemiological studies and comparative trials. To decide whether the service needs modifying, review of access criteria and outcomes has to be undertaken regularly. This process is summarized in Table 4.1.

The principles of action research are a valuable way to structure the process of monitoring and evaluating CT services. A group would need to formulate a pertinent question such as 'how can we develop clinical quality assurance?', 'how do we organize a risk management strat-

Table 4.1 Using Maxwell's criteria for service quality

Maxwell criteria	The questions	The methods
Acceptability	• Which conditions are poorly managed by conventional methods? • Are there categories of patient who find CTs particularly acceptable?	*Practice review* • What do doctors say they need? • Have they used CTs previously? • How? • What do other practitioners need? • What do patients think?
Appropriateness	• What evidence is there for using a range of CTs in these conditions and categories of patient?	*Assessing the evidence* • Review various evidence bases (see resource section) • What do CPs and GPs believe works? • What is their experience? • What do patients say?
Accessibility	• How could access to potentially effective complementary therapies be organized?	*Designing the service* • Which therapies to include? • Selecting coworkers • Structured collection of data: referrals, treatment and outcomes
Effectiveness	• Does access to a range of CTs improve clinical outcomes in the patients and conditions treated?	*Delivering the service* • Action research on structures put in place and processes of referral and treatment • What do patients say about the process? • Reflection on reports of clinical activity
Efficiency	• Does access to a range of CTs improve the practice's use of resources, to produce individual or population health gain?	*Monitoring service outcomes* • Analysis of resource use: GP time, prescribing costs, referrals out • (Plus epidemiological studies and comparative trials would be needed)
Equity	• Is a range of CTs accessible to all those who might benefit?	*Modifying the service* • Review access criteria and outcomes • Adapting service and intake

egy?', 'how can we collect reliable data about our work?' or 'what do we need for better clinical governance?'. Once the priority aims are clear, an action research group can try out different approaches and, providing it can assess and reflect on the outcomes of changes brought in, it will begin to learn and develop until the goals are achieved.

Table 4.2 summarizes the principles of this process here.

Cost effectiveness

A key issue in delivering CTs is whether they can reduce the cost or improve the quality of healthcare. There are six linked problems around evaluating CAM cost effectiveness:

• conditions treated are often chronic or relapsing
• treatment is unlikely to be standardized
• outcomes are often difficult to quantify
• CAM effectiveness depends on practitioner's knowledge and skill
• cost-effective CAM in the NHS will depend on how well it is integrated into organizations
• the quality of a service is multidimensional, and depends on its accessibility, acceptability,

appropriateness, equality, effectiveness and efficiency.

Components of cost and quality can be summarized as in Figure 4.2.

An essential baseline consideration is whether CTs are going to be an *additional* expense or whether they can *substitute* for current spending. Patients are spending their own money on CTs, and currently this brings additional money into healthcare, on top of NHS expenditure. The figure for private spending on CTs could be in the region of £1 billion, compared with an overall NHS expenditure of £40 billion.

One major problem is how to evaluate the benefits of CTs. Whereas reductions in drug costs, referral rates, revisits to the GP and adverse events can be costed, many of the benefits that CTs are commonly declared to produce are intangible and cannot be easily measured. The latter include patient preference, patient empowerment, the process of the consultation, lifestyle changes with delayed health benefits, quality of life including improved stress management, the value of having other options for help available when orthodox treatments have failed, and the preventive aspects of the therapies themselves.

Table 4.2   Developing clinical quality assurance

Question	Aim	Method	Processes	Outcome needed	Benefits
Why develop clinical quality assurance?	to establish quality standards: 1. structures/resources needed 2. processes to be enacted 3. outcomes wanted 4. review and tracking procedures	1. clinicians' meetings 2. agree issues 3. achieve consensus on best practice	1. clinical audit 2. action research	documented standards for practice and evaluation	transparent documented standards, accountability, clear management
Why have a risk management strategy?	establish: 1. safety procedures 2. competencies 3. clinical red flags 4. critical incident procedures	1. clinicians' meetings 2. agree issues 3. achieve consensus on best practice	develop documented procedures for guidelines, review reporting and action	1. patient safety 2. practitioner remediation 3. organizational accountability	transparent documented standards, accountability, clear management procedures
Why collect data about our work?	collect minimum data set: 1. demographics 2. clinical data 3. outcome measures	1. networked computers 2. relational database 3. common data set	facilitate clinical audit by reflection on intake, treatment and outcomes	1. learning organization 2. interprofessional learning 3. add value to joint working	reflective practice, clarity and quality assurance
What do I need for clinical governance?	1. documented intake criteria 2. evidence base 3. treatment protocols 4. evaluation cycles 5. learning cycles	develop above structures, processes and outcomes	1. consensus on standards 2. data collection 3. learning loops	ensure clinical services are: 1. needs led 2. evidence based 3. quality assured	ensure that CT services are: acceptable, equitable, accessible, effective, appropriate, efficient

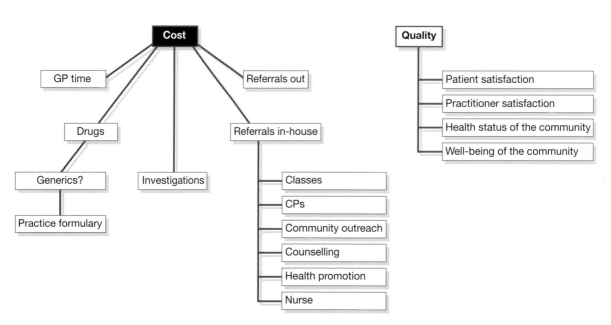

Figure 4.2   Effectiveness and efficiency: what can be improved acceptably? The central issue is whether the integration of CT into mainstream healthcare can be shown either to increase the overall effectiveness of treatment or to decrease its cost. A parallel issue is whether integration improves patients' quality of life or health status. An additional possibility is that an integrated service may increase levels of patient satisfaction or make working in a healthcare team more satisfying. In each of these cases, there is potential cost-benefit. (Classes include relaxation, yoga, breathing; the MHC 'practice formulary' includes a range of OTC products including homeopathic remedies, herbals and nutritional supplements as well as a range of self-help leaflets on diet, exercise and stress management; CPs = complementary practitioners.)

EXAMPLES OF INTEGRATED DELIVERY IN PRACTICE 121

At the end of this chapter we summarize findings from studies that have been done so far on economic evaluation of CTs.

EXAMPLES OF INTEGRATED DELIVERY IN PRACTICE

Marylebone Health Centre delivery

The patient management file

We chose to structure our CT service around condition-based guidelines. Producing guidelines is relatively easy compared with the difficulties inherent in putting them to work. Moreover, at the MHC we had added further challenges such as a more rigorous approach to tracking referrals and assessing everyday treatment outcomes, and implementing a programme of patient information and unfamiliar approaches to data management. Nor, in the days before the Smith Project, which allowed us to initiate these changes, had it been easy to understand the way different healthcare 'tribes' interact with one another. Yet by the early 1990s there was some grounding for a shared sense that, in the name of good management, transparency and quality of service, all these aspects of our integration project had to be addressed simultaneously!

To help all practitioners run the project on a day-to-day basis a file of basic information was kept in each clinic room. It contained:

- the list of guidelines on conditions to be referred (Box 4.3)
- a series of reminder cards about each condition
- guides to:
  — the process of referral
  — the use of MYMOP
  — the use of the computer within the CP consultation
- reference copies of:
  — the referral form
  — the MYMOP form
- therapy leaflets for patients.

(Examples of information sheets, MYMOP guides and forms, and service delivery forms are included in Ch. 6–8). The file also contained information on the contraindications to treatment and possible side-effects of each CT (see Box 4.1, p. 113), to be discussed with the patient at the time of referral to a CP.

The MHC CT referral, treatment tracking and outcomes computer database system

The system is built on a FileMaker Pro application package. We chose this widely available software as it can be used on both PCs and Macs.

Box 4.3 MHC complementary therapy guidelines for chosen conditions

Criteria we used for deciding on guideline development:
- conditions where some research-derived evidence of effectiveness exists
- conditions GPs stated they would want to refer
- conditions GPs had referred to CPs previously
- conditions where CPs declare effectiveness or a strong interest in treating
- therapies available in MHC.

Conditions considered for complementary therapy:
(pilot only: possible order of relevance)

	A	B	C	+'self-care'
asthma	acu	hom	nutri	SM
IBS, non-specific dyspepsia	nutri	acu		SM/diet
migraine	acu	hom	ost	SM/diet
eczema, rhinitis and hay fever	nutri	hom		SM/diet
musculoskeletal pain including:				
back and neck pain (acute)	ost	acu	mass	exercise
back and neck pain (chronic)	acu	ost		SM/ exercise
osteoarthritis	acu	ost	mass	exercise
rheumatoid arthritis	nutri	acu	hom	SM
myofascial pain	acu	ost		SM/ exercise
FMG syndrome	acu	ost		SM/yoga
menstrual and perimenopausal problems	hom	acu	nutri	SM/diet?
complex chronic illness including:				
chronic inflammatory diseases	nutri	hom		
persistent pain	acu	mass		SM
persistent fatigue	hom	mass	nutri	SM
stress-related and transient situational conditions (e.g. bereavement, anxiety, pain, insomnia)	mass			SM

Consider the complementary therapy option if:
- new diagnosis of above conditions
- conventional treatment of above conditions proving unsatisfactory
- side-effects of conventional treatment of above conditions
- patient request for non-conventional treatment of above conditions
- advice on a complex case (Dear CP, might your therapy help?).

When the system is used by GPs and CPs on a computer network, the entire system is password protected to maintain security and confidentiality. The GP's referral entry screen creates a CP case note. The CP finds this using a simple search programme and can return to these underlying case details each time the patient is seen. Whenever the patient consults the CP, a new treatment record is triggered at the touch of a button and here CPs can enter treatment details, self-care advice, MYMOP data and a variety of comments either for their own use or for GPs' attention.

GPs can access these notes any time through the network, just as if they were looking through a paper patient file. If rapid contact with the CP is needed then a note can be emailed directly from the system. The great advantage of a computer record over paper systems is the database's ability to generate a number of standard reports analysing case loads and outcomes (see Ch. 5, p 153–156). The second advantage is speed of entry, since the screens use multiple drop-down menus that can be clicked on to fill in the various field. The third is consistency, because the system actively reminds clinicians to enter a minimum data set, thereby increasing the chance of gathering complete data about a consultation episode and its outcomes. Also, because information is entered from drop-down lists, consistency in sorting and reporting is enhanced.

Figure 4.3 gives some examples of the computer screens available.

Using a patient-centred outcome measure

We chose MYMOP as our evaluation tool because it is a reliable within-patient measure that puts the patient at the centre of the evaluation and is simple to administer. Our early research with patients suggested that it did not seem to detract from the quality of the consultation. However, the CPs found themselves on a steep learning curve when they began to use it consistently with patients during clinic sessions. Changing habitual working practice is difficult. Introducing the use of MYMOP was the biggest change to the consultation that the CPs were asked to make, even more so than the introduction of the computerized data collection system.

The questions they raised included:

- How can I best introduce MYMOP into the consultation?
- What will be the consequences if I forget?
- Will it alter my relationship with the patient?
- Will I have enough time?
- Will the patient find it acceptable?
- How might using MYMOP affect working with the patient over time?

When the MYMOP process was in regular use similar concerns to those of the patients emerged. During one massage session, for example, the practitioner was left with the dilemma of scoring the level of pain where the right side was better and the left side was worse! When difficulties arose the team spent time in the CP meetings and CP/GP meetings discussing how to optimize use of MYMOP with patients.

Our experience of using MYMOP as an evaluation tool can be summarized as follows.

- When choosing what to enter in the space 'Does this symptom stop you doing anything?' (e.g. my back pain stops me sitting comfortably) it is preferable if the patient picks something that is quantifiable. (We call this the 'tracking symptom'.)
  - The question 'How do you think you would tell whether you were getting better?' may help with this discussion.
  - The problem needs to be something *not* directly affected by external circumstances (e.g. if breast feeding a baby were affecting the quality of sleep then 'better sleep' would not be an appropriate indicator).
- Patients may need some assistance on the first session with their notion of 'as bad as it could be' to be able to establish the first score.
- Naming a condition that has multiple symptoms (e.g. migraine or IBS) will not be specific enough. Pain/vomiting/duration of pain/frequency of attacks will prove easier for the patient to score.
- Avoid if possible all-or-nothing problems (e.g. fertility).
- How do you score problems when a condition changes throughout the interval between treatment?
  - For example, in homeopathy syndrome shifts are expected as old symptoms recur or as deep-seated health problems are replaced by more superficial symptoms. The homeopath decided to enter and score baseline tracker symptoms according to what the patient says initially and then put a comment in MYMOP notes as symptoms change. However, if the agreed tracking symptom score has changed then this should also be noted.
  - For change after treatment that doesn't hold—put a comment in the Notes box. If this seems to be a regular occurrence you can create two MYMOP fields for the same problem: (1) ask for an estimated score for the period soon after last treatment; (2) have another score for the symptom at today's treatment
- Emotional states are hard for the patient to put a value to. Symptoms associated with 'stress' or 'anxiety' are easier to gauge—for instance, dry mouth, lump in throat, palpitations, stomach churning, mind racing, etc.

Use of the recording system

Some examples of the use of the comments box and notes about the MYMOP observations on the treatment form are given in the box on p. 125.

The CP team have now been using MYMOP within each clinic session for 4 years. In the first year of the project we asked practitioners for their observations. These are recorded in the section on Feedback in Chapter 5 (p. 149).

Meetings: development and decision making

We have found the difficulties that surround the referral process and the various misunderstandings that interdis-

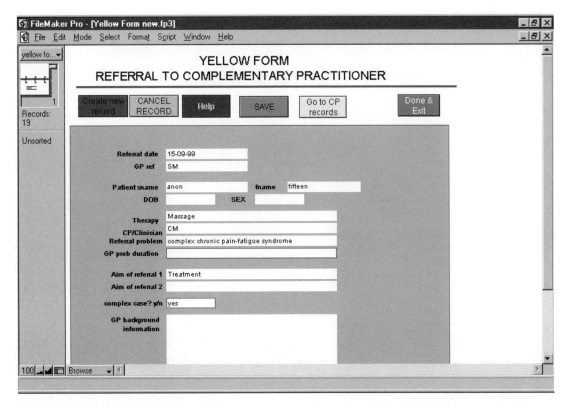

Figure 4.3A Computer screen examples: referral screen;

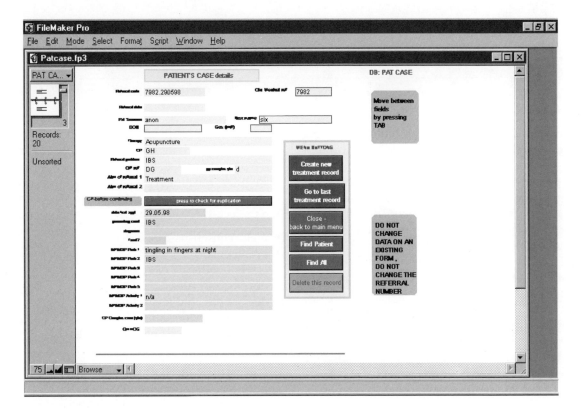

Figure 4.3B Computer screen examples: CP case note screen

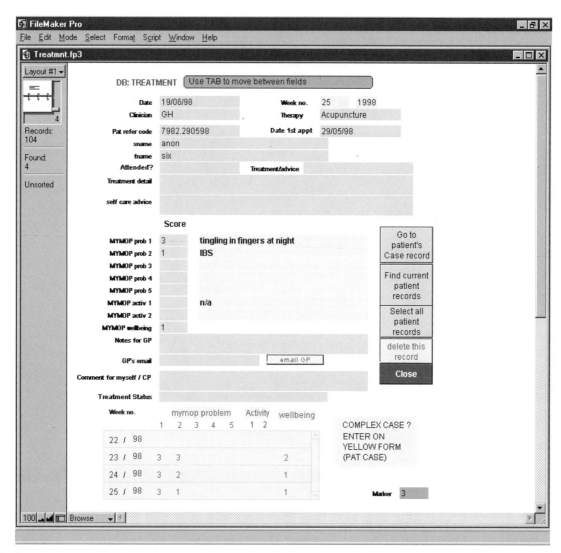

Figure 4.3C Computer screen examples: CP treatment screen.

ciplinary communication can entail are central problems in CP/GP collaboration. They have to be worked through gradually as part of the interprofessional development of the extended team but the time needed for team building and sharing of ideas and information is considerable. Our group feels it needs at least an hour of groupwork each week, even when no joint research project is under way, so that practitioners can share lunch and discuss ideas about patient management, receive support with problems arising and explore each other's knowledge bases, attitudes and beliefs.

However, our CPs work at the Centre on a part-time basis, so finding the resources for overstretched GPs and CPs to meet regularly in an always busy general practice has never been easy. If CPs are taking time out from their own private practice, having already accepted a considerable reduction in hourly income in order to establish a foothold in the NHS (perhaps with the aim of demonstrating the value of their therapy, and because they want

to collaborate with doctors), then opportunities for authentic coworking must be built into any truly cooperative project (see Ch. 5).

Regular meetings operating on an 8-weekly cycle underpin the development and ongoing management of the project. We needed a system that would allow us to:

- make consensus-based decisions
- problem solve
- work together
- develop our ideas
- deepen our understanding of CTs
- develop specific skills
- consider the needs of our patients.

Clinical meetings (fortnightly, 75 minutes) The practice's counsellors and nurses also attend this meeting and reflect on their own caseload. At these meetings CPs can also bring cases to discuss patients the GP is unsure about

Comments on complexity:
'Complex case, depressed woman.'
'Atopic eczema since birth and asthma since 2–3 years; very complex case—can I even help at all?' 'Patient very motivated.' (GP)

Comment on referrals:
'No follow-up appointment, inappropriate referral.'

Comments related to progress:
'This girl does need help but is too chaotic at the moment. Her job is exacerbating her problem but she says she has to continue.'

Comment on patient management:
'Massage has given only very temporary relief. To return to GP.'

Comments regarding other treatment:
'Radiotherapy started since treatment with CT commenced.'

Changes in the patient's circumstances:
'He has been evicted from his house since last session.'
'Wife died 2 days ago.'

Changes in medication:
'She has not had any other treatment since starting acupuncture, and has not needed to take diazepam (sleep).'

Monitoring non-attendance and cancellations:
'Cancelled the previous appointment (first one).'

Use of notes box: MYMOP observations
Comments from patients not reflected in the scores:
'His scores seem the same but he says that he would have had an outbreak by now and is anxious to continue.'
'Although his scores have not changed the patient is very happy with treatment as usually by this time in the year he has suffered a relapse and/or increased medication.'

Unsuitability for use:
'The patient could not use MYMOP today as too distressed.'

referring or where the CP wants to talk about a patient's progress. Case meetings may emphasize clinical issues or be more focused on organizational or interdisciplinary difficulties that have arisen.

CP team meetings (monthly, 75 minutes) These deal with any issues that concern the CPs, including those related directly to the project, patients, or working within the health centre.

CP/GP meetings (8-weekly, 2 hours during development phase) During the 3-year cycle of practice development these meetings were essentially about problem solving and ratifying materials as they came onstream. Invariably, however, these meetings went beyond these purely organizational concerns into discussions, for example, about the nature of health and illness, the limits of treatment, and what can possibly be achieved within a resource-constrained service. At these meetings we learnt to work together and it was usually here that any clashes between the worlds of conventional and complementary medicine would occur. Passions would occasionally run high as we grappled with the often-complex task of understanding one another's perspectives. It was also the place where issues relating to treatment of complex patients arose time and again.

Academic meetings (monthly, 75 minutes) Academic meetings create the opportunity for all clinical staff to get together and share ideas, expertise and in-house research. Each year they have a theme and each team (GPs, nurses, counsellors, CPs) or an individual member is encouraged to host a session. The theme during the first year of the project was patient participation, in the second the therapeutic relationship, and in the third chronic diseases.

Staff development half-days The topics for these training and development sessions included the use of MYMOP, the delivery of the service, the development of the audit cycles, and learning about CTs.

Using a reflective process to modify the developing CT service

When all the structures, processes and written materials were in place a series of reflective cycle meetings were set up. It was agreed that the following areas would be a useful basis for these cycles. There were a total of five reflective cycles, embracing the central issues that emerged through our collaboration:

- the structure of the project
- the process of the project
- the quality and usefulness of written material
- MYMOP data from patients
- development of self-help activities for patients
- health/cost efficiency
- the next step—what we need to do now
- future research (building on what we have already learnt)
- collaboration between CPs and GPs.

Cycle one *Theme*: assessing baseline activity; emphasis on the referral process and outcome measures:

- who was referred for treatment in the past? (review of previous 2 years' data)
- how did GPs decide who to refer and what have we learned about referring?
- which patients do GPs/CPs *not* give leaflets to, and why?
- how can we standardize the administration of MYMOP?

Cycle two *Theme*: treatment outcomes; ethical issues involved in use of computerized records.
Further work includes: GPs to record expectations of improvement on referral forms.

Cycle three *Theme*: the format for reports to be presented to the team.
Further work includes:

- producing discharge summaries about patients
- recording: are there outstanding issues for the patient?

Cycle four *Theme*: continuity of care—planning and managing the ending of treatment with a CP.

Further work includes: What GPs want to know when they look at episode reports:

- did the patient get better?
- did the patient continue with the treatment?
- number of DNAs?
- post-treatment arrangements/management plan?
- outcomes of treatment?
- CP evaluation?
- long-term self-care advice given to patients?

Cycle five *Theme:* GPs' use of the condition guideline cards when referring patients.
Further work includes:

- make cards simpler (layout and contents) for ease of use.

Closing the current inquiry loops

- How do we describe what we do/don't do?—'CT is not intended as symptom-based medicine.'
- Has there been a shift in patient awareness and self-care?
- How do you evaluate how empowered people are?
- Do we prescribe less conventional medication?
- Is cost the only issue: what about quality of care that is valuable and valued?

Quality assurance

Our understanding of quality assurance related not only to the outcome of treatment with CTs but also to all aspects of the delivery of service and health centre contact with patients. We arrived at a list of the areas we felt it important to include for regular review and the methods we employed to review them. Some components have yet to be evaluated—for example, the policy for discharge has been in place for only a short time. The quality assurance of all aspects of the service will form the basis for our future work together.

Communication with patients Discussions in CP/GP meetings revolved upon the consultation process for both GPs and CPs, and informed choice/patient participation in the decision-making process. Topics included:

- how to introduce the self-help material to the consultation
- how to describe the therapies
- information on the limits of the CT
- how to make an appointment with a CP
- introducing the evaluation process to the patient
- using MYMOP with patients
- managing the ending of the course of treatment with the CP
- negotiating future care.

Staff development half-days dicussed more complex matters such as:

- how to manage the consultation process from the initial consultation with the patient to making an appointment to see the CP
- developing a written guide to the consultation process
- developing a procedure for ensuring patients are well-enough informed
- review of an evaluation undertaken in a BSc student project with patients on:
  — the process of giving patients the self-care advice within the consultation
  — the process of introducing MYMOP into the consultation
- using the GP MYMOP to link the GP and CP consultations
- developing a discharge policy for CPs.

Management of the referral process Tasks included:

- the compilation of the evidence base for treatment
- the development of guideline cards for GPs
- increasing GPs' knowledge of who would make a suitable patient for each therapy. (A Therapy choice questionaire was developed to assist in this process—see Ch. 8.)

Under the heading of quality assurance the following were addressed:

- continuous upgrading of the evidence base for treatment
- half-day staff development on the use of the guideline cards within the consultation
- reviewing the guideline cards—the subject of an audit cycle meeting
- developing written guidance on side-effects and contraindications for each therapy.

Topics relating to the quality of written material included:

- self-help leaflets
- patient evaluation—this was the basis of a student project (see Ch. 5).

Appropriate use of MYMOP This was also the subject of a student project (see Ch. 5).
Arrangements for discharge and follow-up This was the subject of a reflective cycle meeting, leading to a procedure for discharge.
Evaluation of long-term effects of treatment We introduced the use of the Glasgow Homoeopathic Hospital Outcome Scale (GHHOS). This is an easily administered tool for the assessment of outcome with CTs post-treatment. We used it with one in ten randomly chosen patients between 3 and 6 months after their treatment

with a CP had ceased. It involves a short telephone conversation with a patient (whom we have asked in advance if they are willing to participate).

Interviewers were given a training session on the use of the form and a written protocol for conducting the interview. When introducing this procedure we employed three people to conduct the interviews. There was no significant difference in the range of scores they recorded, although the numbers were small: 15 patients each.

The N.W. Thames study

One of us undertook a project to explore how a general practice would change its management of back and neck pain if it had access to a locally provided osteopathic service. The project was structured around a series of six rapid audit cycles in a NHS fundholding practice in West London over a period of 8.5 months

A previous study at the MHC[4] had revealed definite problems with the way GPs use a CT service, among them establishing congruence between referring doctors and CPs about the most appropriate and effective use of NCTs,[5] developing communication between clinicians who use substantially different knowledge bases, and acknowledging the complex unspoken issues that tend to distort the processes of referral and communication.[6-8] We believed that if we could solve these problems it would make the CT service more appropriate and effective. If this could be achieved, GP and patient satisfaction would improve and increased effectiveness would be reflected in a reduced referral rate to hospital-based musculoskeletal specialties.

Setting up the service

A practice was found that could provide figures on previous years' referrals and that had a system for monitoring its use of resources. Accommodation for the clinic was found at a nearby osteopathic training college who provided two adjoining treatment rooms and a waiting room for the service.

Knowing that an unfamiliar clinical resource was likely to seem threatening to patients and confusing for doctors, we tried hard to ensure that everyone involved would feel comfortable and familiar with the service as quickly as possible. With these problems in mind, a series of leaflets and forms for use by the referring GPs, administrative staff and patients was prepared in advance. These important structural elements not only ensured the service's acceptability by patients and GPs but also supported its efficient delivery.

A series of seven review meetings were set up to provide an opportunity for reflecting on the referral process and evaluate the data that were being collected. They were

scheduled for once a month at lunchtime to make the best use of the limited time available for discussion and they focused on a monthly activity report summarizing the previous month's activity. At an initial meeting, the GPs had been able to reassure themselves that the service would be delivered in a competent and professional manner. At the first of the review meetings, GPs' expectations of the service were discussed and referral criteria agreed. The main aim of the subsequent reviews was to enable the service to adapt to GPs' needs in the light of the data emerging about the referrals and the outcome of treatment.

The clinics

Clinics were held two mornings a week, 3 days apart (Monday and Thursday), to allow twice-weekly treatment when necessary. Because we predicted the practice might refer as many as 100 patients during the 6 months of the project, two adjoining rooms were made available to deal with the anticipated high throughput of patients.

A GP who had trained as an osteopath ran the clinic (DP). He had also treated patients with medical acupuncture in both general practice and hospital settings for 15 years. In addition, intra-articular[9] and trigger-point injections[10] as well as stress management methods,[11] including relaxation techniques,[12] were used in the clinic from time to time.

Over the first 6 weeks, the booking schedule provided a maximum of three 30-minute appointments for new patients and six 15-minute follow-up appointments. Initial consultations were booked at half an hour, and patients had time beforehand to complete an extensive history and symptom questionnaire. An emergency appointment was also kept open at the end of the session. The clinic generally ran from 9.30 a.m. to 1 p.m. with time allocated at the end of the clinic to update the patient's notes on the clinician's laptop computer.

Meetings

Six audit meetings were held, each one focusing on the report of the previous month's work. The aim was to monitor the use of the service continually and evaluate outcomes. Inevitably, questions arose about aetiology, expectations, referral criteria and the value of treatment. The ensuing discussion, in which the researchers acted as facilitators, helped achieve consensus about these issues and agreement on how the various problems that arose could be solved (Box 4.4).

Data collection

Because the GPs needed a quick and easy way to refer patients, a tick-box proforma for GPs was produced. This

---

Box 4.4   Some central issues that arose in a collaboration between GPs and an osteopath

- *Referral criteria*
  Is it possible to define a typical patient who will benefit from musculoskeletal medicine's approach? If so it would help GPs refer effectively

- *Prognosis*
  Can a musculoskeletal clinician assess at an early stage whether a patient is likely to benefit; and how quickly?

- *Aetiology*
  Whether to attribute any clinical improvement to psychosocial elements in the consultation or to a biomechanical component

- *Mind or body?*
  How to judge whether a patient's pain is best understood biomechanically or as an expression of psychosocial distress

- *Tolerating uncertainty*
  Since no absolute solution to these questions could be found, how would an effective working relationship be achieved and uncertainty tolerated?

- *Expectations and outcome*
  It had initially been assumed that the musculoskeletal clinician would 'fix' patients. But it soon became clear that GPs also wanted help with chronic problems ('maintain') and also with patients whose pain and distress had an important psychological component ('contain')

- *Fix, maintain or contain?*
  How much of a musculoskeletal medical clinic's time should be devoted to 'fixing' mechanical dysfunction at the expense of meeting GPs' need to refer more problematic, chronic (and therefore time-consuming) problems?

- *Cost effectiveness*
  Cost–benefit becomes even more of an issue when a long series of appointments is required (e.g. nine patients did unexpectedly well but had nine or more appointments). The possibility of creating dependency in such patients could also be significant.

---

asked for details of patient history, presenting complaint, the referring GP's expectations, relevant investigations and what other treatment approaches the GP might have considered had the service not been available. The completed form was faxed to the clinician the day before the clinic, along with a copy of the appointment sheet, which reception staff kept at the practice.

A visual analogue scale (VAS) was used to assess pain and function. Function was also tracked using an inventory of 12 common activities. Patients updated these scales in the clinic prior to each consultation, so that pain and function could be tracked as a continuously updated graphic presentation.

The clinician's database allowed clinical information— the provisional diagnosis, treatments used, changes in patient condition and relevant comments—to be entered after each consultation. The Filemaker software produced monthly summaries for GPs (see Ch. 5, p. 153); these became the main focus of discussion at each audit cycle meeting.

On completion of a treatment episode, patients filled in a service evaluation form. Sometimes this had to be posted on to them. GPs also completed a follow-up form when the patient next consulted them.

Since CT consultations are often considered too time consuming for the public sector, the feasibility of working within stringent time constraints and of including an evaluation element was an essential part of the study. As far as possible, the necessary tasks, including entry of all relevant clinical data, had to be fitted into the 3.5 hour clinic session. Analysis of the data was carried out prior to each audit meeting to produce a short report comprising graphs, tables and bullet points.

What happened in the audit cycles?

First meeting: 'the name of the game' This was the first time the two researchers met the GPs and we were aware that we needed to be clear about the project's aims and how we intended to achieve them. The GPs also needed to be assured of our research and clinical abilities. It was important to discuss both our and the GPs' expectations of the project and agree some initial referral and management guidelines that we could all work with.

We all recognized that whatever guidelines were adopted had to ensure an adequate flow of referrals and also avoid the clinic being swamped. The assumption was that they should exclude patients for whom treatment would be contraindicated and aim to focus on those most likely to benefit. Unfortunately, there is no such profile of the ideal patient for non-conventional treatment of musculoskeletal pain. However, as it has been shown that osteopathic intervention for acute mechanical back pain is best given between 2 and 4 weeks after onset,[13] this was offered as initial guidance. It was also suggested that patients with long-standing structural degeneration should not be referred and agreed that those with pathological pain and acute prolapsed discs should be excluded.

We had given considerable thought to the kind of information that might be most helpful: the project's short duration meant that all concerned would need to feel comfortable and familiar with the resource as quickly as possible. Anticipating this we had prepared a leaflet for patients, explaining what they could expect from the clinic and how to get there, and a more detailed explanatory leaflet for GPs (see Ch. 6). Much of the meeting was taken up with explaining the booking and data collection forms that had been circulated beforehand. Following the meeting, further background material in the form of a back pain management protocol, a short paper about osteopathy[14] and two exercise leaflets for patients was sent to the GPs.

First review meeting: 'parachuting in' We knew from the practice's records that referral rates to all specialities were relatively low. This continued to be the case throughout the project and extended to GPs' relatively sparing use of the osteopathic clinic itself. Because all four GPs involved (the practice has a trainee) viewed back and neck pain as usually self-limiting they tended, at first, to refer only the more chronic and unremitting cases; it seemed that they had been saving patients with difficult backs and necks pending the start of the clinic. (Other osteopathic practitioners have noted a similar referral pattern in the early stages of establishing a service for GPs.[15])

Another early observation was the high incidence of associated psychosocial distress and depression amongst the first group of patients referred. Both these points were raised at the first review meeting and were confirmed by the data presented and by GPs' comments about individual patients. A series of broad exclusion criteria had been set up, namely no very acute pain, no self-limiting pain, no chronic degenerative conditions and now, in addition, no psychogenic pain. The result of this swingeing restriction on referral was predictable.

Second review meeting: 'accepting uncertainty' The initial spurt of new referrals rapidly tailed off to the extent that by the second meeting only six of the 24 new patient appointments available had been taken up. Of the 20 patients referred during the first 2 months, eight had been discharged either because they were a lot better or because treatment appeared not to be helping. At this stage, the clinician (DP) was still trying to discharge patients as quickly as possible in anticipation of more new patients.

The remaining 12 patients were a difficult group and progress as tracked by serial VAS was very variable—a reflection of diverse and, in some cases, long-standing conditions. Amongst them were two patients with posturally mediated recurrent pain; one patient with several months of severe, resistant, non-discal referred pain; two Turkish patients with long-standing pain: one dorsal, one sciatic; at least two patients depressed and somatizing; one patient with a prostatic bone secondary (not treated); another with a possible prolapsed disc and three patients with what appeared to be mechanical back pain but was nonetheless resisting treatment. Not surprisingly, levels of distress in this group as a whole were high. Consequently, a recurring issue in the audit cycle meetings was to what extent neck and back pain represents a disorganized symptom of psychosocial distress. Linked to this question was the idea that improvement could be attributable to non-specific effects of touch and attention. The possibility that the associated depression and anxiety might be the primary problem or be secondary to the effects of the musculoskeletal pain and disability was

also discussed. All were agreed that the interaction of subjective symptoms and objective signs could often be difficult to interpret.

At this point, the attempt to define guidelines had excluded many of the patients GPs might have wanted to refer. On the other hand the definition of what was an appropriate referral was still not clear. This truly reflects the central problem where GPs and CPs collaborate. GPs recognize the need for extended clinical services but CPs for their part are often unclear about how to define their clinical role. It seemed that GPs are most likely to refer patients with relatively undifferentiated illness. From the clinician's point of view, the pressure to discharge patients was far less since new patients were not appearing. This made it easier for the clinician to offer this very difficult group further appointments and he therefore suggested to the GPs at this review that they could be less constrained in who they referred. Referral rates immediately increased back to their former levels.

Third review meeting: 'the search for solid ground' Prior to the third review meeting, we reflected on the issues that the project had brought to light. Once GPs had been encouraged to take the initiative on referrals rather than try to create exclusion criteria, new patients appeared in the expected numbers. Our attempt to produce effective guidelines and avoid inappropriate referrals had caused confusion but it was not clear why. It seemed that GPs had their own reasons for referral that were only partially open to strict guidelines. We therefore decided to look at their basic assumptions about neck and back pain, how they thought about it and managed it. We wondered, as well, what happened to those patients who presented with back and neck pain but did *not* get referred to the clinic? It was agreed that a brief questionnaire would be circulated to GPs to establish how they each managed back pain and that we would process the results in time for the next meeting.

Fourth review meeting: 'where have all the patients gone?' At the fourth meeting the results of the previous month's GP questionnaire were presented. Responses suggested that the GPs generally attributed *acute* back/neck pain to non-traumatic muscle tension and spasm. This was in line with the model of musculoskeletal pain presented at the initial meeting. However, there was little agreement about the relative importance of other causes. There was even less consensus on chronic neck and back pain. We were all surprised to discover that two of the GPs estimated they were seeing at least one patient with back/neck pain every day. The third GP estimated two patients a week while the trainee saw only one patient a month with back pain. This meant that, even with the clinic offering six new patient slots per week, it would have been able to cope with only half the patients who were presenting to GPs with neck and back pain. Yet in the period between the two review meetings

(4 weeks) only seven new patients had been referred out of a possible 24 new patient slots. If, as the GPs said, their clinical experience led them to expect spontaneous remission in 75% of cases between 1 and 4 weeks after onset, then the clinic could expect 12 new patients to be referred each month as opposed to the seven who were. Just what, we wondered, was holding GPs back from referring? Had our questionnaire raised anxiety levels to the point that GPs had, once again, become uncertain about whom to refer? Had the act of reflection itself had some inhibitory influence? Now, with summer on the way, the level of cancellations and 'did not arrives' (DNAs) began to increase and new referrals were barely one a week.

In order to confirm that the GPs were actually seeing the estimated 24 patients with back and neck pain each month, we designed and distributed a diary. Our further intention was to follow up those patients not subsequently referred. Were they perhaps consulting osteopaths independently?

At this meeting, we reviewed all 38 patients referred so far. We were beginning to realize that there were three distinct groups attending the clinic.

Fifth review meeting: 'the beginning of the end' It had been 2 months since the last audit meeting. Over the summer, only 12 new patients were referred of whom four failed to attend the first appointment. It is worth noting their diagnoses and the outcome of the remaining eight. Two patients were typical osteopathic dysfunction—one dorsal pain, the other sacroiliac pain—and both did very well; one elderly woman had acute hip pain that was responding to acupuncture; one young woman had an acute coccydynia that initially responded to local steroid infusion; a woman with chronic 'pain all over' had begun to attend for acupuncture after a traumatic domestic incident; one unemployed man with a history of occupational back pain came twice then failed to return; an anxious young woman with relapsing upper back and neck pain was beginning to learn how anxiety, breathing and posture affected her condition.

At this review we presented the list of patients according to how often they had been seen and whether they had done well. The patients, we realized, could be categorized into one of three groups: 'somatizers'—that is, patients in whom pain was a manifestation of psychosocial distress, 'long-term mechanical pain and dysfunction'; and 'typical osteopathic cases'. We began to explore with the GPs an emerging pattern that appeared to offer a useful way of interpreting the clinic's caseload, treatment methods used and their outcomes.

The clinic was to run for only 6 months, so this was the last lunchtime audit meeting held before the service ended. The difficulties around the clinic's ending were acknowledged by the GPs and ourselves, with GPs hoping they had not raised patients' expectations for future access to CT. With only 6 weeks left, it was agreed that no new referrals should be made after the end of September.

Sixth review meeting We looked at the total referrals and DNAs, the categories of patients seen, treatments used and the outcomes (in terms of changed pain score > 6). The results were better than we had anticipated. The stimulating discussion that developed during the course of this meeting brought back to the surface many of the issues raised in previous review meetings (see Box 4.4, p. 127).

The questions raised included: the balance between mechanical and psychosocial influences on pain and pain management, how to identify suitable patients for referral, how musculoskeletal clinicians can assess early on in the treatment who is likely to do well, and how to convey this information to the referring GPs. We realized that our struggle with these questions about aetiology, selection, treatment/assessment and communication were at the heart of our collaboration, but we accepted that no certain solution to these questions had been found. However, a comfortable working relationship had been achieved whereby this uncertainty could be tolerated. Incorporating an unfamiliar approach to managing patients presenting with often undifferentiated painful symptoms appeared to have been useful in three different ways: a referral might imply 'please fix this', but often it meant 'please keep this person going (mechanically)' and sometimes 'please keep this person going (psychologically)'.

We discussed the implications of this simple insight. How much of the clinic's time should be devoted to 'fixing' mechanical dysfunction at the expense of meeting GPs' need to refer more difficult and therefore more time-consuming problems? To a surprising extent, improvements in pain levels were possible even in patients with long-term mechanical degeneration or psychogenic disorders: six patients in whom the clinician recognized significant somatizing tendencies did well, as did three more patients with osteoarthritic joint degeneration. However, this highlighted important cost–benefit issues, as well as problems of dependency, which have to be addressed when dealing with such patients, because a long series of appointments might be required (nine patients did well but received nine or more appointments). Had the clinic received the expected number of referrals, it would not have been possible to offer more than six follow-up appointments.

(The patterns of musculoskeletal service at MHC are summarized in Box 5.1, p. 165)

Was the project a success?

The GPs valued the clinic precisely because it met a number of definably different GP needs. It was on these grounds alone (no information about its cost–benefit or influence on referral patterns being available when the project ended) that GPs initially judged the clinic to have been a success. Improvement in pain levels was often possible even in patients with long-term mechanical degeneration or disorders with a significant stress-related component. About half of the patients seen were assessed as having responded well (change in pain on VAS > 6 on a scale of 10).

Responses to questionnaires completed by GPs and patients indicated a high level of satisfaction with the service. Only one-third of all patients had been initially diagnosed as 'typical osteopathic cases'.[10] Such a small proportion of 'fixable' patients seemed unlikely to make much overall impact on the practice's use of secondary referrals. Generally, the practice made relatively few secondary referrals in comparison to available national figures.[16] Consequently we had thought that access to the new clinic was unlikely to reduce them. However, when referrals were analysed 6 months after the clinic ended, orthopaedic and rheumatology referrals had been halved during the project and over the half year following, while those to physiotherapy remained the same, compared with those for the year before. This drop may have been partly due to a non-specific effect; perhaps by increasing GPs' level of reflection about musculoskeletal problems the project in some way inhibited GPs' urge to refer. However, two features make this unlikely: first, responses to the referral questionnaire indicate that in many cases (> 80%) referring GPs stated that they would have sent the patient to a hospital outpatient department had the musculoskeletal clinic not been available; secondly, the practice's overall use of non-musculoskeletal specialties did not significantly vary between the 2 years reviewed. The effect could be due to a non-specific effect: perhaps by increasing GPs' level of reflection about musculoskeletal problems the project in some way inhibited GPs' urge to refer. It could equally be due to the very concrete and accessible presence of a musculoskeletal specialist 'in-house'.

We believe the project confirmed that, when CTs are being introduced into conventional medical settings, implementation and evaluation need to go hand in hand. The value of rapid audit cycles is that they help manage an unfamiliar collaborative process, while simultaneously allowing a consensus on service use and outcomes to develop in an area where there is little experience to draw on, nor much firm evidence to act as a guide. The project thereby enabled appropriate use of resources and established an essential interprofessional interface.

The next example evaluates our experience of using a computer-based clinical management system to improve effectiveness of a CT service in a fundholding general practice.

The CT service at MHC: an example of a reflective approach to implementation

Objectives

The project's aim was to develop ways of enhancing the effectiveness of a range of CTs in the primary care setting, first by making the collaboration between GPs and CPs explicit and secondly optimizing service delivery by using computer-based data collection in a multidisciplinary primary care team that includes an acupuncturist, a massage therapist, a homeopath and an osteopath/naturopath. The team believed this would entail improving communication, establishing intake and outcome criteria and ways of closing learning loops.

The primary care team explored the problems of developing a rational and quality-assured CT service through a series of meetings. This led to the defining of data collection structures and processes needed. The researchers designed and supervised their implementation and evaluation through a series of action research cycles.

Setting up the study

The clinicians group (four GPs and five CPs) had been meeting fortnightly for several years to review clinical problems. Several members of the group had worked together throughout that time and had already analysed and audited their work.[4,17] In addition the group met for 2 hours every 6–8 weeks to reflect on developments, to discuss the emerging questions and the necessary actions to be taken. For the purpose of the study, the group's convenor (DP), who has previous experience of audit, was made responsible for taking action on the basis of these discussions. A project officer was appointed (GH) to organize and document the work, which took the homeopath's practice as its initial focus.

Structured approaches to referral, collection of consultation data and assessment of treatment outcomes had to be developed and implemented. Over the course of the 3-year study, a GP referral form, a computer program using a relational database and a practical outcome measure were developed and modified. A database was designed that allowed the clinicians to track interventions and outcomes using MYMOP. Patterson's original study suggested that the method is valid and a responsive measure of patient outcomes and is applicable to CT practice.[3]

Critical incidents were brought to fortnightly clinical meetings and methods were continually adapted as problems arose and new options emerged at 6-weekly audit meetings.

Cycle 1: needs identification Why does the health centre need a CT service? It was agreed that the criteria for guideline development of the practice's CT service as a whole should be naturalistic, reflecting conditions which GPs stated they would refer, and conditions where CPs declared they could do effective work or expressed a strong interest in treating. Questions and methods of addressing them for each reflective cycle were as follows:

Question

- For what conditions do GPs believe conventional treatment is inadequate?
- What do GPs think CTs are appropriate for?
- What do the CPs think they can achieve?
- Are there patients or conditions that clinicians want particularly to exclude or include?

Method

- Questionnaires and discussion
- Discussion of available research evidence
- Consensus development

A list was derived from the International Classification of Primary Care. GPs were asked to identify conditions they might refer to CPs who in turn identified conditions they believed they could treat. After three cycles of data collection and discussion a consensus was reached on the conditions whose treatment the team wanted to improve. Various reviews of the evidence for CTs were also taken into account as a possible basis for guideline development.

Cycle 2: mapping intake and expectations The initial aim was to document how a range of CTs had been used at MHC in order to see whether the list of agreed conditions accurately reflected GPs' actions. Questions and methods of addressing them for this cycle were as follows:

Question

- How have GPs used the CPs?
- And what did they expect of CTs?
- What sort of symptoms do patients initially present to CPs?

Method

- Analysis of data from referral forms in notes
- Analysis of data from current GP referral forms
- Analysis of data from MYMOP forms

One year's CT activity (1997–1998) was reviewed retrospectively. A research assistant entered data from the referral form filed in patients' notes. Forms were then analysed in terms of conditions and GP expectations recorded. This list was then compared with the condition list generated in cycle 1.

Cycle 3: evaluating CT referrals and practicality of outcome measures Questions and methods of addressing them for this cycle were as follows:

Question

- Can patients use MYMOP?
- Are these patients in some way distinctive: e.g. complex psychosomatic, high levels of distress, poor levels of well-being?
- Can the CPs make use of MYMOP as a method of evaluating clinical progress?

Method

- Semistructured interviews
- Analysis of data from MYMOP referral forms
- Reflective cycles on use of MYMOP

After 1 year, when data was being gathered more consistently and a clear description of the centre's use of CT was available, another retrospective sample (May–September 1998) was analysed to see what conditions GPs were referring and what they expected to achieve by the referral. Also, because the team was unsure whether patients would accept MYMOP, a sample of patients who had seen the CPs was asked what they thought about using MYMOP and whether the MYMOP results accurately reflected their experience.

Cycle 4: tracking and evaluating patients through a series of consultations Questions and methods of addressing them for this cycle were as follows:

Question

- Can the CPs use MYMOP as a method of evaluating clinical progress?
- Is it practical within a single clinical session to enter this data and other necessary information about referral and treatment on to a computer database?
- Do the activity/outcome reports provide a useful audit focus for managing database and adapting the service?

Method

- Continued reflective cycles on use of MYMOP
- Develop and pilot use of clinical database
- Reflective cycles on use of clinical database
- Pilot of audit meetings to evaluate and consolidate use of the database

Our experience

It was possible to establish the basic elements of the required learning cycle. Initially, decisions had to be made about which conditions to refer to CTs and about how to evaluate outcomes. There can be no absolute grounds for these decisions. However, once decided, their validity could be studied pragmatically using action–reflection cycles.

Results of cycle 1: needs identification An agreed final list was broad enough to be useful in primary care. It included common conditions plus broad categories that allow treatment of undifferentiated illness to be explored. Conditions included:

- asthma, IBS, migraine
- eczema, rhinitis and hay fever
- menstrual disorders, perimenopausal problems
- viral respiratory tract infections, catarrh
- transient stress-related and situational conditions (presenting, for example, as anxiety, pain, insomnia, tiredness, or digestive disorders)
- recurring infections, urinary tract infections (UTIs), urinary–reproductive tract infections (URTIs), herpes, etc.
- musculoskeletal pain including back and neck pain, osteoarthritis, rheumatoid arthritis and myofascial pain
- complex chronic illness including skin diseases, chronic inflammatory disease, persistent pain and chronic fatigue.

CPs were asked about which conditions they were particularly interested in treating. For example, the homeopath's list of appropriate conditions included patients presenting with psychological distress and children with special needs. Several GPs shared this conviction and the retrospective analysis confirmed that such conditions had been referred for homeopathy in the past.

Results of cycle 2: mapping intake and expectations A sample of consecutive referrals to CPs were analysed for complaint, GP expectations (treat, diagnose, advise patient, support patient, advise GP), MYMOP problems and their severity, and well-being scores. The sample of homeopathy patients comprised patients with the following conditions:

- dermatological (8)
- gastrointestinal (4)
- migraine (2)
- (atypical) pain and altered sensation (11)
- cardiovascular (2)
- sweating (on treatment for Ca prostate) (1)
- gynaecological (13) (includes infertility 3, menopausal symptoms 2)
- tension, anxiety, tiredness (7)
- other psychological (2)
- recurrent infections/catarrh conditions (10).

It became clear from this sample that patients referred for homeopathy had chronic complex problems.

The available MYMOP forms were analysed to create a list showing primary and secondary main complaints and (where entered) patients' self-assessed levels of complaint severity and well-being. The analysis also showed that there was often some incongruity between GPs' reasons for referral and patients' accounts of their need. Referrals to the homeopath reflected the main guideline categories, yet many of these patients in particular often had unusual syndromes, often had above-average consultation rates in the past, and their MYMOP scores suggested high levels of distress and low levels of well-being. This preliminary analysis suggested that homeopathic patients might be more complex than, for instance, those sent for osteopathy in the same practice.

Results of cycle 3: evaluating CT treatments In order to see whether MYMOP was an appropriate way of assessing progress, semistructured interviews were conducted with 18 patients. Of these, 11 felt the method accurately reflected the progress of their condition. The interviews tend to show that physical problems are easier than emotional problems to label and relate to a number. Also it seemed that for patients whose difficulties are significantly psychological the use of the word 'symptom' could be problematic: they preferred to use the word 'problem'. The analysis tended to confirm practitioners' impression that many of the patients referred presented with complex symptom patterns, and expressed high symptom severity scores and poor well-being. The analysis suggests that patients referred for homeopathy in particular tended to experience their problems as severe and their well-being as relatively poor. Despite this, many patients rated the medical outcomes of homeopathic treatment as having significantly improved their daily life.

Results of cycle 4: tracking patients through a series of consultations CPs began to use the computer database as a way of summarizing information gathered during the consultation and, although initially hesitant, they eventually found this approach both practicable and helpful. The computer system had by now (after 2 years of development) reached a stage when activity reports and tables illustrating clinical change could be produced for audit meetings. Although interviews suggested that patients and clinicians found MYMOP a practical way of tracking clinical outcome, it sometimes failed to reflect the clinician's impressions: MYMOPs would commonly not improve even when patients said they felt better. A sample of patients was therefore selected and these were written to and subsequently given a short, structured telephone interview (using the GHHOS). The results are included in Table 4.3.

We found overall that:

- GPs tended to refer to acupuncture, homeopathy and massage (but not to osteopathy) those patients who do not fit easily into biomedical disease categories

Table 4.3 This report samples the range of conditions referred to homeopathy. It illustrates case mix and GP reasons for referral. MYMOP scores indicate patients' perception of their problem and its severity. In general these scores are high, suggesting severe symptoms and poor well-being. This particular report structure does not include changes between initial and final MYMOP scores, but notes the Glasgow Homoeopathic Hospital Outcome Scale (GHHOS) scores where they have been recorded

Complaint	GP reason for referring					Patient problem					
	Treat	Diag	Adv pt	Suppt	Adv GP	MYMOP prob 1	M1	MYMOP prob 2	M2	WB	GS
dermatological					1	chronic dermatitis	1	sinus probs	3	3	
dermatological	1					sore face	2	pain in left shoulder	5	4	+3
dermatological	1					spots	3	stress	3	2	
dermatological						psoriasis	6	pityriasis rosea	4	4	+2
dermatological	1		1		1	rosacea	3		6	3	
allergy	1	1				acne	5	rash	4	4	+4
IBS, gastrointest, lower limb	1		1			ulcerative colitis	5	acne	3	4	
IBS					1	aches & pains	5	lethargy	5		
gastrointestinal	1		1			not recorded	4	not recorded	5	4	0
menstrual prob.						PMT physical	0	PMT emotional	4	4	0
gynaecological, dermatological	1					infertility		depression periods			0
gynaecological	1		1			PMT	5				
gynaecological	1			1		hot from waist up	6	shaking cold	6	3	0
infertility	1		1			cough	5	repeated colds/flu	0	4	
infertility			1			infertility	6				
infertility						husband infertility	6	depressed, sleepless	5		
menopause						hot flushes	5	indigestion	6		+3
menopause	1					hot flushes	3	energy	3	2	0
migraine	1					migraines	5	stress	2	3	
migraine						rhinitis	5	migraine		2	+3
pain, altered sensation		1				insecurity/anxiety	4	feet	6	4	
pain, psych, gynaecological	1 1		1			sleepless	6	pain (whole body)	3	3	+2
pain, stiffness, depression, dermatological, gynaecological						bladder	5	skin	5	3	+3
musculoskeletal						sciatica	5	muscular aches	5		0
altered sensation in neck, dorsal and lumbosacral	1		1	1		IBS	5	deafness/dizziness	3		4
pain and stiffness in hands		1				pain in joints	3	digestive	5	3	+4
pain, stiffness, altered sensation, tiredness	1		1			rash	3	osteoarthritis	3		2
pain, tension, respiratory, IBS	1		1		1	IBS	4	tiredness	4	4	
pain, stiffness				1		migraine	6	depression	5		
CVS	1		1		1	not recorded		not recorded			0
CVS, tiredness	1		1		1	not recorded		not recorded			+3
sweating++ (on Rx f or Ca prostate)	1					heat	6	urine	6	3	−1
tiredness, chronic catarrh	1		1			rhinitis, sinusitis	2	back pain	2	3	+4
tiredness, respiratory, support		1		1		not recorded	5	not recorded	4		+2
depression			1	1		sporadic depressions	5	relationship with mother	3		
confusion, allergy, psych	1		1			allergy/hay fever	4	shaving rash/spots	5	4	
mother–baby probs, dermatol	1					wakefulness	4	eczema	4	4	+3
catarrhal baby						sticky eyes		ears			+3
chronic sinusitis	1					sinusitis	1	asthma	6		
recurrent cystitis	1		1		1	cystitis	0	constipation			

Table 4.3 (*contd*)

Complaint	GP reason for referring					Patient problem					
	Treat	Diag	Adv pt	Suppt	Adv GP	MYMOP prob 1	M1	MYMOP prob 2	M2	WB	GS
respiratory			1	1		croup	0	general health	0		
respiratory						hay fever		dry eyes			+4
respiratory, nasal discharge	1					nasal congestion backache/	5	chesty cough	4	4	+3
recurrent cold sores	1	1				flu-like		tiredness/pregnant	3		
recurrent colds and coughs						producing phlegm	4	blocked sinuses	4		+3
recurrent URTI				1		constant catarrh	4	repeat cough/colds	1	2	

Treat = treatment, Adv pt = advise patient, Diag = what is your diagnosis?, Suppt = support patient, Adv GP = advise GP, MYMOP prob 1 = patient's main problem, M1 = (Lickert scale 0 good, 6 severe) severity of problem 1, MYMOP prob 2 = patient's second priority problem, M2 = (Lickert scale 0 good, 6 severe) severity of problem 2, WB = MYMOP well-being, score (Lickert scale 0 good, 6 very poor), GS = Glasgow Homoeopathic Hospital Outcome Scale (+5 = cure, –5 = severe exacerbation) at 3–6-month follow-up.

- patients referred for these CTs tend to self-rate themselves as experiencing notably poor well-being
- MYMOP has to be used skilfully with CT patients, especially where psychological distress is identified as one of their main complaints.

Conclusions

Intake and outcomes At present the MHC guidelines for CT referral are broad and GPs' referral patterns and their reasons for referring suggest that they should remain so. Guidelines based on named conditions may be convenient, but CT perspectives take as their focus patients' own experience rather than named diseases. So it is interesting that in this study many patients referred for CT fell into a group of complex patients who in many cases do not conform to biomedical categories, who have high levels of distress and poor well-being. Furthermore, because health beliefs are diverse, one patient's affinity for a particular CT is bound to differ from another's. These three factors—complexity, distress and patient preference—will influence not only GPs' decisions about whom they refer to CPs, but also the outcome of CT treatment. How should they then be taken into account when using any guideline for referral and in assessing outcomes? For instance, are outcomes better among patients who 'believe in' or prefer CT treatment? One study suggests this is (suprisingly) not the case.

It may be that GPs want CTs as a resource for patients whose problems are difficult to label. We have concluded at this point that, in our setting, GPs value CTs not so much as a way of curing but rather as a way to help maintain function or contain distress in patients with ill-defined health problems whom they would otherwise find it very difficult to deal with. However, even if CTs were to meet these CP expectations might not always be revealed numerically on a MYMOP graph; discrepancy between MYMOP outcomes and subsequent interview scores gave cause for concern. However, overall outcomes were usually better than satisfactory. Preliminary findings suggest that the MYMOP process requires practitioners to guide patients carefully toward an appropriate symptom that is likely to be a fair indicator of clinical change.

How many treatments? Problems are likely to arise in a CT service where intake criteria and outcomes are undifferentiated. To a certain extent this is unavoidable, but how then are we to define what we mean by 'appropriate use', 'effectiveness' and 'cost–benefit' particularly in an NHS CT service? For example, should a patient whose chronic problem is not improving be discharged, or should new approaches be tried and the treatment extended? Must the number offered be capped even if CT is producing temporary remissions or would a longer-term maintenance series be a possibility? The audit system we have developed makes such issues explicit and review meetings allow chosen solutions to be tested out. Further reflective cycles could establish whether an efficiently functioning CT service could actually be cost effective: for example, by reducing repeat visits to GPs and avoiding expensive secondary referrals and investigations. (The example of such an economic argument for a service based at Glastonbury Health Centre (p. 138) illustrates this.)

What has been the impact of the study so far? The reflective method we used allowed the development of a system for organizing data collection and for reflecting and acting on it. The aims of collaboration between GPs and CPs became clearer and the pattern of delivery more defined through using a computer-based data collection system. It has been possible to evaluate the outcomes of the CT service in a practical way, and to use the data to improve practice and integration through action research based around a series of reflective cycles. This approach to service management allowed increased understanding of

CTs' role and their impact on patients and on practice resources. We started from the assumption that the effectiveness of CTs in a NHS GP setting would depend on how well they can be integrated into the work of the primary care team. Our system enabled this process to happen and we believe its further development will enable CTs to play an increasingly effective part in a primary care team's work.

An example of how to develop a local CT service for GPs*

In June 1994 an innovative project was launched within the Lewisham Hospital NHS Trust in south-east London. The project introduced complementary therapy (acupuncture, homeopathy and osteopathy) into the NHS in the context of an evaluation programme.[17] The launch followed approximately 4 years of working towards raising the profile of complementary therapies within the hospital through study days, workshops, and establishing a massage and osteopathic service for staff within the hospital. The author established a steering group to draw together a proposal for funding the service. This was followed by setting up, organizing and managing the service once it was funded, and evaluating the outcome of the service.[17–20]

Local background

Publications by the British Medical Association[21] in 1993 and the National Association of Health Authorities and Trusts (NAHAT)[22] had indicated a desire, from within the NHS, to begin to incorporate complementary therapies into conventional medical practice. A number of staff within Lewisham Hospital had established a complementary therapy special interest group and, with the support of the Medical Director, felt that they were in a good position to explore the potential for providing such a service. In February 1993 the author established a steering group to identify how an NHS-funded complementary therapy service could be provided to the local population.[18] The steering group included a number of complementary therapy practitioners, key personnel from with the hospital (such as the Director of Contracting and the Medical Director), two local GPs and a Consultant in Public Health Medicine from the local health authority.

The steering group decided that the way to proceed would be: (1) to seek local health authority funding (Lambeth, Southwark and Lewisham Health Authority;

LSLHA) to provide a service for the local population; (2) to evaluate the service that was provided; and (3) once the service was established, to seek funding to conduct a number of RCTs. It was anticipated that service provision would focus on a small number of therapies for which there was some evidence of effectiveness, and from which referring medical staff thought patients would benefit. As the planned service provision was to be provided on an outpatient basis, it seemed most likely that the referrals would be generated by GPs. It was therefore important to establish the level of interest in CT provision within the local GP community.

Surveying local interest

A survey was conducted during May 1993. It included a covering letter outlining the intention of the steering group to put a proposal to the health authority for funding for a complementary therapy service. The 200 GPs surveyed had been defined by the hospital Director of Contracting as falling within the catchment area of the hospital. A total of 200 questionnaires were sent to local GPs and 71 (36%) were returned. Despite a low response rate, it was clear that 65 of these 71 GPs were in favour of CT provision within the NHS. There was no pattern by practice observed in the responses. Twelve local GPs reported that they already had access to CT within their practice, with the majority having access to acupuncture (10) and osteopathy (5). Fifty-nine (83%) GPs reported that they did not have access to CT within their practice. Sixty-five GPs (92%) reported that they would refer patients to a CT service provided by Lewisham Hospital. The therapies they were most likely to refer to were acupuncture, homoeopathy and osteopathy.

Figure 4.4 shows the therapies that 65 GPs said they would be most likely to refer patients to if services were to be provided by Lewisham Hospital.

The results of the survey of GPs local to Lewisham Hospital were consistent with evidence from the NAHAT report suggesting that the therapies GPs were most likely to support for NHS provision were acupuncture, homeopathy and osteopathy. It was agreed by the steering group that any CT provision within the hospital should be limited (at least in the first instance) to these three therapies. Further, it was clear that in order to control what could prove to be a demand for services that exceeded planned provision (and funding), referral guidelines would have to be established.

Developing referral indicators through a consensus conference

Before submitting a proposal to the health authority, a consensus conference was held at which local GPs and complementary practitioners developed a set of referral

---

* This example has been provided by Dr Janet Richardson, Research Director, School of Integrated Health, University of Westminster, London, UK

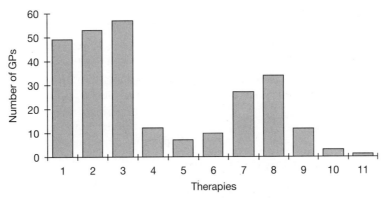

Figure 4.4   Complementary therapies for which GPs would refer patients. 1, homeopathy; 2, acupuncture; 3, osteopathy; 4, spiritual healing; 5, Shiatsu; 6, reflexology; 7, chiropractic; 8, therapeutic massage; 9, aromatherapy; 10, herbal medicine; 11, meditation

indicators. An evidence-based approach to determining service provision and policy is desirable; however, where health providers face the problem of trying to make decisions in situations where there is insufficient information, consensus methods provide a means of synthesizing the available information.[23] Two consensus methods are commonly used in medical, nursing and health services research: the Delphi process and the nominal group technique.[23,24] Eddy[24] suggests the combination of (a) an outcome-based approach that describes the evidence and estimates the outcome, and (b) a preference-based approach that incorporates patients' preferences. The choice of method used to develop policy guidelines should be determined by what it is meant to accomplish, and should be explicit, in order that others can review the process.[24] In the absence of a large body of good-quality evidence regarding the effectiveness of CTs, the development of referral guidelines was based on a consensus conference that brought together local GPs, hospital doctors, CT practitioners (acupuncturists, osteopaths and homeopaths), and representation from the health authority.

The aim of this consensus conference was to develop indications for referral to an outpatient service of acupuncture, homeopathy and osteopathy. The referral guidelines were developed through the application of a modified Delphi technique (Box 4.5) which brought together 'expert witnesses' in a consensus conference discussion. The initial conference was attended by 27 healthcare professionals and chaired by the hospital's Medical Director. It began with a presentation of the intention of Lewisham Hospital to provide a limited CT service on the basis of a block contract with LSLHA. The results of the GP survey were presented and this was followed by a brief presentation of the evidence for effectiveness based on published reviews available. The main work of the conference took place in small groups with the specific brief 'to develop referral indicators for an outpatient service providing acupuncture, homeopathy and osteopathy based on the following: (i) the evidence of effectiveness currently available; (ii) conditions

GPs feel may benefit from the treatments; (iii) conditions which the complementary therapy practitioners feel that they can treat effectively'.

The guidelines agreed through the consensus development process (Table 4.4 & Box 4.6) were included in the funding proposal submitted to the health authority to support the service. Once the contract had been awarded, the guidelines were distributed to all local GPs and hospital consultants within Lewisham Hospital.

Submitting the proposal

The steering group formulated a proposal to provide an osteopathy, acupuncture and homeopathy service, on

---

Box 4.5   Using a modified Delphi technique to develop agreement about referral indications

- Presenting evidence from systematic reviews of clinical trials.
- Small groups included both GPs and complementary therapy practitioners.
- Each group appointed a chair to ensure that the group worked to the brief and reported back.
- Groups worked for 2 hours.
- Each group drew up a list of the conditions for which they would refer patients.
- The groups were asked to split the conditions into two lists: list one for conditions they would definitely refer and list two for conditions they might (but would not definitely) refer.
- The groups came together and presented their lists of conditions to the whole group.
- Further discussion enabled the individual groups to develop two lists of agreed conditions: those for which they would definitely refer (list 1) and those that they might refer (list 2). List 1 was drawn together on the basis of agreement by more than 75% of participants.
- Following the consensus conference, the two lists of conditions were typed and circulated to participants, who were given the option of agreeing to the lists or changing the conditions from one list to the other. However, they were not allowed to add more conditions at this stage. All participants responded to the second consensus round.
- The final list of referral conditions was based on the agreement of at least 85% of participants for conditions for which they would definitely refer. Only 15 participants (56%) agreed on the conditions for which they might (but would not definitely) refer.

Table 4.4 Agreed indications for referral to the service, and contraindications

Condition	Therapy	Contraindications
allergies	acupuncture, homeopathy	
arthritis (RA/osteo)	acute: acupuncture, homeopathy	
	chronic: acupuncture, homeopathy, osteopathy	
asthma (acute/chronic)	acupuncture, homeopathy, osteopathy	status asthmaticus
chronic obstructive airway disease	acupuncture, homeopathy	
disease of upper respiratory tract	acupuncture, homeopathy	
rhinitis (allergic/infective)	acupuncture, homeopathy	
back pain (acute/chronic)	acupuncture, homeopathy, osteopathy	exclude motor deficit and/or underlying pathology
chronic neurological conditions	if presenting with pain: osteopathy	
	supportive: acupuncture, homeopathy, osteopathy	
palliative care	acupuncture, homeopathy, osteopathy	certain cancers: osteopathy
digestive disorders	IBS and reflux oesophagitis: acupuncture, homeopathy	
disabled (non-functioning limbs)	acupuncture, homeopathy, osteopathy	
eczema	acupuncture, homeopathy	
emotional disorders (excluding somatization)	acupuncture, homeopathy	
eye and mouth disorders	acupuncture, homeopathy	
gynaecological problems	prolapse/endometriosis/menstrual: acupuncture, homeopathy	
	infertility: homeopathy	
headaches (stress/fatigue)	acupuncture, homeopathy, osteopathy	
insomnia	acupuncture, homeopathy	
hypertension	acupuncture, homeopathy	consider homeopathy during pregnancy?
musculoskeletal problems	acupuncture, osteopathy	exclude organic pathology and inflammatory conditions
stroke	acute and rehab: acupuncture, homeopathy, osteopathy	
tinnitus	acupuncture, homeopathy, osteopathy	
viral conditions	acupuncture, homeopathy	
common childhood disorders	homeopathy	

Box 4.6 The Lewisham guidelines for referral to complementary practitioners: acupuncture, homeopathy and osteopathy

Acupuncture
Acupuncture is a branch of Traditional Chinese Medicine that uses an integrated system of diagnosis incorporating tongue observation and pulse reading. Developed over 2000 years ago, it is based on the principle that the stimulation of certain areas of the body influences the functioning of the physical organs. The treatment involves the use of sterilized, disposable needles.

Homeopathy
Homeopathy is a system of healing that treats the whole person, not only the presenting symptoms. It is a gentle treatment using highly diluted forms of natural substances to treat people with physical and emotional problems. Useful in acute and chronic conditions, it can also be used to treat patients constitutionally to help prevent the recurrence of an illness.

Osteopathy
Osteopathy is a healthcare system based primarily on the reciprocal interrelationship between structure and function in the human body. Dysfunction of either will result in altered physiology, which may manifest as symptoms and/or illness. The treatment, consisting of manipulation, adjustment of posture and exercise, aims to improve circulation, restore muscle tone and maintain joint integrity.

All treatments can be used together with, or independent of, conventional medical treatment. Discussion between practitioners and referring physicians is encouraged. Patients are encouraged to continue their medically prescribed drugs, which should be reduced only in consultation with the referring physician.

The referral guidelines can be used to identify which therapy is most useful for the patient's condition. Where two or more

therapies might be used the following guidelines might be helpful:

- patient preference or history of use
- needle phobia (rules out acupuncture)
- patient may not like being touched (this may rule out osteopathy and acupuncture)
- patient is unable to attend weekly (this may rule out acupuncture and osteopathy).

an outpatient basis, taking referrals from GPs and hospital consultants. The proposal outlined the service that was to be provided, including the referral guidelines. It also included details of how practitioners would be chosen to provide the services, including relevant qualifications, registration with professional bodies and insurance/liability cover. As a pilot scheme, a full evaluation of the project was to be included in the service, with plans to develop the service according to the evaluation results.

In September 1993 this proposal was submitted to LSLHA, and in April 1994 the health authority agreed to fund the service for the 1994–1995 financial year. Rooms within the hospital were refurbished and staff recruited so that the Lewisham Complementary Therapy Centre could begin treating patients on 4 July 1994. The service evaluated positively, showing improvements in health status as measured by the SF-36 health survey.[36] It was fully occupied with referrals from local GPs until its demise in 1997 when the health authority withdrew funding.

The Glastonbury study*

The Somerset Trust for Integrated Health Care was established to support an integrated CT and conventional medical service within a three-partner NHS primary care practice (initially in Glastonbury). Between 1994 and 1997, it undertook a systematic evaluation of the benefits patients received from the CTs and what the service contributed to the overall running of the practice. It subsequently undertook a cost–benefit study with a subsample of the patients (those with long-term health problems). The aim of this was to determine whether, in this group, CT treatment resulted in any reduction in costs, in terms of reduced referrals to secondary care and reduced usage of other health services (e.g. prescriptions, visits to the GP and diagnostic tests such as radiography). The stated aim was to demonstrate that: 'this approach is more beneficial to patients, and at least as cost effective to the NHS, as the present system based entirely on conventional medicine. Our aim was to establish a model of integrated primary health care that is clinically effective, cost effective and transferable to other GP practices.'[25] This second stage was completed in May 2000.

The CT programme

Patients were offered a total of 3 hours of treatment, usually split between four to six appointments, in one of the following CTs: acupuncture, herbal medicine, homeopathy, massage and osteopathy. Patients were referred from the GP, and were assessed before and after their course of treatment.

In the first phase of the project the programme was funded by Somerset Health Authority as part of the Health Promotion Initiative, and then as a health authority research programme. This enabled the practice to offer CT treatment for free. When this funding ended in 1997, alternative funds were needed and two mechanisms were established to provide these. First, patients were charged £6 a session for treatment—the price being set at a level considered manageable by most of the patients themselves; however, this was below the actual cost to the practice for providing the CT (£9–12 a session). Secondly, a practice-based charitable trust was set up: the Somerset Trust for Integrated Health Care. This currently subsidizes the CTs by about £6 per patient appointment.

---

* Summarized from Hills D, Welford R 2000 Complementary therapy in general practice: an evaluation of the Glastonbury Health Centre complementary medicine service. Website: www.integratedhealth.org.uk

The number of sessions received by patients was kept flexible to accommodate the different requirements of each therapy. In osteopathy, patients received an initial 1 hour appointment then four half-hour appointments; in massage they received four three-quarter hour sessions; in acupuncture, herbalism and homeopathy there were six half-hour treatments. Initially, all sessions apart from those with the herbalist were booked to be once weekly. Later, this system became more flexible, CPs arranging their own appointments after the initial appointment.

Between 1994 and 1997, around 600 patients were referred to the service (around 17% of the practice population). The majority (71%) were patients with long-term, chronic health conditions, most commonly musculoskeletal problems (59%)—particularly long-term back or joint pain. Another significant group (15%) had psychosocial problems related to anxiety, stress or depression. The remainder had nervous, respiratory, genitourinary or gastrointestinal problems, and many had multiple problems. Two-thirds of patients described their problems as either 'severe' or 'very severe', while a significant proportion (34%) were referred because their problem had failed to respond to more conventional treatments.

GPs referred patients to CT for a variety of reasons, frequently because the patients themselves had requested it. Patients were more likely to request CT when suffering from long-term problems, and when their problem was not musculoskeletal or psychosocial in nature; they were most likely to request herbalism or osteopathy.

Management of the system

Running a CT service alongside other primary healthcare activities placed a considerable extra burden on the administrative resources of the practice, and a special system of appointments had to be initiated. The problems were that the numbers of sessions available each week for each therapy were quite limited; each CP was available for just half a day each week, and the number of sessions varied from therapy to therapy. To ensure patients had continuity of treatment once this had been started, appointments were booked on a block basis of between four and six sessions at weekly intervals. This, however, was a considerable challenge to the normal reception service and the computerized appointment system, so an administrator was made responsible for handling the CT service. Later in the project, the computer appointment system was adapted and a terminal set up in the CPs room so they could make appointments directly with their patients.

As a result of the popularity of the service, lengthy waiting lists built up, particularly for osteopathy and acupuncture. Patients sometimes had to wait for up to

4 or 5 months for appointments. This made referral for short-term problems pointless. A priority system instituted for 'acute cases' simply added to the length of wait for those with less-urgent problems, which discouraged GPs from referring acute cases. This was particularly unfortunate given that one of the project's findings was that patients with shorter-term problems showed the greatest improvement following treatment.

Various steps were taken to reduce waiting lists, including closing the lists for a couple of months when they become too long. When charges were first introduced the waiting lists reduced rapidly, but built up again as these became accepted, though not quite to the former level.

Meetings

In the initial stages of the project neither the CPs nor the GPs knew much about each other's work. In order to overcome this lack of knowledge, each practitioner was asked to write a brief description about his or her therapy, and the conditions for which it was particularly appropriate.

In addition to this, there were regular lunchtime meetings at which CPs and GPs met, which took place every 3 months. Their main aim was service administration, and any research activities attached to this. In addition, there were occasional evening meetings set up specifically for professional exchange.

Aims and research methodology

Discussion amongst members of the practice, CPs and the health authority had produced the following research questions:

- What contribution can CT make to primary healthcare?
- Which patients can benefit from CT?
- What are the advantages and disadvantages for the practice of having a CT service?
- Can such a service be cost effective?

To answer these questions, several methods were used. First, GPs and CPs completed referral forms on all referrals to the service. These forms included information about the patient, the illness, the treatment selected and an outcome assessment. Secondly, questionnaires were given to patients on referral, on completion of the course of treatment and 6 months after referral. The questionnaires used were: the SF-36 to measure overall well-being, the Functional Limitation Profile (FLP) Index to assess pain, and patient satisfaction forms. Lastly, interviews were conducted with a sample of patients, with practitioners and other health service staff.

Outcomes were measured by patients' self-assessment of improvement, CPs' assessment of change and changes in scores on SF-36 scales between referral and completion of treatment. The questionnaire completed by patients included questions about the impact of treatment on their problem management and coping strategies, and their satisfaction with treatment.

Evaluation of outcomes

Response rates on the questionnaires were reasonable initially, but subsequently fell off: 82% of questionnaires were returned following referral, 76% on completion of treatment and 56% at 6 months after referral. Only a small proportion of patients completed all three.

Analysis of these revealed 85% of patients to have reported some or much improvement in their condition after treatment, which the majority ascribed to the treatment itself. A similar number reported they were either 'very' or 'mostly' satisfied with their treatment. This contrasted with the ratings of CPs, who considered 11% of the problems treated to be very much improved or resolved, and a further 57% to show some improvement. Scores on the SF-36 health and well-being scale also showed a significant improvement for the majority of patients. Treatments seemed to be most effective in those with more severe symptoms, or with problems of shorter duration, and in the relief of pain in those with musculoskeletal problems, or of social and emotional distress in those with psychosocial problems.

In general there was reasonable agreement between patient- and practitioner-assessed outcomes, but a low level of correspondence between patient-assessed outcomes and SF-36 scores. This discrepancy may be partly due to the variability in the patient population, as a breakdown of scores according to different patient groups (by main symptoms) revealed a closer correspondence between self-assessed outcome and SF-36 scores.

The SF-36 scale proved to be quite a sensitive measure, nevertheless. There were significant improvements on all dimensions (apart from the general health dimension) between referral and completion of treatment, with most dimensions showing a continuing, though lesser, improvement at 6 months.

Patient satisfaction The CT service is popular with patients: 75% described themselves as generally or very satisfied with their treatment and 96% said that they had found the treatment useful. This level of satisfaction is perhaps surprising given the frequent apparent mismatch between patients' expectations of treatment and the actual outcome in terms of improvement in condition, or of explanation and understanding. However, generally patients had modest expectations of CTs. Only a small proportion expected full recovery after treatment, and less than a third of those with long-term problems (of a year or more) expected any major improvement whatsoever, while patients with emotional problems had significantly lower expectations than did those with primarily physical problems.

The main cause of dissatisfaction was the number and length of sessions: 65% thought that there had been too few sessions, and 33% felt that the sessions themselves had been too short. Some felt that they were just beginning to see some improvement when the sessions came to an end and, although it was possible to ask for further referrals, actually this often meant going to the end of the waiting list, resulting in a break of several months between sets of sessions.

Which patients benefit from CT?

There is currently very little information available on those patients, and conditions, most likely to respond best to a particular therapy. However, one finding was that those who had their problems for over a year showed significantly less change in their condition following treatment, compared with those referred with shorter-term problems. This suggests that if CT were used more for patients with acute and short-term problems, the results in terms of patient improvement may have been even more marked.

Conclusions

The annual costs of providing CT were approximately £17 000 (these included CP time, administrative time and additional costs such as herbal medicines or acupuncture needles but not practice overheads such as room rent, heating, lighting, and so on). These costs must be balanced against those of providing conventional treatment.

For instance, the subsample of patients (41) with long-term problems received, between them, 48 sets of referrals to CT; the cost of treating them with CT would have been around £2600. Following their initial CT treatment, there was for most a marked reduction in the use of other health services for the problem referred, the largest reduction occurring in those who had been the heaviest users of other services prior to referral. Visits to GPs dropped by around a third, the largest reduction coming from the 11 patients who had visited their GP most often prior to referral. The reduction in the number of prescriptions was even more marked, and again it was in the high-user group that the largest reduction took place.

A similar reduction was seen in the numbers of further referrals, tests and other treatments required by the group for the condition referred, particularly in referrals for physiotherapy and X-rays. Since the service had been

set up in 1992, it had received around 1000 referrals. The majority of these (around 650) were for musculoskeletal problems, with a further small but significant group (around 120) with psychosocial problems; patients with such problems are generally referred to physiotherapy, consultants in orthopaedic surgery and rheumatology, or the community mental health team. In the Glastonbury practice referrals of this kind were generally quite high. However, examination of their records revealed that referrals for orthopaedic surgery and physiotherapy had reduced since the setting up of the CT service, whereas psychiatric referrals, after an initial increase, had levelled off. This contrasted favourably with the rise in similar referrals elsewhere, and supported the findings that the availability of complementary medicine had reduced demands on other health service resources.

The researchers subsequently analysed the savings made from the reduction in the use of other health services. It was estimated that the average costs to the NHS of this subgroup of patients (assuming, for example, an average number of sessions for physiotherapy, complementary medicine, etc. or an X-ray of average cost) were slightly over £4000 in conventional treatments in the year prior to referral. After treatment these costs reduced to just over £1500—a saving of around £2500. Table 4.4 summarizes the estimated costs before and after CT treatment.

Although in the practice secondary referral costs are very unevenly spread (referrals to the mental health team for counselling and referrals to consultants being the major expenditures) the savings made by this group of patients in the year following CT referral more or less covered the cost of the CT provided (approx. £2570). If this group is representative of the subgroup of patients with long-term problems, the amount saved per annum would be around £7500, which is almost half of the annual cost of providing the service.

This result is supported by the analysis of referrals to secondary care. When costs were estimated, the results suggested that the overall saving in secondary referrals in the year 1995/96 was over £18 000 (Table 4.5).

The results from this 3-year experiment indicated that CT was widely welcomed by patients, and appeared to be effective in a wide range of health problems, particularly for short-term, severe conditions and for musculoskeletal conditions, even though most referrals were patients with longer-term health problems.

The cost-benefit study of the use of the service by a subsample of patients with long-term health problems indicated that cost savings had been achieved through a reduction of referrals to secondary care, and a reduction in usage of other health services (GP time, prescriptions, radiographs and other tests) in the year following complementary medicine treatment. Cost savings from these sources almost matched the cost of the treatments

Table 4.5 Total costs before and after complementary therapy

	In year before treatment		In year after treatment		
	No. of sessions	Total costs (£)	No. of sessions	Total costs (£)	Difference (£)
medication		691.69		309.22	382.47
GP sessions (£7.62)	128	975.36	88	670.56	304.80
physiotherapy (£63)	7	441	2	126	315
counselling (£520)	2	1040			1040
X-ray (£17.50)	8	140	4	70	70
blood/urine tests (£7.50)	4	30	3	22.50	7.50
consultant referrals (£195)	7	1365	5	975	390
Total		**4683.03**		**2173.28**	**2509.77**

FromHills D, Welford R 2000 Complementary therapy in general practice: an evaluation of the Glastonbury Health Centre complementary medicine service, with permission.

Table 4.6 Comparison between referral costs from Glastonbury and from other practices in Somerset*

Type of referral	Difference between actual and hypothesized referrals in 1995/96*	Hypothesized cost savings (£)
Orthopaedic consultations (£195)**	70.9	13 825.5
Rheumatology consultations (£195)	−7.4	−1 443
Physiotherapy (£63)	91.7	5 777.1
Total	**155.2**	**18 159.6***

* From Hills D, Welford R 2000 Complementary therapy in general practice: an evaluation of the Glastonbury Health Centre complementary
   medicine service, with permission. These figures are adjusted for the increased size of the practice in 1991/2 and 1995/6
** This price is only for consultations, and not the cost of surgery, hospital bed, physiotherapy, etc.

provided by the CT service. Therefore, this study provides evidence that a CT service is at least cost neutral, as its costs are balanced by savings made elsewhere in the primary care service, and may be cost effective.

CAN COMPLEMENTARY MEDICINE BE COST EFFECTIVE?*

In the Glastonbury study, CTs appeared to stabilize secondary referrals to orthopaedic, rheumatology, physiotherapy and psychiatry, whereas the average for the county rose by 30% over the same period. When the researchers analysed the patient records, they surmised there was effectively a fall in orthodox healthcare costs resulting from CT use, and this largely covered the cost of providing the CTs. This was only limited evidence, however, as there was no control group to indicate what would have happened *without* CTs.

Do other studies concur with this conclusion? There are currently very few studies addressing this question. In a report of 10 models of provision of CT in primary care, GPs had the impression that CTs paid for themselves. It is revealing, however, that these GPs were not prepared to purchase any more CTs unless additional funds were available (i.e. they did not consider CTs to be self-funding).[26]

* This section draws on material presented by A White in the paper 'Are complementary therapies cost effective?' presented at the NHS Alliance conference on primary Care Groups and complementary medicine, University of Exeter, 2 September 1999.

Some studies have looked at the effect of providing a single CT. For instance, one primary care practice made homeopathy available for specified conditions, and found that subsequent GP consultations fell from 3.1 to 0.9 per annum.[27] However, the conclusions that can be drawn from this study are limited as the results were calculated in only a subgroup of patients.

In another primary care centre, acupuncture was offered for musculoskeletal pain to carefully selected patients, and an analysis was made of the costs of providing this service, including treatment purchase costs and estimated alternative referral costs if acupuncture had not been available.[28] The researchers concluded the average costs per patient to be £182 for acupuncture and £352 for alternative referral. However, once again because of criticisms that may be made about the study design only limited conclusions can be drawn.

It is the manipulative therapies that have been the subject of most economic analysis. Meade and coworkers[29] compared chiropractic and hospital outpatient treatment and concluded that extending the provision of chiropractic throughout the UK would increase health costs by £4m per annum. Three other controlled trials of spinal manipulative therapy that included economic analysis also concluded that manipulation does not reduce health service costs of back pain.[30–32] One of these indicated that the highest total direct outpatient cost per episode of low back pain was for chiropractors.[30] One obvious reason is that, on average, chiropractors use more consultations per episode of back pain than other professionals.[33] However, studies with other designs sometimes provide the opposite results.[34]

Herbal medicines likewise are becoming accepted as effective, but not necessarily cost effective. *Hypericum* for moderate depression and *Gingko biloba* for intermittent claudication appear effective,[35] but not demonstrably cheaper, than the conventional alternatives. However, saw palmetto for benign prostatic hypertrophy is both effective and may well also be considerably cheaper than conventional drug or surgical treatment, although long-term studies are still awaited. (This leaves aside the salient question of whether there is any difference in side-effects of the alternative treatment options.)

So, do CTs save money for healthcare systems? At this stage it can only be said that there are some positive indications, but that no definite conclusions are yet possible, as most of the rigorous studies do not provide clear evidence that it does.

NEW DEVELOPMENTS IN THE MARYLEBONE PCG: DISSEMINATING THE APPROACH

Marylebone Primary Care Group is developing a locality-based CT service. With equity rising to the top of the NHS modernization agenda it seems that one way of protecting public sector CT services is to ensure that they become more widely available. So the local practices where CTs are available have agreed to open their doors to patients of other GPs—10% of all our CP appointments in the first year and 20% in the second year. Fortunately the PCG has found some new money to increase our CP sessions. We think the key to appropriate referrals is the linked education programme for GPs—two 3-hour sessions discussing with the CPs involved what they can and can't do, and to help the GPs get to grips with the information and audit system we are putting in place, which will be much the same as the MHC system. But still the service will be under a lot of pressure so, with the numbers of eligible patients growing suddenly from around 10 000 to 80 000, even though we have tightened up our intake guidelines and capped the number of sessions at six per patient, we expect waiting lists to swell quite quickly.

We expect the osteopathy and acupuncture services to be in greatest demand. We are relatively well supported here though—a locality back pain clinic with physio, osteopathy and a psychologist, plus the GP-based roll-out involving six osteopathy sessions a week. The acupuncture provision is growing to five sessions a week too, along with as many homeopathy sessions. Practitioners have stipulated that they want to focus on common conditions where these therapies seem particularly likely to be helpful so we intend to use the MHC guidelines as the service expands. In addition there will be classes for people with chronic degenerative and inflammatory disorders who want to explore the naturopathic approach to nutrition and exercise.

SUMMARY

Quality assurance and cost effectiveness have become crucial issues in the purchasing and evaluation of health technology and they imply a need for rationing and prioritization, and possibly also suggest that real-world health gain will become an important consideration. These are important messages for CTs in the public sector, so how we as practitioner–researchers respond will determine whether they survive in this sector. The four accounts given in this chapter as examples of service integration and evaluation demonstrate that it is possible to introduce CT provision into primary care in ways that are transparent and accountable. At the present stage of development these services have the capacity to keep track of clinical activity in ways that allow sample outcomes to be assessed. Various measures of CT's effectiveness can be continually evaluated, and early impressions confirm clinical benefits and high levels of patient satisfaction. There are also grounds for suspecting that these approaches might effect significant reductions in demand on other healthcare services.

REFERENCES

1. Hammond C 1995 The complete family guide to homeopathy. Penguin Books, New York
2. Maxwell R 1992 Dimensions of quality revisited: from thought to action. Quality in healthcare 1:171–177
3. Patterson C 1996 Measuring outcomes in primary care: a patient generated measure, MYMOP, compared to the SF36 health survey. British Medical Journal 312:1016–1020
4. Peters D, Davies P, Pietroni P 1994 Musculo-skeletal clinic in general practice—a study of one year's referrals. British Journal of General Practice 44:25–29
5. Reason P, Chase HD, Desser A et al 1992 Towards a clinical framework for collaboration between general and complementary practitioners. Journal of the Royal Society of Medicine 85:161–164
6. Reason P 1991 Power and conflict in multidisciplinary collaboration. Complementary Medical Research, pp 144–150
7. Peters D 1994 Collaboration between complementary and conventional practitioners. In: Sharm U, Budd S, eds. The Healing Bond. Routledge, London, pp 171–192
8. Pietroni P 1992 Beyond the boundaries—the relationship between general practice and complementary medicine. British Medical Journal 305:564–566
9. Cyriax J 1982 Textbook of orthopaedic medicine, vol 1, 8th edn. Baillière Tindall, London

10. Travell J, Simons D 1983 Myofascial pain and dysfunction, vol 1. Williams and Wilkins, London
11. Linton S J 1986 Behavioural remediation of chronic pain: a status report. Pain 24:125–141
12. McCauley J D, Thelen M H, Frank R G, Willard R R, Callen K E 1984 Hypnosis compared to relaxation in the outpatient management of chronic low back pain. Archives of Physical Medicine and Rehabilitation 64:548–552
13. MacDonald R S, Dell C M J 1990 An open controlled assessment of osteopathic manipulation in non specific low back pain. Spine 15:364–370.
14. MacDonald R S, Peters D 1986 Osteopathy. Practitioner 230:1073–1076
15. Bradlow J, Coulter A, Brookes P 1992 Patterns of referral. Health Services Research Unit, University of Oxford
16. Peters D, Davies P. Rapid audit cycles: an approach to introducing and evaluating a complementary therapy service into general practice, in preparation
17. Richardson J 1995 Complementary therapies on the NHS: the experience of a new service. Complementary Therapies in Medicine 3:153–157
18. Richardson J 1995 Complementary therapy on the NHS: a service evaluation of the first year of an outpatient service in a local district general hospital. Lewisham Hospital NHS Trust, London
19. Richardson J, Brennan A 1995 Complementary therapy in the NHS: service development in a local district general hospital. Complementary Therapies in Nursing and Midwifery 1:89–92
20. Worth C, Richardson R 1995 Complementary therapies—a real alternative? British Journal of Health Care Management 1(10):494–496
21. British Medical Association 1993 Complementary medicine: new approaches to good practice. Oxford University Press, Oxford
22. Cameron-Blackie G 1993 Complementary therapies in the NHS. Research paper number 10. National Association of Health Authorities and Trusts, London
23. Jones J, Hunter D 1995 Consensus methods for medical and health services research. British Medical Journal 311:376–380
24. Eddy D M 1990 Practice policies—guidelines for methods. Journal of the American Medical Association 263(13):1836–1841
25. Hills D, Welford R 2000 Complementary therapy in general practice: an evaluation of the Glastonbury Health Centre complementary medicine service. integratedhealth.org.uk
26. Luff D, Thomas K 1999 Models of complementary therapy provision in primary care. University of Sheffield, Sheffield
27. Christie E A, Ward A T 1996 Report on NHS practice-based homoeopathy project. Society of Homoeopaths, Northampton.
28. Lindall S 1999 Is acupuncture for pain relief in general practice cost-effective? Acupuncture in Medicine 17(2):97–100
29. Meade T W, Dyer S, Browne W, Townsend J, Frank A O 1990 Low back pain of mechanical origin: randomized comparison of chiropractic and hospital outpatient treatment. British Medical Journal 300:1431–1437
30. Carey T S, Garrett J, Jackman A, McLaughlin C, Fryer J, Smucker D R 1995 The outcomes and costs of care for acute low back pain among patients seen by primary care practitioners, chiropractors, and orthopedic surgeons. New England Journal of Medicine 333(14):913–917
31. Cherkin D C, Deyo R A, Battie M, Street J, Barlow W 1998 A comparison of physical therapy, chiropractic manipulation, and provision of an educational booklet for the treatment of patients with low back pain. New England Journal of Medicine 339(15):1021–1029
32. Skargren E I, Carlsson P G, Oberg B E 1998 One-year follow-up comparison of the cost and effectiveness of chiropractic and physiotherapy as primary management for back pain. Spine 23:1875–1884
33. Shekelle P G, Markovich M, Louie R 1995 Comparing the costs between provider types of episodes of back pain care. Spine 20:221–227
34. Stano M, Smith M 1996 Chiropractic and medical costs of low back care. Medical Care 34:191–204
35. White A 1999 Are complementary therapies cost effective? Paper presented at NHS Alliance conference on primary care groups and complementary medicine, University of Exeter, 2 September 1999
36. Richardson J 2001 Developing and evaluating complementary therapy services. Part 2. Examining the effect of treatment on health status. Journal of Alternative and Complementary Medicine: Research on Paradigm, Practice and Policy (in press)

Chapter 4 REFLECTIVE LEARNING CYCLE AUDIT

1. **What did you need to know?** *(clarify learning objectives)*

2. **What did you notice?** *(key points)*

3. **What have you learned?** *(learning evaluation)*

4. **How will you apply it to practice?** *(clinical relevance)*

5. **What do I need to do next?** *(reflective educational audit)*

6. **Proceed to next area of interest / section you have identified.**

5

Reflecting on and adapting the service

INTRODUCTION

So far we have described how we approached the integration of CTs, how they were introduced and how we assessed their impact on patient care. The final stage in the action research cycle involves adapting the service. Once outcomes have been evaluated and it is worth spending some time reflecting on them, and on experiences, events and questions that have arisen during the course of delivering the service. Feedback from all the participants is helpful. Information from study results, personal reports, review meetings, and general reflection upon events and issues can be used to shape the next phase of design, implementation and reflection. In this chapter we use the example of how our team had to reflect on our experience at the MHC, and decide how to take the next steps.

FEEDBACK ON THE SERVICE
The MHC Project summarized

Our original mission statement had three key elements:

- to provide high-quality integrated health and community care in the face of continuing NHS policy change and declining resources
- to aim for a sustainable level of collaboration and interprofessional practice
- to maintain a focus on reflective practice and innovative approaches to healthcare delivery in the context of the needs of individuals, families and the community.

The Marylebone Project has tried to meet patient needs through integrated care pathways, and to deliver them effectively and through sustainable multiprofessional practice. Throughout our 15 years of working at the centre, patients and doctors alike have continued to express considerable interest in integrating CTs into a primary care setting.

Our core questions about CT use included the following:

- What needs are being met?
- How can we work collaboratively?
- What is the evidence base?
- What are the most appropriate referral procedures?
- How are treatments selected?
- What quality assurance procedures are relevant?
- How are CT practice and the necessary reflection time to be funded?

At the start of the Smith Project GPs and CPs had been working together at MHC for 10 years—enough time for good working relationships to be established. During this time there has been a growing emphasis within primary care as a whole on: evidence-based care, cost effectiveness, assuring quality of care, increasing patient participation, and introducing computerized databases. There has also been an enormous increase in the interest and demand for CTs within both public healthcare and the private sector. So by the mid 1990s the time was clearly right to design and deliver a CT service fit for this new climate and one that could serve as a generally useful model for CTs in primary care settings. The service was not intended to be comprehensive, but rather to find ways of using CTs that are appropriate to the public sector with its many constraints. The project therefore became implicitly a way of gathering evidence to support wider provision of effective CTs in the NHS. The project had to develop a generalizable approach, which could be used as the basis for implementing CTs in other centres. Though the project entailed mainly reactive, practice-based work, we also explored possibilities for proactive healthcare delivery in the local community and emphasized the use of the role of 'self-help' techniques in the management of chronic problems. We have had to consider how we work collaboratively and how our respective clinical theories, roles and practice are affected by working in an extended primary care team. A great deal of time was taken up consolidating multiprofessional learning and working, but this has allowed us to develop trust and a sense of team cohesion. This has meant challenging some assumptions about the desirability and practicability of shared working. We have learned that we can progress from working alongside one other to really working together only by first understanding each other's working worlds.

Working together

Some basic questions about the nature of the collaborative work kept recurring:

- Who is complementary to whom?
- How are we complementary to one another?
- Why should we complement one another?
- Do we want to work together?
- Is it possible to complement one another?
- Are we complementary in name but alternative in nature?

The following important clinical management themes emerged:

- the difficulty in maintaining continuity of patient care
- whether it should always be a GP who directs clinical activity
- how to find a common professional language to formulate diagnoses and clinical objectives
- practitioners' and patients' inflated expectations of integrated treatment and management
- the difficult dynamics of multidisciplinary intergroup power, rivalry and envy.

We now have in place the basics for delivering a quality-assured computer-based CT service, which makes effective use of limited resources and aims at fully involving patients making informed choices about their CT care. We have also organized a developmental process revolving around regular discussion and decision-making meetings and a staff development programme that helps team members to acquire new knowledge and skills. Reaching this point has involved a series of reflective learning cycles, the essential components of which included:

- involving everyone concerned in decision making
- building on our experience
- working to short-term achievable goals
- agreeing long-term goals
- a willingness to contribute to cross-discipline decisions
- a willingness to listen and understand the points of view and difficulties of other health professionals
- patience and tolerance
- coping with uncertainty (and, at times, confusion and frustration)
- a willingness to learn and use new skills
- time for reflection (always in short supply).

Cooperative action meetings

Reports produced by the data system became the focus for regular discussions. Lunchtime weekly meetings were a chance to consider both organizational issues and interprofessional dynamics, and though these could be challenging we were nevertheless encouraged to continue our project. Everyone involved in this work at Marylebone regards it as 'work in progress'.

Our findings

We have found that:

- practical guidelines were acceptable to doctors, patients and practitioners
- it was possible to introduce rigour into the provision of a CT service in general practice
- it is feasible to introduce a patient-centred outcome measure into the referral and treatment cycle
- clear lines of communication can be established between CPs and GPs
- structured action research can be used to manage CT 'packages of care'
- in a resource-constrained system such as NHS practice, treatment numbers have to be rationed
- a computer-based, networked data system is essential.

Feedback from different groups

It is valuable at this stage to obtain feedback from each of the different groups that are participating in the CT service, including the patients.

The GPs' experience

Some comments from the GPs involved in the MHC project were as follows:

I have worked alongside alternative and complementary therapists in one way or another since I first became a GP principal in 1976. I have always valued having access to the widest possible range of treatment options for my patients, for my family and friends, and for myself.

I welcome treatments that are safe and effective and conventional medical and surgical treatments are of course often neither safe nor effective. I welcome also the attitude that is often (though not always) inherent in alternative and complementary therapies, an attitude that embraces holism, respect for the individual, the subtleties and complexities of illness, and the need for listening and time. Many of these approaches draw on vast bodies of knowledge and experience.

I regularly refer to osteopathy, acupuncture, homeopathy, naturopathy and massage therapy. I have also seen people benefit from a range of other therapies, from Alexander technique, dance therapy and herbal treatments to qigong, tai chi and yoga. Often these treatments complement conventional treatments; sometimes they are true alternatives.

I try to combine open-mindedness with a healthy scepticism about both conventional and alternative treatments. Cost is always a consideration. I support the current drive towards evaluating all treatments and regulating all practitioners as long as the evaluation and regulation are fair and well informed.

The wide range of approaches to helping human distress is endlessly fascinating. Cross-fertilization between different approaches is increasingly common. I cannot now imagine working without having access to such a broad palette of possibilities. In purely practical terms both staff and patients seem to benefit.

Richard Morrison

The chance to develop a way of auditing our CT service seemed like a very exciting idea at the time. It was obvious that we should be making some attempt to assess patients' perceptions and practitioners' perceptions about the use of complementary therapy in the primary care setting.

But I found it surprisingly difficult to get going with the paperwork. It took me a long time to familiarize myself with what I now feel to be a very simple process. We started the project at a time of increased pressure in the consultation. Increasing use of the computer and generally less time meant that we are under enormous pressure to fit everything in within a 10 minute consultation and having to think about criteria for referral and then asking the patient to fill in the MYMOP form felt like one thing too many. Although I wasn't always conscious of it, I am sure for a while this project actually reduced my referral rate to complementary therapy because of these factors.

Now I am in a different place. Having rather obsessively learnt how to use the tool and make a quick and efficient referral, I am somewhat dismayed to find that my colleagues are using it erratically, and not only that but as ever there are resource constraints which make it very difficult to get the maximum analysis and use out of the data that we have so laboriously collected.

Sue Morrison

I think my knowledge was very minimal, my knowledge has increased because of speaking with the complementary therapists and asking if a particular thing would be useful if it was referred and if it was treated. We produced some leaflets about the therapies which I think are fantastic and I find useful to give to people to look at before they come back to me.

Assistant GP

The CPs' experience

What has been the impact of the development work on the CPs so far? Not surprisingly they feel the process has put them and their discipline under a microscope. Fortunately their sense of colleagues' goodwill and support has made this bearable. All the CPs describe the learning process as having encouraged rigour and enabled reflective practice. So it has helped them bring about a greater clarity of aim and greater discrimination about what can be reasonably achieved in a resource-constrained service.

Some general comments were:

Be prepared for the funding to be insecure. Keep abreast of changes in the area of how posts are funded. Have an agenda for things to learn to make the most of the experience. Be prepared to take the initiative communicating with the GPs both about the scope of the conditions that you can treat and in reporting back on the patient's progress. The importance of informal contact with the GPs can't be overestimated. Don't miss out on building relationships with others in the clinic including the nurses, practice manager and receptionists.

Acupuncturist

[NHS] patients may need different explanations of the therapy and what to expect from it than those who seek us out. It is worth spending a lot of time at the beginning of the course of treatments outlining exactly what to expect from treatment both during the session and talking about what outcome it might be reasonable to expect. It is also very important for them to know that you are working together with their GP.

Acupuncturist

USING MYMOP* CPs expressed some dismay that, in this sample of patients (who in the main express moderate to severe symptoms—often with a psychological component—and poor well-being), MYMOP sometimes failed to register improvements despite CPs' clinical impression of benefit. We subsequently reinterviewed patients in order to clarify why this discrepancy occurred; at this point we suspect that the problem often has more to do with the way MYMOP is used than with a lack of actual benefit of the CTs.

Selina Macnair, a final-year acupuncture student at the University of Westminster, did a project on practitioners' experience of MYMOP and threw further light on this question. The first question that was asked was: 'how has MYMOP changed your practice?'. Among the negative responses were that it could interrupt the flow of the consultation, and that it was inappropriate when the patient was distressed. Its positive effects included:

- it helps both the patient and practitioner to stay focused on the patient's concerns and set goals, and helps practitioners be more thorough
- it makes practitioners more unwilling to take on patients who won't get better, i.e. it encourages appropriate referral
- it encourages patients to feel that their opinions and information are valued
- it makes practitioners more aware of an improvement in a patient's condition, giving precise feedback.

The second question was: 'how do you use MYMOP in your session?'. Most of the practitioners had administered the form at the beginning of the session, though this depended on the therapy. All the practitioners said that the time taken was no more than 3–5 minutes. Some patients had needed more assistance than others to fill in the form, however.

The third question asked was: 'in its present form, what disadvantages do you think MYMOP has?'. Practitioners commented that in many conditions it was meaningless to use numbers, especially in patients with emotional concerns, as these measures were purely arbitrary (for instance, can pain be 'worse than 6'?). Also, the symptoms listed did not always represent the condition itself that the patient was suffering from. Information entered about the immediate conditions of a patient was

not relevant in some conditions—for example, cyclical conditions like PMS. Some patients had also found it hard to score their condition consistently from session to session, as they could not remember what the severity had felt like on previous occasions.

Practitioners had found the system to be inflexible in some respects—for instance, how do you score someone who has improved and then got worse since the last session, or got worse and then got better? Also, in certain therapies such as massage the form did not cater for external factors that were involved in the treatment.

Other criticisms related to the negative effect on the patient–practitioner relationship. Some practitioners commented that they found using MYMOP could close down communication. It had also led to increased patient disappointment, as patients were more aware of any lack of improvement. Finally, some practitioners found that the MYMOP process put extra pressure on them to succeed (or appear to succeed).

The last question practitioners were asked was whether they had any suggestions for how the MYMOP form could be improved. The most notable suggestion was for space to be made available for free text comments, as this would allow any external circumstances that affect treatment to be taken into consideration.

One therapist commented:

The patient comes first. Instead of being able to deal with how a patient has been this week there is a pressure to get on with MYMOPing. I try not to interrupt the flow too much and I can now sort of pull a MYMOP out of someone without disrupting the flow. When someone has really had the most awful week it's very hard to pull them back from that and ask them what score they would give to their tracking symptom! You have to jiggle around a bit. Some weeks it's fine and other weeks it's a bit shambolic but I think we've done our best.

Massage therapist

The patients' experience

Our patients liked the fact that CTs were being made available from within the public health system. It particularly gives those patients who cannot afford to pay for complementary treatments the opportunity to receive them. Patients also appreciated that there are alternatives to conventional therapy that may be able to help them and that there is also a wide range of self-help information available where there is choice about what might help and what they might like to try, and suggestions that do not rely on taking additional medication. Those patients who are already interested in following guidance on healthier living will engage readily with proven health-enhancing activities. Those patients who have less experience, or have less confidence in their ability to help themselves, may be encouraged to try exercises, dietary

---

* Selina Macnair contributed this section on MYMOP discrepancies.

changes or simple supplements (e.g. peppermint for IBS) that fit with their health beliefs and address their experience of illness and attempts at coping with it.

We also wanted to obtain patient views on whether the number of treatments they received was adequate for treating their complaint, if there was any reduction in their use of medication or frequency of illness episodes, or change in coping strategies.

Below are some responses from a small group of patients who were interviewed because their MYMOP outcome scores had indicated little or no change in their main complaint but post-treatment they expressed improvement when the Glasgow Homoeopathic Outcome Score was administered.

Number of treatment sessions

As I understand it, most treatments consist of six sessions—whether it's homeopathy or acupuncture or whatever. But the reckoning is that you get six treatments. And therefore you will see an improvement or not in that time. But I think that as far as I'm concerned, that was nowhere near long enough and maybe the scale is geared to that number of sessions and not to 15 sessions or 12 sessions or whatever—which some people might need. In my case, it was not going to be shown to be better or worse in six weekly sessions. And it didn't happen that way but it did over a long period of time, simply by dint of experience that didn't recur, which has been the cause of my taking it in the first place.

The treatment which I had was allowed to go on which I felt was good thinking because I felt that there was something to be got from it but it was not going to be got in 6 weeks. I feel that the pattern that has happened with me may well not have been possible to try out on other people and that there may be other conditions where a longer series of treatment is really what you need rather than the quick fix thing. I'm not saying that 6 weeks is a quick fix really but by the scale of things it is. I'm immensely pleased with the progress that I've made, because it has made a difference to me. So I'm perfectly willing to cooperate in this interview if it helps other people to learn and to adapt the treatment so that we think more widely about the scope that might be necessary rather than be constrained into a very rigid pattern.

This patient was one of a small number for whom we decided to provide extra treatment as a pilot study for the next phase of our research.

Evidence of improvement with treatment

Man with asthma:
And what happened was that I gradually became aware that the problems had diminished. And both my wife and my friends said, 'look you're getting better'. I certainly wasn't going back asking for more antibiotics by then. And the thing that made me absolutely convinced was that whereas in the winter 1998–9 I really had a bad time, coughing I spent a lot of time coughing. This last winter, I went through the entire winter without getting a cold or flu—these were the things I'd had the previous winter. And I have seemed to have sort of got a resistance to the infections. And having got that far I thought it has to be the acupuncture that's done it.

Man with dermatitis:
The treatment I got I did notice a difference. I did do the course and I think later—I came back a couple of months later—I had been quite a lot better, I feel. It didn't go, but it had calmed down quite a lot. And then a milder course the next time to take, if I felt the trouble starting up, which I did.

And I think it's contained it rather than eradicated the problem completely.

Comments on drug usage

Man with asthma:
I take Becotide at a regular dosage without being able to improve it, so it doesn't go up. But layered on top of that is how much I use the Ventolin. And on the MYMOP score where I went really down it was because in the middle of my treatment I suddenly had a really quite bad attack and so on that occasion I had to start using my Ventolin a lot and so I felt 'I'm really down on this'—I can't pretend otherwise. But then I was able to stop using that and at the present time hardly use it at all. So it has helped. With the Ventolin it has helped a lot. I used it a fair amount when I first started treatment. And at the moment I'm barely using it at all. So that aspect of it has improved. Indeed the last few weeks or so I have gone out and come home and not even thought about the Ventolin and thought I didn't have it with me, did I? It didn't matter.

Man with migraine:
I think it's certainly true that the frequency of the headaches is less. And that's reflected in fact that I've been using less sumatriptan than I was. I think the last lot I got lasted me 6 months whereas normally it lasted me about 3. I don't think I had the sense of kind of instantaneous or very short-term relief from the attacks. I was using more or less the same amount of the medication while I was having the treatment then afterwards it seems to have tailed off. Which is why, I suppose, it is difficult to decide whether the two were actually connected.

Mother of small boy having recurrent infections:
So we started with X and I think the antibiotics went down dramatically and in fact I find that it's all part of giving the child time to mature, his own system or in this case his lungs, to allow them to grow. And now he's much more—he deals with colds and coughs on his own, we don't even have to give him any homeopathic medicine and that so I find that is really an achievement.

Treatment makes patient feel more in control

In this course of treatment I feel much more in the position that I am in control of what's happening to me. I was losing control before I came here on this particular treatment.

Well in my experience one of the things which was quite important with treatment with X was that she really involved us in the whole treatment. What she did was she tried to give us some sort of tools for how to deal with specific situations on our own, which I suppose was also responsible for us being so aware sometimes, and only come when we really need advice. It doesn't mean that my child hasn't had a cough or a crisis or whatever. That means that we can cope with it on our own and when it gets out of hand we come for guidance.

Treatment has lessened frequency of attacks of illness

Well I was warned actually that it might actually get worse. And I did seem to have one or two particularly nasty headaches at that time. And I suppose I must have been about once a week or once a fortnight having a session. And since then the frequency of the headaches has been less.

General comments from patients who had expressed improvement with treatment

The treatment was very good. I saw the osteopath over a period of a few weeks and have had no more problems since that time. There's not much I can change. I am 78 years of age. I take a lot of medication but for other problems, not the reason for seeing the osteopath. I used to need a walking stick but now no longer do. It has certainly improved the quality of my life. I would say to people go along it worked for me. I would like more but luckily at the moment I don't need it.

The treatment I received was excellent. The GP referred me because of back pain, the only limitation was that I could only have four treatments. At the time treatment was really beneficial. Now 6 months later I need more. I didn't use much medication in the first place. I chose to register with MHC in the first place because of the complementary therapies. I got some good advice. I do it and get a great deal from it. The lack of ongoing treatment is a problem for me, I would love some more.

I am very pleased with the service at MHC. Very beneficial—I had very bad backache, I was in a state. It didn't vanish, but I feel much better, I know I'm not going to be cured completely but I am much better. I am happy. My quality of life is much better. I would recommend anyone to have acupuncture. I would love to have more if it was possible.

Treatment at MHC helped in the main part and carrying on with the self-help treatment at home. I have made a full recovery—minus the odd crick—the self-help exercise really loosened up my neck. I didn't take much medication anyway. The changes I have made have been through using the exercises. I only needed to have massage therapy for a while. I had enough treatment to start me off.

Patients' perceptions of using MYMOP* During the pilot phase of the project a small sample of patients (17) who had experienced the use of MYMOP were asked for their opinions. We wanted specifically to inquire into:

- the reliability of the MYMOP instrument
- the appropriateness of its use during consultations.

On the question of reliability, patients felt MYMOP was a good representation of how they felt both when they were asked and when they were shown their MYMOP graph at the end of a semistructured interview. The majority felt they were easy to use. It was found, however, that people experiencing emotional problems felt it was more difficult to fill out. For instance, the word 'symptom' was seen as problematic to those with emotional problems and they preferred to use the word 'problem'. Those with physical problems found these easier to label and also easier to pick two symptoms. Some patients with intermittent problems also found these hard to score. The wording of the form favoured those

who saw CPs weekly. The comments below underline such patients' perceived difficulties, many of which were already becoming apparent to the practitioners (see previous section). Because of this we used the results of this research as the basis for a staff development session with practitioners using MYMOP.

Some of the comments on MYMOP reliability included:

- *Emotional problems were more difficult to choose:*
'With a psychological problem sometimes people cannot put their finger on exactly what is wrong with them . . . they know they don't feel OK but they cannot quite pinpoint what the problem is. . . . '

'I found it very difficult to define a specific problem. I went to see (my CP) just generally not feeling well and that made it hard to define any one or two symptoms that I really wanted treating.'

- *Difficulty in scoring the problem on a numbered scale:*
'If I said to you ' "how are you feeling this morning on a scale of 1–6?" how would you answer? You'd have to think for a minute or two.'

- *Difficulty in choosing between numbers:*
'Difficult to get the balance of these gradations...to distinguish between 2 and 3, you know, and 4 and 5. So it was all very much hit and miss.'

'Sometimes the differences are very minimal, you can't really move from one number to another.'

- *Use of numbers was irrelevant to their problem:*
'Fertility is an issue of all or nothing; the numbers are irrelevant.'

- *Intermittent problems were more difficult to score:*
'My emotional problems would come in one big burst and then in between I would be as happy as Larry, so it probably depended on what I was feeling at the time.'

On the question of appropriateness for use during consultation, only one patient said that filling in the MYMOP form took any significant time away from the consultation. There was some valuable feedback obtained on how patients had experienced the process of filling out the form. They felt it was important to:

- have the impression that MYMOP is an important part of the consultation
- be reminded of the reasons they are being asked to use MYMOP; some patients were not remembering the explanation and didn't therefore know that MYMOP might also benefit them directly as well as contributing towards the 'greater good'
- understand why they are being asked to fill out the form
- be given a very clear explanation of the form

---

* This piece of research was carried out by Harriet Landenburg, a medical student taking part of her course with us.

- be given enough time to think about their answers; some patients felt they wanted to fill the form in themselves—this helps cut out practitioner bias, and patients could spend more time on the form
- fill out the form at the beginning of the consultation.

Experiences of using the self-help leaflets MHC patients were pleased that we had written a set of leaflets specifically for them. (Although these were general in nature, as they were given to patients only within the context of their consultation the advice could be tailored to each patient as needed.) Patients did suggest some improvements to the leaflets, however, including:

- they should contain less information
- instructions for exercises should be clearer and contain more diagrams and pictures
- visually there was too much text.

We are continuing to develop and strengthen the self-care arm of the service. Leaflets, classes and groups are part of an ongoing attempt to engage with and motivate patients with chronic and relapsing problems. We also feel certain that in any service where CTs are in short supply they have to be seen as part of a package that aims to identify the key areas health improvement and self-management.

Meetings and reports

Regular audit meetings have become a necessity. At these meetings, case mix and outcomes can be reviewed and they provide an opportunity to identify recurring themes that emerge from time to time (see Ch. 4). Ninety minutes once a month is enough time to achieve this, providing practitioners receive aides-mémoire prior to the meeting. Whereas other meetings (see Ch. 4) allow the team to learn about the process and dynamics of working together, the audit meetings have to be more structured, given the amount of data generated in each episode of care. They therefore rely on aides-mémoire produced by the computer system; see Figure 5.1 for the report menu screen. These comprise summary lists and audit reports:

- A summary list for each GP reminds them of who has been newly referred and who is having ongoing CT treatment during the review period (see Figure 5.2).
- A summary list for each CP reminds them of who has been newly referred to each of them and who is having ongoing CT treatment during the review period (see Figure 5.3).
- Each GP is sent a linked audit report (see Figure 5.4) summarizing their patients' treatment series and its outcomes.
- Each CP is sent a linked audit report summarizing the treatment series of patients they have seen and their outcomes (Figure 5.5).

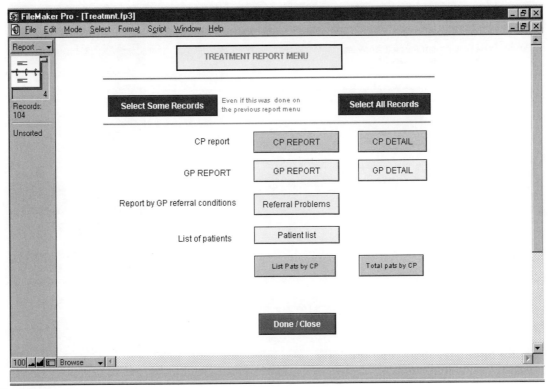

Figure 5.1   Report menu screen.

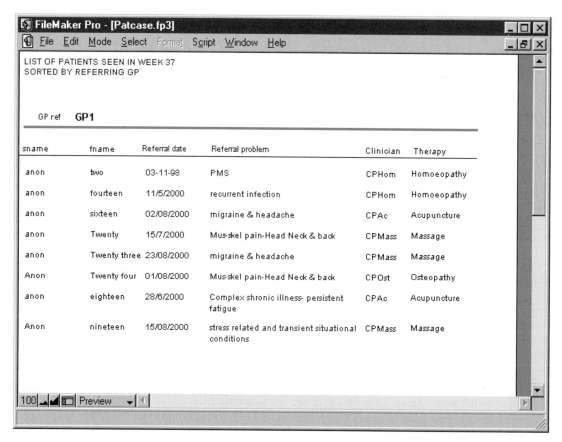

Figure 5.2 GP summary of patients referred.

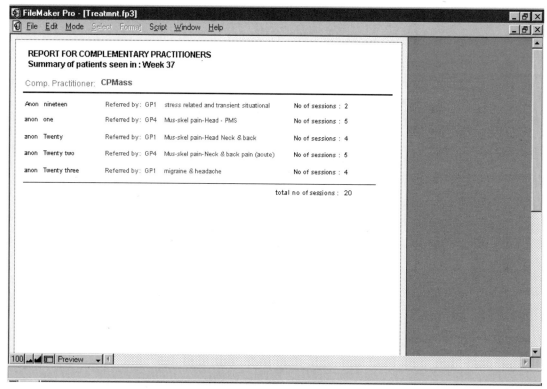

Figure 5.3 CP summary of patients seen.

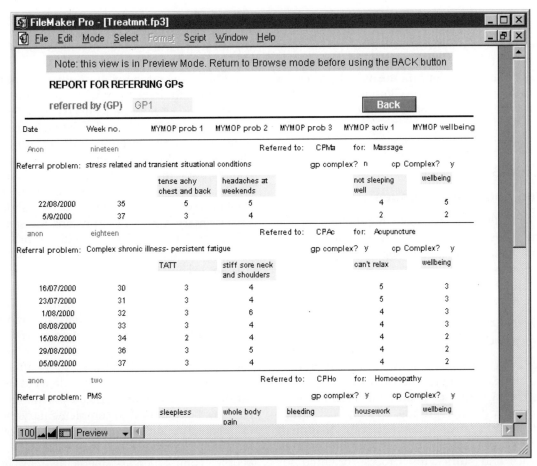

Figure 5.4   GP detail of patient tracking report.

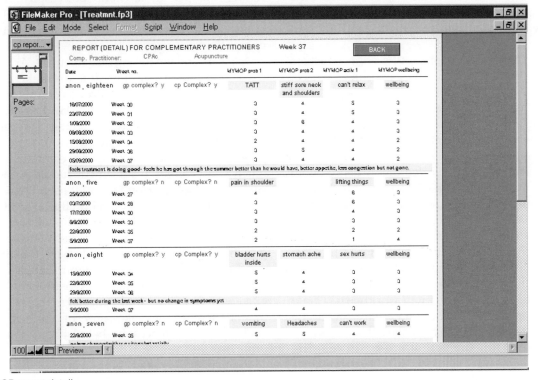

Figure 5.5   CP report detail.

The reports can be produced at the push of a button by the audit secretary, who then distributes them every month. CPs can use the system during consultation, to tag brief comments on to their reports. The comments generally raise questions about the treatment process or outcomes and serve to remind the CPs and GPs involved of details of patient management that need to be discussed.

REFLECTIONS
Unresolved and difficult issues

A number of difficult issues were highlighted in the course of the study. Some of them were immediate and practical, and we tried to work through them during the course of the project; others prompted wider questions, reflecting different notions about the nature of the service. Some remain unresolved.

Team dynamics and potential problems

In Chapter 2 we discussed some basic differences between the clinical concepts held by doctors and CPs. These have the potential to distort the working relationships between the two groups. GPs and CPs groping towards collaborative integrated care treatment have to find a set of ideas and images scientific enough for the medics and sufficiently process oriented for the CPs but they will also have to overcome their prejudices about their colleagues. This section explores some of the potential for misunderstanding and conflict.[1]

Stereotypes: CPs are unscientific, GPs are pill-pushers One way of defining CTs is that they are those ways of treating health problems not included in conventional medical education and practice. Pietroni has pointed out that this is like labelling all nations other than one's own as 'foreign'! Clearly the term fails to differentiate, and is vaguely derogatory, but at the same time the definition also reveals a real, barely concealed ambivalence about doctors' relationship with this other strange culture: a mixture perhaps of fantasy and envy, that colours all relations between different cultures. The biomedical paradigm can seem so all-pervasive, and its image of the human being so unsustaining, that people feel compelled to return to more traditional ideas about healthcare. In turning away from conventional medicine are patients sensing CPs' allegiance to a different worldview? Could it be they find in CT approaches and advice something more in tune with their own health beliefs than a doctor's biomedically framed offerings? Doctors' developing interest in complementary medicine may be sparked by a wish to work more 'holistically', to encourage homeo-

stasis and respond appropriately to patients' changing health beliefs. But CTs can also represent a way of searching for new kinds of 'magic bullets', or of avoiding professional depression.

Because several, possibly conflicting, attitudes may be operating simultaneously when CPs and GPs are working together, we suggest teams try to acknowledge them. Otherwise a secret ambivalence will be around, perpetuating the communication gulf, creating obstacles to shared clinical management and potentially sabotaging collaboration unless it can be explored—and laughed at. For example, though medicine is often stereotyped as applied biotechnology practised by dehumanized doctors, primary care is by no means the same as biomedicine. CPs joining a family medicine practice learn this very quickly if they can sit in on some sessions with a GP.

Great expectations Doctors' inability to 'cure' most of the problems presenting has made them curious about whether complementary medicine could provide an effective (and less potentially harmful) and practical way of manipulating the self-regulatory process. Many people do report satisfaction with CTs in a wide range of common illness and diseases even after conventional practitioners have failed to provide what they perceive as satisfactory treatment. Perhaps practitioners, as well as patients, hope to find in complementary medicine a way of reconstructing the clinical transaction—and, at a time when patients tell us they want to be seen as whole people, complementary medicine may have come to signify the person as mind–body–spirit. Health and wholeness have become synonymous in our postreligious times. These are high expectations and may be unrealistic.

Collusion and not risking disagreement And clearly our framework, though it aims to address the interdependency of mind, body and culture, is contingent and negotiable, not real common ground. We have to deal with overlapping models, ways of telling and being able to hear more or less relevant stories about our own and our patients' experience. There is only common ground in as much as we can reach agreement and trust one another's subjectivity. So our group found it useful to reflect on the clinical care of patients at weekly clinical meetings. These problem-oriented sessions allow practitioners to share their different impressions and discipline-specific interpretations. This is where we have learned to disagree and cope with most problems of communication and the challenges of joint decision making. Occasionally we still find ourselves tumbling into 'paradigm holes' where one practitioner cannot make sense of another, or clashing over basic differences in belief about diagnosis and prognosis.

Therapeutic ambition Not everyone can be 'fixed'. Many GPs, especially those influenced by Balint's psychoanalytic ideas about the GP role,[2] see the 'being with' aspects of practice—the 'doctor as drug'—as their main strength. Disputing in particular the idea that primary care is about removing symptoms of 'unorganized illness', they see the GP's task as being to accompany patients through ill health, managing problems that arise and helping contain distress. Such 'listening GPs' realize that patients set great store by a practitioner's 'being with' skills, as do many CPs. So there might appear to be considerable common humanistic ground between CPs and GPs. A particular problematic phrase is 'treating the real or underlying cause', a term that, depending on the practitioner's orientation, might imply a food intolerance (naturopath), a short leg causing a persistent pelvic tilt (osteopath), a deficiency of 'Kidney Qi' (acupuncturist) or an inherited chronic 'miasm' (homeopathy). There were also 'real causes' (e.g. an impossible marriage, a traumatic childhood, homelessness or redundancy) that both the GPs and CPs would not expect to influence in a very short course of treatment. This was difficult for the CPs to deal with, as in private practice they might treat and support a patient through very difficult times over a period of years, and there may be an expectation that the treatment itself can support the person to make changes in their lives. This has been a core issue for our team, and we have found that using a language that emphasizes the *management* of patients rather than their *cure* avoids inappropriate expectations. If patients can be helped to feel and function better for a time then we feel a referral from GP to CP is justified.

Trying too hard and trying to please We have had to question our emotional attachment to outcomes and our personal investment in any favoured mode of treatment. Feelings of omnipotence and therapeutic ambition are a complicating factor (although they can be a powerful therapeutic factor too at times) spurred on if practitioners are convinced that, although they may fail, their espoused therapeutic system is inherently infallible. We have had to put such idealism aside and be more pragmatic about producing significant change in chronic health problems. Gradual improvement is possible (see: Fix, contain, maintain, p. 166). However, the therapeutic nihilist would insist that we could only track the inexorable exacerbations and remissions of chronic conditions, offer support and limit damage. A recurring theme in our CP/GP collaboration has been how to find a middle way between the manic defence of the idealist position and the depressive position of the nihilist. Whether or not diverse CT *techniques* actually encourage homeostasis, CP time certainly makes available the attention, touch and sense of integration that biomedicine so often lacks, plus lifestyle advice and support for lifestyle change. We should be quite clear though that these approaches are not a cure for severe acute or life-threat-ening diseases and that biomedicine can often palliate in serious disease where CTs alone would fail.

CP/doctor working groups are microcosms of our culture and they probably generate even more difficult dynamics than other interdisciplinary working groups. Our culture has been profoundly intertwined with the values and beliefs of biomedicine, and if, as some authors have suggested,[3] the rise of complementary medicine is part of a wider cultural upheaval then we can expect that where the languages of new and old healthcare subcultures collide there will be conflict. Perhaps it is the aspect of complementary medicine as counterculture that makes the problems of collaboration so particularly potent and focused. Collaboration creates unconscious, conceptual and organizational turbulence. The discourse about health is inevitably about human nature itself, and the validity of developing new metaphors or different languages in healthcare raises issues of paradigm power.

Clinicians from different disciplines clash because, while they may agree about what the patient needs, they interpret those needs through different frameworks, and bring to the situation fundamentally different assumptions about what an intervention may do. Beyond the interpersonal disagreements and the structural differences, something else is around (although these superficial conflicts will multiply the effects of the deeper ones). People will suddenly find themselves in conflict they did not expect. They will not be able to express themselves in words clearly. They will feel their world is taken over. I think this might well be called 'paradigmatic power struggle'.

Practitioners' unconscious beliefs are significant aspects of the intellectual and emotional investment they make in their work as practitioners, important features of attachment to their clinical worldview. They make us partisan for certain approaches, and so create sensitive areas that potential collaborators may feel they need to protect. As in any team, professional pride will sometimes be seen as arrogance or provoke confrontation. For example, in one joint consultation a doctor who had studied homeopathy was discussing, with an acupuncturist, a patient whose high blood pressure in the lungs was caused by a structural chest disease. When the acupuncturist, a senior practitioner with an extensive grounding in psychotherapy, began to talk about the possibility that Chinese medicine could influence this structural circulatory disorder, the doctor quietly exploded with disbelief and ill-concealed scorn. His CP colleague, incensed by this reaction, accused the doctor of intellectual arrogance. The doctor paused, surprised by the vigour of his own response, but only grudgingly accepted that he had no definite basis for refuting the acupuncturist's assertion. Even if he had, the confrontational style he had learned on hospital teaching rounds (where it might have passed unnoticed in the cut and thrust between two medics) was actually quite inappropriate and a somehow shocking way of transacting a clinical discussion with a peer clinician from a different 'tribe'.

What had been revealed was an unconscious lack of respect for another's worldview. The ensuing argument, and the practitioners' eventual reconciliation over a period of several months of working together, was reminiscent of a clash between disciples of opposing religions who, having recognized the potential for harm implicit in their irreconcilable positions, struggle to find a way of coexisting and so grow into an authentic regard for one another. This is no easy journey, but it is a way that has to be travelled if we are to explore the sometimes-confused subject/object relations that all clinical work, but especially collaborative work between systems of medicine, throws up.

Without close working relationships the dialogue between complementary medicine and the mainstream becomes difficult because of two commonly witnessed attitudes. The first position—denial of the conflict—has contributed to the creation of an autonomous complementary medicine subculture that pays lip service to the idea that complementary medicine and biomedicine complement one another but avoids exploring how, when or why. Second, and worse, is the projection of blame—for the failure of biomedicine's theory and practice or for the folly of its practitioners—on to conventional medicine. This has produced antimedical elements in complementary medicine's subculture that would deny biomedicine any relevance whatever.

Tension between individual and group nature defines the human psychic territory; so we are simultaneously fascinated and appalled by similarities and differences. Consequently the third way, towards coexistence with the powerful forces of conventional healthcare, will remain by far the most difficult route for CPs to take, and it may prove impossible unless our kind of MHC clinical pluralism can be validated. Controlled clinical trials alone will not facilitate cooperation, and close collaboration between doctors and CPs—stimulating and clinically innovative though it can be—will continue to be the exception until more doctors and CPs attempt to work side by side. In order to do this they will not only have to find the resources and learn to tolerate the difficulties, but also learn how to explore the important meaning behind the discomfort, uncertainty and anxiety that working together will sometimes engender.

The GP–CP interaction When issues arose that involved the clinical interface between team members we aimed to address them at clinical meetings. We have also tried other methods, including sitting in with colleagues—which, though helpful, calls for considerable

trust, careful preparation and sensitivity; videoing consultations (though we have as yet seldom succeeded here)—which can be less threatening; and accepting a treatment from a colleague—which may be difficult, but one can learn a lot from the experience. The team have also explored (in some depth!) the difficulties of collaboration. Prior to the Smith Project we organized two separate 1-year cooperative enquiries. These linked projects involving all the CPs and GPs explored our ways of working together. One project looked into the particular problems arising in a clinic where patients referred themselves for a consultation with a multidisciplinary group. Both involved group time where discussion of theory and practice related directly to the patients we had seen together, a problem-centred approach that allowed free exploration of these issues in a relatively unthreatening way. The inclusion of an experienced facilitator in the second project greatly improved the team's ability to make sense of itself, to unravel and describe its own internal processes and to manage its work better.

We believe the issues revealed—problems of power, resource allocation, differing clinical models, communication and the logistics of the referral process itself—are an inevitable part of the territory of CP/GP collaboration. Because they hinder effective collaboration they are relevant to other groups planning similar work, since the seeds of interdisciplinary rivalry are easily sown and misled by fantasies of power (GPs' historical and statutory power versus CPs' unfathomable expertise) and privilege (GPs' eminent legal status versus CPs' 'otherness'). These features of medical/complementary therapist cooperation are not unique to healthcare teamwork, but rather represent exaggerations, at times bizarre, of problems that are typical of interprofessional and interagency work.

Why refer for CT?

The referral process involves many detailed issues that require collaborative management. A referral to a CP might be made in order to gather information from the practitioner but, given the lack of any common clinical language and the uneven spread of power between doctors and CPs, how can information be exchanged or joint management be made to work? If the CP is to take over care, then how does that square with GMC regulations about the doctor ultimately carrying responsibility? In fact GPs' joint working with CPs is defined as a delegation of tasks for which the doctor maintains clinical responsibility. All the more important then for doctors to be sure that their CP colleagues are competent and fully insured and to make the flow of information about contacts and outcomes as easy, consistent and reliable as it can be. That was our plan.

When GPs refer to CPs working outside their practice, the expectations are probably similar to those they would have of a conventional specialist: probably 'please fix this' or 'my patient believes you can fix this and has asked to see you'. In house, a wider exploration of one another's working models and style of work is possible. This encourages a more broadly based referral inquiry. Examples from our working together include:

1. 'What would *your* system call this syndrome/illness/ disease?'
2. 'I think this is a psychosomatic problem, but what do you make of it?'
3. 'Can your therapy possibly offer anything for this patient?'
4. 'Can your therapy offer anything for this condition?'
5. 'Have a go and let me know.'
6. 'Can you look after this patient for a while? . . . I'm worn out.'
7. 'I need a break from this patient—can you support him/me for a while?'
8. 'I am curious about your therapy's potential for this patient; shall we explore this together?'
9. 'I have been treating this patient without much success; would your approach help?'

In our work together we have accepted that a certain pragmatism is unavoidable in CP/GP collaboration; for example, since there is a dearth of well-researched referral criteria, all referrals are actually requests for a trial of treatment. Furthermore if, as it is said, each complementary medical treatment is individually prescribed, then every treatment becomes a trial in which $n = 1$. This can make selection of suitable cases difficult—the more so if CPs feel a need to impress medical colleagues with good results, in which case even the most challenging referral is unlikely to be refused. But such indiscriminate acceptance of all-comers is likely to produce poor results.

We have found that the usual factors already influencing referrals include the following:

- patients' wishes to see a CP because of their own, another's or a reported experience
- GPs' knowing of a previously successful treatment of a similar condition
- or of a previously successful treatment of a certain type of patient
- CPs' reported conviction that they can successfully treat certain conditions
- published or conference reports of the relevance/ effectiveness of a CT
- GPs' conviction that they cannot treat certain conditions (e.g. 'I'm no good with backs')
- no conventional treatment options exist/remain/are acceptable
- GPs' intuition

- GPs' or CPs' wishful thinking
- GPs' workload or frustration.

Typical problems arise in the process of referral. We have recognized some in our own work, and identified reasons for them. The absence of any referrals might, for instance, indicate 'I don't understand what you do', 'I don't believe what you claim', 'I don't recognize the need for your contribution' or 'I don't trust you'. Too many referrals could signal 'I don't understand what you do', though it might also indicate 'I am trying to discover your limits' or 'I can't deal with patients with x, y, z. I hope you can'. It could also suggest the organization or individual GP is overstrained or that for some other reason GPs are not 'gatekeeping' adequately. Impossible referrals are sometimes made, not always unwittingly: perhaps when a GP feels disempowered, deskilled, passive–aggressive or overoptimistic. Obviously if opportunities for adequate feedback from CP to GP are not in place, then inefficient use of a CP resource and inappropriate expectations will be perpetuated. Even the best-equipped extended team will usually find that patients with 'thick notes' nevertheless confound practitioners attempts at 'cure', and there are always going to be some patients who move from one CP to another, straining the limits of the team's patience, competence and time.

'Complex cases'

A recurrent theme in our GP/CP meetings has been the treatment of what came to be known as 'complex' patients. The conditions that doctors could refer to the CP team had been previously decided, namely:

- conditions in which CT treatment had the best evidence base
- common conditions whose conventional treatment is commonly unsatisfactory
- conditions that CPs said they could treat effectively.

These categories were, however, specifically designed to be broad enough to reflect the reality of general practice and the needs of the GPs and patients. GPs had a great deal of leeway when it came to deciding which particular patients with these conditions they should refer. In fact it became apparent during the study that one perceived benefit to GPs of having in-house CPs was that they could share the load of treating 'frequent attenders' and other sorts of challenging patient. One GP summed this up by saying: 'Why would I refer someone I can treat myself?'. However, though difficult and complex patients were often seen, we also observed that CTs often proved most effective with patients who have newly diagnosed conditions.

One emerging question is whether access to CT actually improves the management of patients who, for a variety of reasons, GPs find it hard to deal with. Among them are patients with chronic and relapsing conditions, some with named diseases, others lacking definitive diagnoses, perhaps displaying symptoms of 'undifferentiated illness' or exhibiting 'somatization syndromes'. Especially if they have been labelled 'high-rate consulters', 'difficult patients', 'heart-sink' or 'thick-note' patients,[4] these patients are likely to draw heavily on a range of more or less inappropriate resources. However, it is never easy to evaluate the multidimensional approach to treatment that everyday family medicine entails, particularly in conditions that are chronic or relapsing. Here, GPs' typical interventions and treatments tend to be neither standardized nor specific. Though CTs, like general practice, entail specific therapeutic techniques, they also employ generalist features; these non-specific but potentially therapeutic elements are determined perhaps by practitioners' beliefs, their attitudes, or kindness and communication skills. At this stage of our enquiries we have made no attempt to control for these factors, or for variations in advice given to patients.

As clinicians we know distress may express itself as illness, though often in ways that do not conform to biomedical explanations. There are diverse ways of labelling such marginal presentations—some of them listed in the previous paragraph. Experience suggests that many patients referred for homeopathy, acupuncture and massage at MHC fall into such a category. It could be said that CTs reach into this marginal zone of uncertainty. Homeopathy and TCM in particular apply 'outsider' medical models that extend the possibility of non-psychological interventions in such patients. So at this stage of our understanding it seems reasonable to inquire pragmatically into their role and their impact in a GP setting using naturalistic approaches, rather than adopting an experimental design or imposing exclusive intake criteria. Consequently GPs did not constrain their use of CTs to distinct diagnostic categories, even though we intended that this should be our overall strategy for ration(aliz)ing the CT service. To do so would have been to predetermine the outcome of what had to be a pragmatic and qualitative study. So our guidelines recognized that patients' interest in a particular CT vary and that health beliefs are diverse. These factors not only influence GP decisions about whom they refer to CPs, but will also be a significant factor in determining the outcome of treatment.

Several types of multiple consulter can be recognized.

• *The consumer.* These patients are keen to shop around and get the most out of the system.
• *The desperate mechanic.* These patients believe there must be an external solution for their condition/distress: an intervention that will fix them. Because of CAM's

pragmatism, its air of omnipotence and the 'have a go factor', a CP may be tempted to rise to the challenge even though this therapeutic ambition ought to be minimal.

• *The heart-sink patient.* These patients will always feel the latest practitioner is not good enough, and will compare any available practitioner with some idealized figure. Encountering such patients, one senses their problems are overwhelming (for them as well as for you) and, knowing that one will not be good enough, one's heart sinks. These patients always have thick files, having previously been referred to every available resource because they and/or their GP have been driven to desperation by their problem. It may be that better teamwork, with a jointly agreed management plan and an agreed key worker, can contain these patients' distress. Many of the patients who present with persistent unorganized illness may be depressed or anxious (perhaps with unrecognized hyperventilation syndrome), with problems of daily living. If these problems can be recognized and dealt with among the team members such patients can become less dependent on multiple consulting. The role of CT though is less clear.

• *The iatrogenic multiconsulter.* These patients, on the other hand, form a category, possibly overlapping with any of the above, whose consulting behaviour has been engendered by doctors. These are difficult patients who are repeatedly referred by their doctors, perhaps under pressure from the patient, or because of GPs' own anxiety or problems of daily doctoring, or because they still hope against the odds to find a specialist who will be able to help. Patients like these may benefit from complementary medicine but very careful choice is neccessary, i.e. where the CP can make a clear and definite differential diagnosis of the person's problems according to the principles of their therapy. This allows the practitioner to assess very quickly with the patient whether treatment is helping, avoiding a prolonged course of treatment with little expectation of change. Some patients in this category may need to be protected from referral to any specialist of whatever ilk, conventional or otherwise. Our experience suggests that there is a more than theoretical danger that when complementary medicine becomes more widely available some of these patients would simply come to rely inappropriately on regular visits to CPs. One solution is to cap the number of treatments that any patient can receive, together with an end of treatment review to be taken back to the team, ensuring that decisions for continued management can be made taking into account the last treatment experience and any insights that the practitioner might be able to contribute to future care.

A core issue for collaborative research in this area is whether what appears 'unorganized illness' to a conventional practitioner is, from the perspective of a complementary medical system, a recognizable pattern, and whether the appropriate CP on this basis can exert specific therapeutic leverage. For example, recurrent mechanical back pain—to conventional medicine an apparently unorganized condition that is difficult to grapple with—is apparently well dealt with by chiropractors and osteopaths. Might there be parallels in other systems where CPs recognize distinct syndromes and treat them effectively even though doctors see there only chaotic signals of distress?

Will the project validate GPs referral of 'complex' cases to CTs? At the present time the guidelines for CT intake remain broad and our current understanding of GPs' referral patterns and needs suggests they should remain so. Further data gathering and reflective cycles will clarify GPs' intentions and allow us to redefine the most appropriate conditions and categories of patients who benefit by being referred for different CTs. It may transpire that a lack of definition is itself an important indicator of GPs' need to use certain CTs (especially homeopathy and acupuncture) as a resource for patients whose problems are difficult to label. Whether such 'complexity' will eventually become a criterion for a patient's referral or exclusion from these therapies remains at present an open question. In the current action cycle GPs have begun to note on the referral form whether they believe a patient is 'complex'. But good outcomes from, for example, homeopathy in these 'complex patients' would confirm that such referrals are valid.

The CPs, whilst very willing to work with taxing patients in partnership with the GPs, were still concerned that they could be asked to see a disproportionate number of such patients. Patients who are challenging to GPs either because of relationship difficulties or owing to the severity and length of disease could easily swamp our limited CT resources. So it had to be agreed by the team that CPs could offer a course of only six treatment sessions at the most. Therefore questions about the most effective way of using this time and how to make the most appropriate referrals have been inescapable. How, for instance, could CPs do justice to their own skill and experience or their therapy if asked to treat only patients whose condition demanded more time and treatment to have a hope of change? Moreover, the need to evaluate the outcome of each treatment episode with the patient can add to CP anxiety; what would the consequence be if the MYMOP scores showed no improvement at the end of a course of treatment?

Questions about the CT role in general practice included:

- Should CPs be thought of as 'generalist' or 'specialist'?

- Do we expect CPs to 'fix', 'contain' or 'maintain' (see discussion on p. 166)?
- Can CPs treat acute problems, thereby improving the quality of life, without working on what they regard as the causes of the problem?
- Can the CT service offer long-term support rather than just a short course of treatment?
- Should the CT service be capped or, like the MHC counselling scheme, develop more flexible patterns of short-, medium- and long-term delivery?

The team recognized the problem the CPs could find themselves in if asked to accept patients with long-term chronic disease and be expected to improve their symptoms within a short space of time. Can it be acceptable or feasible to use resources only for those most likely to show an improvement? What then of the many cases where the GPs needed CPs' help in maintaining patients' function or supporting long-term management?

Having decided on the conditions to be treated the joint team embarked on a long process of deciding which patients could benefit the most. We have found that learning about the strengths and limitations of each therapy and each practitioner's expertise has been central to this process. Equally central has been the issue of 'complex cases'. CPs, on hearing of a case where the patient or the syndrome had a strong match with one of their diagnostic categories, will be much more willing to accept a complex case referral. Conversations on these issues have proved invaluable and have been an important factor in improving the appropriateness of referrals.

Questions concerning the treatment of complex patients included the following:

- What is a 'complex' patient?
- Are all these patients equally 'complex'?
- Which 'complex' patients might do well with treatment with CTs?
- As a GP, how do I decide whether homeopathy, acupuncture or massage might be the best for this particular patient?
- As a CP, just because I have an apparently relevant diagnostic category, does this mean I can treat this patient successfully?
- What should a CP do when a patient presents with a condition that seems simple to the GP but where the initial consultation with the CP reveals more 'complex' problems?
- How can the treatment of 'complex' problems best be documented?
- How can the CPs keep a balance in their work between 'complex' patients and those with more 'fixable' problems?

- What happens at the end of a course of CT treatment when a CP wants to offer a 'complex' patient the opportunity for more treatment?
- Do CPs need to work differently when working within the NHS?
  — Is it possible or desirable to work only with less 'complex' patients?
  — Would this mean that what CPs see as the greatest benefit to patients (working holistically) will be lost to NHS patients?
- To what extent do GPs refer for the therapy or to a therapist?

Many of these questions continue to be raised in our weekly meetings, but in our experience they are often hard to articulate, let alone answer. Yet they certainly cannot be ignored. In any medic/CP workgroup these issues must be acknowledged and somehow addressed, for if such core concerns are not considered then the group will not function as a team.

Feedback on the topic of 'complexity' from different CPs included the following comments.

The homeopath's experience First, people may have had a long history of illness with a minor problem. Even if the patient has a long history of conventional medication it can still be suitable, but if the condition (for instance sinusitis) is really the manifestation of an overflow of rubbish in the system it may not necessarily be treatable or suitable for treatment.

Secondly, someone who is deeply depressed, long-term medicated, psychotic or a 'borderline personality' may not be suitable for homeopathy even though the GP has referred the patient for the treatment of a minor problem.

Thirdly, complex cases that are treatable often have a history of some initiating or underlying infection or inflammation, for instance VD, chronic thrush, cystitis, arthritis (in younger people Reiter's disease) or gout. Patients like these can do very well but need long-term follow-up.

The naturopath/osteopath's experience The kind of 'complex' patients I do well with have been referred for particular aspects of their condition (gut or skin problems, for example) but in addition to this problem I can identify multiple dysfunction, for example in the digestive tract, liver, toxic overload, hyperventilation tendencies and psychological distress. Complex cases like these could take many months or years to improve even under ideal conditions. I therefore have to suggest palliative approaches for practical reasons (sometimes, for instance, financial concern over the costs of nutritional supplements that would have to be purchased) in such cases. Identifying such individuals is not always possible at the first interview and to an extent is something that becomes apparent over time.

The acupuncturis's experience First, 'complexity' can sometimes be determined by whether or not I can make sense of the progression of an illness. Even something that I would say was a deep, long-standing problem with many aspects and manifestations may not be categorized as complex if I can see how the person's condition has come about and progressed. I can then be clear about what I can offer the person, both in terms of an explanation and what acupuncture might do (or not). Conversely a patient might present with a collection of symptoms of short duration and a more superficial nature but, because of their diversity according to TCM diagnostic categories, prove more difficult to treat than the 'symptoms' might indicate.

Secondly, there is practitioner limitation. Sometimes I am unable to make a clear diagnosis, and the patient and the condition do not change.

Thirdly, there is the circumstance where I make a reasonable diagnosis but the patient does not get better. Sometimes a patient's history and circumstances can make a difference. For example, a patient's lack of motivation, unhelpful health beliefs and practices, and adverse life circumstances that may be unlikely to change in the short term can hinder a successful outcome. Sometimes I just do not know why someone is not responding and the situation becomes more complex than I first thought.

The osteopath's experience There are certain aspects of a case that tend to ring alarm bells for me. These include:

- the patient's behaviour prior to the consultation—if the patient has upset practitioners, has seen multiple practitioners, or has a thick set of notes
- patients who react in unexpected or unpredictable ways, whose symptoms are not 'explicable' or 'polysymptomatic', or whose signs are inconsistent
- patients to whom I react in unexpected ways
- if a patient fails to progress, so that it gradually dawns on me that there is 'more going on', psychologically and somatically
- patients who come with certain 'labels', including geopathic stress/ME/chronic candida.

At the beginning of the project the CPs were keen for GPs to indicate whether they considered a patient's condition as 'complex'. Initially this was because it was important to keep track of the number of 'complex' patients in order to avoid impossible caseloads. There has been a shift in the way we work, however, and GPs' and CPs' expectations have become much more realistic. GPs perhaps no longer expect some magical cure but have a greater understanding of the therapies and appreciate the support CPs provide to people with 'complex' conditions. The CPs are more likely to be realistic about what they can achieve within a time-limited service and will work with the patient and the GP on what can be achieved practically.

What is clear from our initial data is that patients designated by both the CP and the GP as 'complex' also have high scores indicating a poor well-being; this is especially so for patients referred to massage and homeopathy. We realize that somatization itself is a complex issue (see below) and we are only beginning to explore the relevance of CTs here. By entering into the process of recording patient-centred outcome and by creating structures and processes for regular reflection, the issue of treating 'complex' patients has become startlingly clear. We suspect that, in any medic–CT service, CP caseloads will need to balance the numbers of fixable and 'complex' patients and consider carefully the question of CTs' role when somatization is suspected.

CT and mental health problems The Mental Health Foundation recently published a report on current research, policy and practice concerning the use of complementary and alternative therapies for a wide range of mental health problems.[5] This report illustrated a high level of CT use by patients with mental health problems.

The field of mental health and CT use typifies the problem of research: there are few RCTs, but if longitudinal surveys, case studies and uncontrolled trials are taken into account then the evidence for a range of effective and appropriate CTs expands. However, even if the evidence is restricted to RCT studies there is a convincing case for the use of CTs in depression, anxiety and a wide range of psychologically mediated functional disturbances (asthma, migraine, IBS, etc.).

Counselling or CT? Are there patients for whom the 'talking cures' are inappropriate, yet who do well with complementary medical treatments? Designing studies to test such a hypothesis would be challenging, for what would be the end-point of such a study? Even if these approaches do not 'cure' patients with hard-to-treat health problems they can, in our experience, be helpful, and our practice's approach to patient-centred outcome tracking is one way of demonstrating this potential. Primary care teams spend much of their time dealing with chronic problems—some of them caused by physical diseases, some by intermittent dysfunction or problems of daily living. GPs are likely to see CPs as a potential resource for managing such patients. In our group, CPs have acknowledged that part of their work is about long-term management of patients who for a time need regular appointments with a CP as part of a strategy to help contain on-going distress or pain. In such cases cure is not the aim.

We are quite clear at Marylebone that CTs are not a substitute for talk therapy. We also appreciate that many patients do not think 'psychologically' and would there-

fore be unsuitable for counselling approaches, which depend on the client's ability to bear the pain of reflection on feelings and to turn their distressing experience into a narrative. Nor should CTs be seen as a routine stage on the way towards counselling; we do not usually expect a patient with a psychologically mediated somatic symptom to move from, say, acupuncture treatment into a talking cure. However, we have found that CT can offer a possibility of short-term support in acute situational disturbance and life crisis.

Somatization Our 'complex' case category includes patients who from the conventional medical perspective would be thought of as 'somatizers'.[6] Some CTs, notably acupuncture and homeopathy, use diagnostic categories that blur the boundaries between 'emotional' and 'physical' symptoms. It makes perfect sense to a homeopath that patients who describe their situation in terms of feeling overburdened, and of being unable to cope with the smallest things, will also have digestive problems. For the acupuncturist the symptoms of being short tempered, having a feeling of constriction in the chest and difficulty in swallowing are all part of one instantly recognizable diagnostic pattern related to 'Liver Process' dysfunction. As there is no split between the body and mind it is perfectly reasonable for one patient to come to the acupuncturist with a physical manifestation of a diagnostic category and another with a mental manifestation of it. Perhaps this can be stated as follows. With some CTs (acupuncture, homeopathy) we are aware that, because their underlying theories do not split the mind and the body, the practitioner can equally well take those patients who present with physical manifestations of psychological distress as those who present with psychological symptoms and can talk about their distress. So one question that has emerged clearly in our team is whether complementary therapies have a role in the treatment of patients labelled as 'somatizers'.

A challenge for our team has been bridging the gap between those whose medicine includes the notion of somatization and those who do not. A concern for the GPs was that if the CPs could successfully treat patients who 'somatize' without the patients having to talk about their feelings then this would collude with somatizing patients' need to express their distress through symptoms rather than language. If so, is this an argument against their use, given that the literature suggests that many patients who somatize do not think psychologically and this is part of the difficulty? However, all the CPs have experienced patients to whom it gradually dawned over the course of a series of treatments that 'tension' or 'stress' was a perpetuating factor. These patients sometimes subsequently changed aspects of their behaviour, or took up exercise programmes or relaxation programmes, and benefited from these. Some even sought counselling. This, for the CP, would often be seen as a direct consequence of treatment, according to their model. The challenge for the CPs was to take on the GPs' concerns and perhaps change their consultation style to give greater emphasis to communicating to the patient the continuing need to give attention to the maintaining causes, even though the physical manifestations of their condition had been resolved.

A remaining question for our team is, given that we feel that self-awareness and increasing a patient's ability to cope with psychological distress are important, do we want patients to have the physical manifestations of their condition resolved without also engaging them in a discussion of the maintaining causes that fundamentally affect them psychologically?

Containment Most mainstream primary care entails either 'fixing' or 'maintenance'. These mechanical metaphors epitomize two different kinds of healthcare activity. Fixing relies on a definitive intervention with a relatively short-term aim, for example giving antibiotics for a bacterial bronchitis. Maintenance is about keeping a patient going during chronic or relapsing illness, for example prescribing inhaled steroids for an asthmatic patient or antirheumatic drugs in RA. A less obvious feature of primary care can be described as 'containment'.[6] This also has to do with long-term health problems, in such cases where a person experiences distressing and unrelenting dysfunction, distress or disability that cannot be 'fixed' and whose 'maintenance' seems, for a variety of reasons, to be unusually difficult. Containment is a complex activity because practitioners have to tolerate the (usually negative) feelings stirred up when dealing with these patients' predicaments. In general practice this kind of activity is particularly associated with Michael Balint's work. Pointing out that the urge to treat or refer can be a defence against anxiety, Balint advised practitioners to limit their 'therapeutic ambition'.[2]

Given the case mix of patients referred to CPs at MHC, it is hardly surprising that 'fixing' is often not the aim. Maintenance with small improvements in symptom scores and general health are more often achievable, nevertheless. The Marylebone team has accepted that CPs have a part to play in containing difficult patients, so we had to consider the CPs' role not only in fixing and maintaining patients, but also in the more complex task of containment. At times this has been the only possible approach to take.

In exploring this task in a practitioner group that included psychodynamic counsellors we came to the conclusion that containment can mean three quite different things, as follows.

1. 'Supportive' containment (providing a safety net). Where we cannot help patients to learn, or to change, or to get better we may still be able to keep them, or their situation, from deteriorating. This entails being available, listening and offering treatment, support, advice or clarification when needed. The patient is nevertheless motivated, but for a variety of reasons (skills, nature of illness/behaviour, lack of resources) practitioners can help only a little.

The various professional groups use this term differently, as follows:

GPs: We think of a person who asks for support during a difficult life predicament: e.g. bereavement, loss and separation, pregnancy and childbirth, dying, chronic disease, psychological illness, disability.
CPs: We think perhaps of patients who acknowledge their complex condition is triggered or maintained by a variety of factors (nutritional, structural and/or psychosocial) but who, because of a lack of inner or outer resources, feel unable to escape these influences or make significant practical changes. In such cases, an initial period of treatment would have revealed the importance of these factors so, having achieved only a little improvement, the CP might offer occasional follow-up appointments for support and review. (This is an example of how CPs work in a 'GP mode' with a chronically unwell patient.)
Counsellors: We think of long-term seriously ill patients with, for example, dementia or severe mental illness.

2. 'Repressive' containment (creating boundaries). This patient continually seeks help, often across a range of services and often in ways that both waste resources and upset staff. In such cases not only is there very little that practitioners can do to help, but also the team will need to limit the wastage and the damaging impact on staff. Understanding does not seem to help; the pattern of contact just endlessly repeats itself.

How the different professional groups use this term:

GPs: These are 'heart-sink patients' and 'difficult patients'; often they are thick-notes patients who have been widely referred to specialists. They are usually frequent consulters (more than 12 times a year). Generally we suspect them of being 'somatizers': of expressing distress (which they cannot put into words) through body symptoms; or of having an inappropriate degree of awareness of normal body sensations; or of needing inappropriate levels of reassurance about minor symptoms; or of being unable to cope with problems of daily living (which might include difficulties related to persistent ill health). But whereas safety-net patients arouse a feeling of 'I must help', heart-sink and difficult patients are more likely to incite an urge to pass them on to someone (anyone!). In responding to this pressure, GPs may be quite unaware of the undercurrents of depression, anger or anxiety that these patients provoke in them.

CPs: Generally these are patients with long-term intractable conditions *without* a clear organic cause or a clear diagnostic category within the CT—perhaps pain or bizarre polysymptomatology (see the acupuncture and massage examples later in this chapter). Although occasionally a CT perspective can enable major changes, perhaps because of a fortuitous mix of the timing of the treatment for the patient, a quick response to the therapy and something in the nature of the patient–practitioner relationship, this type of patient unfortunately may be added to the list of inappropriate referrals. It comes very hard to some complementary therapists that there may be patients who they simply cannot help. There might be a tendency to want to battle on with patients who clearly are not being helped or feel themselves to be helped. The challenge for the CP is to recognize these patients and begin to say 'no' more often to referrals that sound decidedly demanding and confusing clinically. If a team wants a CP to take on such clients, it should be within a supportive structure where management plans and objectives can be negotiated. Without such a structure and opportunities for supervision, the 'difficult patient's' distress is likely to affect the practitioner and disturb the team dynamics.

Counsellors: There are very few of these patients; it mostly occurs only when an inappropriate referral has been made without adequate preparation.

3. *'Transformative' containment (enabling change).* This meaning (which is the most complex), has been substantially theorized by Wilfred Bion. It could be stated as follows: 'These patients seem to want to understand their symptoms/difficulties/behaviour and to grow/change their lifestyle/behaviour, and furthermore we think that with our help they can do so, at least to some extent. Therefore we will take in their communication in some depth and try to understand it, and perhaps begin to help to articulate it. In the process, we will take some of the sting out of the unbearable feelings they are bringing to us, so that it feels safer for the patient to take them back and reintegrate them.'

The various professional groups use this term as follows:

GPs: The patients I would refer for counselling are those who seem to want to make sense of the psychological component of their distress. They have become aware that feelings and memories contribute to their illness or anguish and need to find a language and a voice to express them.

CPs: The ideal CT patient who has a chronic health problem is someone who is becoming aware that complex interweaving factors undermine their well-being. This might even include an appreciation of the part emotions and predicament play in generating symptoms. The practitioner's role is to support appropriate attempts to act on such insights. Within the CT frame of reference this is more likely to entail a cognitive–behavioural change (ideas about and approaches to diet, lifestyle, exercise,

adopting a mind–body method like yoga, qigong or meditation) rather than a psychodynamic intervention. Also within the CT consultation, discussions around the topic of 'energy' and 'spirituality' can offer new frameworks that might allow such patients to re-evaluate or reinterpret their predicament.

Counsellors: This is most of counselling practice.

Some case studies of how these categories are used by massage therapists in the musculoskeletal service at the MHC are given in Box 5.1.

Box 5.1 Case studies from massage (extracted from discharge summaries sent to GPs). The first three are typical of the massage therapy caseload

Maintain
Patient aged 78, female
Hypertension, angina, osteoarthritis.
Experiences recurrent low back pain and sore knees
Treatment given: TLC + back and leg massage—loves to chat
Feels better, but not long term (can only have quota of four sessions)
Lonely and quite isolated, puts on a brave face. Can I see her for long-term sessions?

Contain (support)
Patient aged 51, female, recently bereaved
Says she aches all over and poor sleep (?fibromyalgia syndrome)
Treatment given: massage, stress management, self-care
Some improvement in symptoms
MYMOP 1—throbbing legs 4–4–2
MYMOP 2—back ache 4–4–3–2
But not in Well-being MYMOP 3–1–3–3

Patient aged 62, female, immigrant family of reasonable means
Depressed, osteoarthritis, but pain all over. Has high expectations of what the medical service ought to provide!
Treatment given × 3: full body massage
Very little change in symptoms or well-being

The following cases demonstrate that a combination of therapeutic bodywork (neuromuscular and muscle energy techniques) plus simple behavioural techniques can, when allied to massage, offer effective ways of managing stress- and posture-related pain and dysfunction.

Fix
Patient aged 65, male, benign brain tumour operation 5 years ago
Experiences pain and stiffness in left neck since operation; tinnitus, depression
Treatment given × 4: massage, muscle energy neck and shoulder, stress management, relaxation, breathing, stretches, relaxation tape
Improvement ++ once he had learned how to relax his shoulders
MYMOP 1—neck pain, stiffness 5–4–3–2
MYMOP 1—tension 5–4–3–2
Function—Turn head 5–4–3–2
Well-being 5–4–3–2
(**NB** Letter from ENT consultant confirms my impression of good outcome.)

Patient aged 28, male
Persistent headaches, shoulder pain, 'stressed', health anxiety
Findings: tense short trapezius and posterior cervical muscles. Upper chest breathing
Treatment given: massage and muscle energy techniques to neck and shoulders, breathing, diet, relaxation tape and leaflets, chat re lifestyle
Week 2—headache better, but shoulder pain still bad, using tape and doing exercises
Week 3—done well, stretching neck regularly, relaxing with tape, using breathing exercises
MYMOP 1—4–3–1
MYMOP 2—shoulder pain 3–3–2
Well-being 2–2–1

'Fixing', 'containing' and 'maintaining'—examples in acupuncture treatment Many of the patients being referred to acupuncture with musculoskeletal problems fell into the 'contain and maintain' categories rather than the 'fix' category.

Fix. In acupuncture, examples of a 'fix' patient are difficult to find. This is partly because what Western medicine offers is seen as appropriate and effective and therefore the patient is not referred. But it is also because in making the diagnosis other symptoms the patients has, which can be minor and can in Western terms seem unrelated to the patient's presenting problem, do not allow for the patient to be purely fixed. The concept of 'fixing' is also alien to the way acupuncturists understand how their therapy works, although patients may see their health problems in these terms.

An example from acupuncture of a 'fix' patient was:

A young woman in her twenties presented with a diagnosis of repetitive strain injury (RSI). She had no other major health problems apart from a little PMS. The RSI had come about through overuse and, as the name suggests, repetitive movement. Traditional aetiology explains the pain as the result of overuse having affected the ability of her 'Qi' to flow smoothly through her wrist, causing pain. (The osteopath attributed her pain to a build-up of myofascial tension and subclinically congested circulation involving the whole arm and shoulder—the same concept in different language.) On taking her pulses, observing her tongue and gathering information it was apparent to the acupuncturist that this impairment of her Qi was localized and in acupuncture diagnostic terms the disease was still at a superficial level. As her underlying Qi was strong it did not take very many treatments to effect some change. Had her tension been more deeply psychological and/or had she been exhausted, her RSI would have been more difficult to fix. (Though expressed differently this approach corresponds to the osteopath's concept of preceding and maintaining causes of prognostic factors.)

A shared understanding of the causes of disease with this patient was easy to obtain as it was clear to both the patient and the practitioner that it was due to overuse of a joint. This patient was happy for her PMS—which in TCM terms represented another aspect of the same underlying tendency towards congestion—to be treated in parallel. So, although this had not been why the GP had referred her, it was taken as the second problem on her MYMOP form.

Maintain. Many patients sent to the acupuncturist with musculoskeletal problems fell into the 'maintain' category. In these patients the disease process had impaired their underlying Qi. Some were long-term users of NSAIDs or took regular pain relief medication.

An example of a 'maintain' patient was a woman in her seventies with a long history of pain in both knees and some back pain. Here the TCM diagnosis indicated the disease process was complex. The treatment sought both to provide relief from pain through local work on her knees and to address the long-term deficiency of her underlying 'Qi'. This patient had many creative interests and community activities that gave her pleasure and seemed very happy with life apart from her pain and stiffness. After weekly acupuncture treatments her pain improved and she had more energy after the constitutional work of building up her level of Qi.

However, because of her age and the persistence of the problem (in TCM terms the underlying lack of Qi and the depth of the disorder), it was clear she would need occasional further treatment to maintain the improvement. This was arranged.

Contain. Many cases referred to the acupuncturist were patients that needed support and where the GP wanted help with 'containment'—whether 'supportive' or 'repressive'. In the following example, all treatment was undertaken only with the full participation of the patient at each stage because, as the consultation series unfolded, the focus of the treatment and the likely outcomes of treatment changed. This case underlines the importance of developing a shared understanding of how treatment might work, and what can be realistically expected from treatment. In such a complex case the practitioner must be prepared for the patient's emotional ups and downs and be able to negotiate contingency plans with the patient for dealing with unexpected developments that might, for instance, mean extra support was needed.

A woman in her sixties who was referred for treatment with joint pain had recently been diagnosed with cancer. The treatment did address her joint pain, and this did improve, but this was not by any means the main focus of the treatment sessions.

On an 'energetic' level the practitioner was able to give supportive acupuncture throughout the patient's cancer chemotherapy, but more importantly she also supported her humanly. It became very important to this patient that acupuncture does not split the mind from the body and that her underlying pattern of Qi predicted a tendency to severe anxiety. Acupuncture treatments focused on this aspect and the developing supportive relationship helped her cope.

It is important to understand that this patient's treatment entailed rigorous attention to negotiated informed consent.

Making and dealing with 'difficult referrals'—an example of massage treatment When practitioners from different professions collaborate, they will from time to time be faced with unfamiliar challenges. When this happens members may interpret the group's aims and what is going on in radically different ways. This example illustrates a typical problem.

It had become clear that bodyworkers were experiencing difficulties with certain kinds of patient, but it seemed very hard to make sense of what was going on or to do anything about it. Our massage practitioners were getting tired and angry and felt frustrated that no one understood why. It seemed as though they were somehow trapped in some inescapable pattern and that it had to be someone's fault. In reflecting on this we gradually realized that we were in an uncharted area. We now suspect that this situation recurs cyclically in a CP–GP team, and that it may be an unavoidable aspect of interprofessional group learning processes. If so then being able to recognize it and cope with it, time and again, is necessary work in progress. The observations that follow try to make some sense of these processes.

Why refer for massage? Dealings between conventional medicine and what used to be called 'the fringe' are complicated. They illustrate a mixture of idealization and antipathy that so often characterizes relationships with an unknown other. When CTs are available in house the problems that arise are easier to deal with, and CTs' contribution to managing even serious illness can be explored. Yet unfounded assumptions are still made: the idea that the practitioners involved necessarily understand how best to use such an extended clinical team, or manage the novel problems that emerge, being just one of them.

Our monthly theoretical seminars took up the themes of 'containment' and 'heart-sink and other kinds of difficult patient', and the way the centre's various health professionals—GPs, counsellors, nursing staff, complementary therapists—understand these terms (see Containment above). In the mid 1990s we began to ask why massage practitioners were feeling uncomfortable with certain aspects of their work. It seemed that massage therapists' 'difficulties' clustered around certain kinds of referral where some 'emotional' or 'relationship' component of massage had, either explicitly or tacitly, been requested. In discussing these issues, we asked why such referrals were made and what the primary care team members meant by the term 'difficult patient'.

To understand the massage practitioners' predicament we must first look at the reasons why a GP refers a patient for massage, what the expectations are, and what massage does. It helps to clarify the role of massage if we think of it as making its impact in four ways:

- through a physical impact of manipulation on soft tissue, lymphatic drainage and local blood circulation—this is the most specific effect
- through the induction of a relaxation response
- through its potential to call up emotions associated with touch
- finally, and least specifically, through the practitioner–client relationship.

The other important point to consider in a very general way is the reasons why GPs send patients to other practitioners:

- typically *referral* to a 'specialist' is for a diagnostic opinion or definitive treatment
- possibly because the 'specialist' *gatekeeps* an otherwise unavailable resource (e.g. a hospital bed, a CT scan)
- but most commonly, in a primary care team, GPs *delegate* aspects of care (e.g. nursing, social care, CT) to non-medical practitioners as a way of using time more effectively
- and thereby employ another practitioner's *particular skill*.

It is unlikely that a GP would ask a massage therapist for a 'diagnosis'—and other CPs might have little to offer in terms of diagnostic labels comprehensible in a strict biomedical context, though a chiropractor or osteopath might use concepts more familiar to a doctor—so the therapist is not in that sense a 'specialist'. However, 'referring a body part' (e.g. sending a patient for massage because of a painful shoulder) does look rather like a 'specialist' referral. Yet the intentions and aims are more tentative and exploratory: the GP is actually asking 'can you contribute something to "fixing" this?' Although by implication the GP is also saying 'if not let me know', referrals are in fact seldom refused. In contrast to the 'specialist' referral, a GP would more confidently, for example, involve the massage practitioner when someone needed help with 'tension', whether construed as literal (bodily) tension or as metaphorical (emotional) tension. This amounts to referring a person rather than a part and reflects a 'generalist' role, which conforms to popular ideas about massage and what it can do. In the former example the more 'specialist' referral suggests 'fixing', whereas in the latter 'generalist' type of referral there are overtones of 'maintaining'. Nonetheless, in both instances it is probably certain 'specific' attributes of massage (i.e. the physical effects and relaxation response) that GPs are expecting.

Given the strain of coping with 'difficult patients', it is hardly surprising that GPs sometimes want to delegate their care to someone else; indeed some patients demand it. When the intention is to provide respite for the GP and temporarily contain a difficult patient then delegating this sort of care within the team can be quite appropriate. However, everyone involved has to be clear that the intention is not to use CT for some kind of magical fixing. Inevitably, though, the availability of CTs in a primary care team will at times engender inappropriate magical expectations.

The 'fix' and 'maintain' categories often intertwine. Take the example of a patient with a tension headache: specific musculoskeletal massage treatment could be one intention behind referral, but the element of relaxation would be beneficial too. So the 'specific-specialist' role ('fixing' the headache) shades into the 'generalist' role of 'maintaining' the ability to relax. In addition, the GP may be aware, for instance, of a patient's recent bereavement, and feel that massage sessions will provide support. This is an example of 'supportive containment'. Although for most GPs delegation to a counsellor would be a more familiar step, in our experience referring such patients for massage is justified. This is because we know from our discussions that, as well as touching clients in structured and effective ways that help them relax, massage practitioners also listen to clients and provide in a very tangible way (literally) a sense of being supported and cared for. And, in the quiet tactile intimacy of a massage session, pent-up feelings may surface but, when they do, clients need to experience that they are both literally as well as symbolically 'well held'.

This is where the task of 'containing' can get complicated. Dealing with a client's unbearable emotions is not easy, but at least where transient life events are a specific cause of distress and bodily symptoms the practitioner can understand, identify and empathize, even though it may be anything but comfortable to do so. But sometimes patients come to GPs because of unbearable tension and inexpressible feelings whose source is hidden. Patients like this will perhaps 'somatize' their feelings and be unable to experience them directly and so name them as fear, anger or sadness, still less to express them as such, or to show insight into them. For the massage practitioner to whom the GP might refer, such a patient is likely to be far more troubling. The recently bereaved, redundant or dispossessed patients have been overtly 'wounded', but the distress that somatizing patients experience cannot be attributed to a recent injury or loss; yet their emotions often communicate themselves powerfully, sometimes even painfully, to the practitioner. Probably something resembling what psychodynamic therapists call 'transference' is happening here, but it is less straightforward than the identification we feel when a patient's bereavement resonates with our own experience of grief. In that case, providing we have some degree of insight, we will deal with this process of identification. In the 'difficult patient', however, where the trauma is more deeply hidden or secret, the patient may have repressed or split-off feelings and memories. In this case they are also likely to be defended against and denied by the practitioner, who can experience them only unconsciously. As long as these reactions remain unthinkable, and therefore barely available to be reflected on, the practitioner will in the presence of such a patient come to experience negativity, tiredness or pain also. One way of dealing with this situation if you are a GP is to refer the patient to someone else. Some 'thick-notes' patients are a testament to what can happen if a practitioner is not aware of these feelings and what the sense of 'difficultness' in the consultation means.[4]

Recently, in analysing caseloads, we realized that massage practitioners had been seeing many such clients. This was a cue to examine management policy but also to think through why this type of referral might be happening, and how to recognize when it did. The dynamics involved are elusive, but in a consultation, whether with a general or a massage practitioner, the clue may be the very presence of this sense of 'difficultness', perhaps at the periphery of one's emotional vision. Recognizing this, the question 'whose feelings are these?' is worth asking. What should one do when this happens? The ability to talk about 'heart-sink patients' has given GPs a language that can help articulate the practical and intrapersonal difficulties of managing these patients. It is generally agreed that it calls for strategic containment and, though different approaches may be tried, all are characterized by avoiding acting out the patient's own unconscious splits and projections. The term 'heart-sink' describes a very broad group but it is not a homogeneous one and the 'heart-sink' label probably conceals significant differences. Given that their only common denominator is the 'heart-sink' they provoke, and having some understanding of what 'splitting' entails, we have to acknowledge that darker and less disclosable emotions and fantasies than 'heart-sink' alone are sometimes provoked in practitioners too.

Bodywork for heart-sink patients? Bearing these ideas in mind we should consider the consequences of using hands-on therapies with such clients. What does it do to the practitioners they are referred to? Several questions arise, both strategic and organizational. If, for instance, massage is an appropriate way of working with some 'heart-sink' patients, then which ones, and how might such work be integrated into a team approach? When, on the other hand, might referral to massage represent an inappropriate collusion that splits the patient or the team further? This leads to questions of differential diagnosis: particularly if bodywork as well as being beneficial for many patients could, for a small minority, be contraindicated. Can we for instance discern when various 'difficult' feelings aroused (including 'heart-sink' but other possible experiences of countertransference too) predict that, far from being helpful, massage (and presumably other kinds of manually based CTs—e.g. osteopathy, chiropractic, aromatherapy, reflexology, acupuncture) would be too intrusive and threatening? Perhaps in the independent sector, where people find their own way to bodyworkers, it is less likely that the choice will have to be made. But in the public sector unguided delegation is perhaps more likely to lead vulnerable patients inappropriately into the hands of bodyworkers. But how are we to tell when boundaries are too vulnerable, or perceive when a person is barely able to contain their emotional life and sense of identity? When, for instance, would it be appropriate to massage a patient bordering on breakdown? Perhaps it is only the bodyworkers themselves, reflecting on their reactions to a session, who *can* differentiate. Massage transactions have a different quality to those of GPs, and perhaps it is only while working on someone with one's hands for 40-plus minutes that these kinds of insights arise. But when the GP's referral is in some way a response to a splitting process it should not be surprising that during such long hands-on sessions the massage therapist might begin to experience feelings the referring doctor had (understandably) failed to suspect, let alone recognize or even contain.

We have found that an extended clinical team *can* share the burdens of managing persistently unwell and high-consulting patients. We know that massage can often restore a sense of comfort, even in a patient who is struggling psychologically or whom we suspect is expressing some inner turmoil through the body, but sensitive selection is important. Only an experienced therapist should be asked to work with such patients, and so adequate guidelines have to be developed. How therefore can we differentiate those patients who are not suitable for bodywork therapies, and provide the time, support (and supervision?) the 'bodyworker' might need when dealing with such potentially 'complex' patients?

To explore these issues and help the CPs gain insight into this group of patients, a supervision programme was organized for CPs at the MHC.* Its first aim was to explore the ideas of transference and countertransference and help CPs to use these psychodynamic notions as a way of looking at some of the feelings aroused by certain clients. When working with distressed clients it can be difficult to avoid taking these feelings personally. The essential learning objective was that the therapeutic relationship can be important for the client without the therapist having to become overinvolved and overwhelmed by the emotional maelstrom.

A second aim was to help with spotting cases that were beyond the bodyworkers' expertise. This category included patients who are too fragmented to be able to get any benefit from massage; they are so tense and hostile that they are unable to relax even with stroking, or if they do it is very temporary and may even provoke great feelings of unease in them.

A third aim was to help practitioners protect themselves during and after a difficult session. Discussions of difficult cases helped practitioners learn how best to support each other, and also to disentangle what had actually happened in the sessions. The supervision has begun to help practitioners think much more carefully about ways of transferring patients when they feel they are not appropriate for massage, or if they feel they need a second opinion. Practitioners also said the supervision sessions had helped them to step back to a position where they did not feel threatened but still had something to offer the patient.

A final aim was to make it clear that containment is an active process, but that by becoming more aware of the feelings evoked during a session practitioners could learn to be more receptive to patients without being overwhelmed. Discussions helped the practitioners to under-

stand how different therapists, using different approaches, would deal with similar situations. All the practitioners felt they could benefit from ongoing supervision sessions because these so clearly helped them 'digest' the problems encountered with angry, frightened and needy patients.

'Difficult referrals': ways forward If a referring practitioner is aware of being emotionally 'stirred up' by a patient one can predict that the bodyworker will be too. Once acknowledged, these difficult feelings ought to signal a need to be very clear about the expectations and aims prompting such a referral. And if indeed a referral is made then how would these expectations and aims be communicated? How might massage practitioners in turn communicate their objectives and evaluation back to the GP? We think this type of delegation requires a face-to-face meeting to discuss the case, because this tends to 'contain' the referral and make it easier for the CP to 'contain' the client and help avoid the acting out of 'splits' within the team.

Massage is usually practised in the private sector; NHS family medicine is a significantly different context. For instance, the act of referral itself directs patients who might otherwise not have chosen to be massaged into an inherently complex clinical relationship. Once referred for massage our current policy is that patients, after an assessment session, have a package of four sessions, but then no further sessions in a year. Even if patients feel bodywork has been helpful the unit does not currently have the resources to offer more. The rationale behind this use of massage has been to see it as a way of giving patients a relaxed experience of their body—the hope being that they will subsequently maintain this benefit through self-care, facilitated by leaflets, advice or classes in relaxation, stretching, movement, autogenics, exercise, etc. This policy places bodywork activity firmly in the 'fixing–maintaining' role. If the 'containment' role is to develop we have to decide how a carefully selected and thoughtfully distributed caseload of 'difficult' patients might be managed. Handling beginnings and endings, how to shape longer-term contact, and the definite need to provide supervision for 'difficult' feelings would be essential considerations for any team that wants to develop this role for difficult patients referred in public sector settings. For instance, the way we might extend our own use of massage parallels the use of long-term occasional contact as used in the monthly appointments model of containment used by the counselling unit at MHC.

Although stressed, disturbed, somatizing patients continue to find their way to the whole range of CTs at MHC, we do not see CTs as necessarily a resource for patients unsuitable for counselling. Referral of patients to a CT service such as massage is not always appropriate. To avoid inappropriate referrals our counsellors developed

---

* The following text is based on feedback from massage therapist/nurse Sarah Martin from a supervision course on transference and countertransference.

a simple counselling referral protocol; this was a written system of practice agreed and conformed to by all parties, and subject to regular audit and review. The protocol provided GPs with guidelines for the use of forms and an information leaflet. It also offered a reminder list of criteria associated with successful counselling outcomes and the common reasons for failure. (For example, in order for patients to benefit from counselling and use the scarce time available they *must* be motivated, available and have the capacity to bear some psychological pain and the ability to reflect on their experience and talk about their feelings.) It also provided a simple way to communicate the aims of the MHC counselling service to part-time staff members who were rarely in the building on the same day as the counsellors.

If the patient decides to proceed, the patient must also complete a request form (which is blue for quick recognition), and this is sent or handed in, in a sealed envelope, to reception. The referral box is cleared every week, and a counselling appointment is sent *only* when both GP referral and patient request forms are received. A counsellor guarantees to contact the patient within 2 weeks.

Reducing DNAs on first appointments. Patients referred by GPs to other members of the primary care team commonly miss their first appointment. Good preparation by the GP and appropriate information about the CT service helps avoid unnecessary DNAs. This preparation requires good enough information about the reasons and the benefits, testing out commitment to and congruence with the aims of the referral, and giving some preliminary paperwork in preparation. At the MHC the use of leaflets and the filling out of MYMOP forms has helped to reduce missed first appointments in the CT service.

To facilitate regular review of referral patterns, the counsellors and CPs circulate a list of their current patients and their waiting list once a month, together with a list of any DNAs. This information provides a useful quick check on the progress of current patients in the system. This paperwork also informs the regular audit meetings (see Meetings and reports section, p. 153). If (as now happens less often) a patient does not arrive, the GP has a chance to ask why, and to explain that resources are limited and that the courtesy of making a cancellation is something we expect. Counselling DNAs on first appointments currently stand at only 5%—a cause for celebration. The success of this system prompted the CPs to try introducing a similar system.

Implications for the multiprofessional team. The weekly meetings where doctors, nurses, CPs and counsellors discuss cases and organizational issues provides an essential forum for thinking things through and for forward planning. The above example of sharing innovations with other members of the team is one way we have learned to overcome the different professional groups experiencing defensive blocks. The multiprofessional team at MHC is a constant source of new ideas about interprofessional collaboration and for maximizing the use of scarce resources.

Conclusion and recommendations Our reflections have identified a particular patient group who is experienced by massage practitioners as being 'difficult' to deal with. This made us consider the role of bodywork in 'containing' difficult patients, some of whom fit into the 'heartsink' category, and others who may have more or less overt mental health problems. If referrals are to be made for 'containment', this should be explicitly mentioned and explored face to face. Bodyworkers may need supervision when working with these patients, just as counsellors would. Very disturbed or borderline clients should probably not be referred (even though at times they might slip through the net). We realize that, however good our guidelines are, there have been more problem interactions and problematic endings at busy times when either general or complementary practitioners have been overburdened with patients. Though overload may be less likely as a team expands, the need for clear referral and treatment guidelines and communication— including, for instance, adequate ways of beginning and ending a series of bodywork treatments—becomes greater. We now think that, with a clearer awareness of the issues, we are in a position to develop the guidelines and processes needed.

Marylebone Health Centre was established to explore 'holistic approaches to inner city general practice'. 'Holism'—a response to late modern medicine's tendency to fragment patients and their care—is concerned with integrating the part into the whole and accepting back what has been marginalized. The 'difficult patient' in a certain sense carries the unacceptable. Our deliberations are a reminder that holistic interprofessional practice depends on our willingness to reflect on clinical and organizational integration of CTs into primary care in order to reown aspects of healthcare that have been pushed away. We now suspect that these boundary issues are a key to developing the tools needed to set boundaries and to explore overt critical incidents, and also to take note of and articulate unease when it occurs.

The role of CTs in family medicine

The demand for long-term support of patients with difficult, relapsing, chronic ill health seems an obvious focus for the use of CTs in family medicine. If so, acute cases would in all probability get squeezed out (although chronic patients also have acute episodes and it is at these points that referral tends to happen). To avoid this the approach needs to be well structured, capable of minimizing inappropriate referrals and ensuring efficient use of scarce resources, to make time available for a more broadly based use of a CT service.

When our group first came together our time was, relatively speaking, protected by research funds, which pump-primed our study of the MHC's innovative approach. Consequently no one questioned whether the time-frame of CP private practice was appropriate. Long appointments—typically 30–60 minutes—were the norm. The NHS GPs meanwhile were often seeing six or more patients an hour for up to 5 or 6 hours a day as well as carrying the responsibility for administration and management and out-of-hours cover for patients. Understandably, this differential fuelled conflict about power, responsibility and privilege. GPs felt that long CT appointments strained the resources of a busy NHS health centre. Could CT practitioners therefore adapt to a resource-limited, high-demand system—and if so, how? Perhaps there are lessons to be learned from the failure of psychoanalysis to make much impact in the NHS. There are parallels to be drawn between the way complementary medicine might develop in this context and the way brief forms of psychotherapy developed— particularly in the USA—as a response to resource limit- ation. Can we then imagine 'brief-intervention' TCM, massage, homeopathy or osteopathy, perhaps based on a limited number of short 30- or even 20-minute 'NHS units'? Whether or not this is practical, or even desirable, it is what we had to do in order for the CT service to sur- vive. Why, we had to ask ourselves, should CPs need to see patients for 40 minutes to an hour at each visit? If they do, then few people will have access to them unless many sessions are available. Waiting lists would inevitably become unacceptably long, or CP hourly pay would have to be kept unacceptably low. Yet time and/or touch are important elements in all CTs, so how could a CP consultation be shorter without fundamen- tally undermining the very core of what CTs represent?

Our group has tested out solutions to this problem and, though no definitive answer has been reached, there are signs that CT can be delivered effectively in brief sessions. Our current time-scales are:

- osteopathy/musculoskeletal acupuncture: 20 minutes (using two rooms for overlapping appointments)
- homeopathy: initially 40 minutes, follow-up 20 minutes
- massage: 45 minutes
- traditional acupuncture: 30 minutes (with two rooms and overlapping appointment times).

What have we learnt?

In summary, some underlying themes emerged from our review of our own and similar practices:

- What do GPs expect of CT treatment ('fix', 'contain' or 'maintain'?) for 'complex' patients?
- In some situations a CP sees a case as 'complex' but the GP might not (e.g. miasms).
- Practitioners are concerned that CT's full potential is recognized (e.g. how many sessions?).
- How can one avoid the CT service being overloaded with patients whose conventional labels disguise complex problems or complex maintaining causes?
- How should teams identify patients and conditions likely to be resistant to treatment?
- Is the CP a 'specialist' treating diseases, or a 'generalist' managing illness (e.g. 'I may treat OA then find the patient's migraines also improve')?

The reflective method developed at MHC is based on structured data collection. We believe this approach to service management allows greater understanding of CT's role, including its impact on patients and on practice resources. We think that the effectiveness of CT in the primary care setting depends on how well it can be integrated into the work of the team. The data system's further development and use should ensure that CTs play an increasingly appropriate and effective part in our own primary care team's work. At this point and because this is action research, the conclusions are emergent and determine new questions and methods to be tested out in further cycles.

Many questions have remained unanswered or need revisiting as a practical reality distils out from the early rhetoric. Several major issues still need addressing at practice level and also need to be considered wherever CTs are being commissioned in primary care:

- *Demand*—This needs to be assessed from the position of the user, the clinician and the policy makers. Should CTs be selectively available in public primary care provision?
- *Resources*—How can sensible purchasing policies be developed?
- *Interprofessional issues*—How can complementary and conventional practice develop a viable interface? How can we develop a common language and common language base?
- *Information needs*—What is the overall task? What is the appropriate primary healthcare delivery system? What is the clinical and management evidence base?

The MHC has developed a quality assured integrated healthcare model through the flexibility of a PMS pilot since 1997. The PMS structure in UK general practice was designed to reduce bureaucracy, increase creativity, input quality indicators and outcomes, allow an extended range of clinical services, improve links with the PCG and establish temporary budget certainty.

After exploring some of the interprofessional issues that arose as we began to work together, a research and development project helped define and audit patient-centred health outcomes of complementary and self-care interventions. We are appraising the use of specific complementary interventions in identified conditions (e.g. IBS, back pain, asthma, PMS, migraine) and the ongoing usefulness of patient-assessed medical outcome measures. This work will, we hope, make a significant contribution to the current evidence base and inform efficient ways of identifying the needs and using resources in clinical purchasing. For example, MHC in partnership with another local practice (Cavendish Health Centre) has recently designed a model for provision of CT to its local primary care group. We hope that this will be a generalizable model that can be adapted for other collaborative health initiatives.

Lessons we learned from collaborative working in an integrated primary care team include the following.

1. The guiding principles underlying all the work continue to be partnership and governance:

• this partnership includes intraprofessional partnership within unidisciplines working in a collaborative team
• interprofessional partnership with other healthcare professionals in the team
• partnership with patients through a strong patients' partnership group
• partnership with the community through work with local statutory and voluntary agencies
• partnership with government in responding creatively to new organizational structures for the delivery of primary healthcare
• governance has been achieved through the development of a 'quality referral and outcomes' model; working within this model has highlighted the ways in which accountability and professional development are inextricably linked.

2. Change takes time. No matter how strong the motivation, a reasonably stable team membership and regular staff development, the development of interprofessional working is slow. Particular difficulties can be high autonomy needs held by some practitioners, and uniprofessional tacit assumptions.

3. Collaboration is expensive. Teamworking and liaison take a lot of time; this has both financial and time consequences for participants and the practice.

4. There is a tenuous link with improved outcomes. Teamworking is poorly studied and tools for assessing patient health outcomes and interprofessional learning outcomes are underdeveloped. It has taken a great deal of time to produce our qualitative descriptive study.

How can we measure outcomes that are not formally codified?

5. Collaborative working entails new interprofessional dynamics. Power, rivalry and competition have been mentioned previously. Working in teams is difficult, and a collection of professionals does not necessarily make a team. Some members belong to several teams, within as well as outside the MHC.

6. Practitioner intentions and outcome assessments need to be clarified. The team had already established that referral to a CP does not necessarily mean 'fix this problem' (see discussion in Complex cases, p. 159). So it appears that GPs might see in CTs a possibility not always of fixing, but of maintaining function or containing distress, in patients whom they would otherwise find difficult to deal with. However, such an extended range of expectations even if met might not be revealed as a quantifiable outcome on a MYMOP graph, particularly if only a limited number of consultations can be made available. So we may have to rethink what 'effectiveness' and 'cost–benefit' might mean in a NHS CT service.

7. There needs to be an understanding of the problems practitioners face when introducing new approaches. We have identified a number of these; they are summarized in Box 5.2.

Finally, as a result of our experience we have formulated a number of key questions that GPs and CPs need to consider when considering setting up a CT service. These are listed in Box 5.3.

LOOKING FORWARD

Our immediate aim for the future is to keep going. We have operated and improved our integrative approach and its systems for the delivery, management and evaluation. And we intend to work with other centres to implement similar ways of capturing and reflecting on data. The work of the last 3 years has also focused our minds on work with 'complex' patients, using a range of self-care materials for patients, learning each other's skills and improving our ability to work multiprofessionally. Development of the MHC delivery system further will involve more work in these areas too.

Our underlying principles of partnership and governance will best be achieved by education in its broadest sense, and in particular interprofessional learning. We intend the MHC in the next phase of our work to develop as a teaching and research unit. In our work with the University of Westminster we will be producing information and a range of short courses to practices and individuals who want to build more integrated primary care services.

Our experience has generated a host of new questions and emerging lines of enquiry. These are summarized in Table 5.1.

Box 5.2 Some problems practitioners need to consider before introducing new approaches

- Conventional medicine provides some perfectly adequate treatments for many common conditions: e.g. acute bacterial RTI, congestive heart failure, and glaucoma. Where this is the case, no alternative or adjunctive treatments are really needed.
- Many common health problems are not easily 'fixed', however: e.g. relapsing mechanical back pain, migraine, asthma, IBS, RA, OA, etc. The continuing management of these patients is a daily challenge for general practice and the cost in both human and financial terms is high.

  Accepted modalities currently available to family practitioners (e.g. nursing, physiotherapy, specialist referral, and counselling, prescribing drugs) do not necessarily meet the expressed needs of patients whose problems are not 'fixable'. But are the potential collaborators convinced that CTs are relevant to these problems?
- The management of some patients may involve 'containing' them psychologically (viz. Balint[3]) in order actively to help them avoid an endless succession of specialist interference. Others have long-term relapsing structural or functional disorders whose medical treatment is often less than satisfactory and which understandably, both doctor and patient hope might be improved.

  The boundary between the patients whose high consultation rates are due to somatization disorder or high trait anxiety and others with chronic disease is inevitably blurred.
- Consumer surveys show that patients usually cross over from conventional care to CTs for help with conditions already being treated conventionally, and that they express satisfaction with the outcome of a combined approach.

  This suggests a market for multiprofessional practice. But does this observation necessarily support development of integrated CTs in the public sector?

Box 5.3 Key questions that GPs and CPs should ask themselves before setting up a CT service

Key questions for GPs
Patient involvement:
- What do my patients want?
- What do they need?
- Is this the same?
- How do I find out?

What do you want CTs to provide for you?
- Attract new patients to practice?
- Offer safe and effective alternative to conventional treatment?

What do I want specific CPs to provide?
- Specific service for conditions conventional medicine not good at treating?
- Support for GPs with complex patients/difficult cases?
- Maintaining treatments for those with chronic conditions especially pain?
- Flexible approach to conditions of recent onset linked to patient request and where Western medicine offers little?

As a GP how much do I want to do for myself?
- What can I learn and easily use?
- Has a good evidence base?
- That I can use in conjunction with my existing skills and knowledge?
- That my patients find acceptable?
- That I can fit into a 10-minute consultation?

What would I like my patients to do for themselves?
- A range of self-care measures?
- Attend local health-focused classes?
- Obtain additional support to help themselves?
- How much time can I devote to supporting them?

Resources:
- What resources do I have already?
- What is the minimum that I need?
- Where will these come from?
- How much time would the project I have in mind take?
- How much time can I devote?
- Who do I need to involve?
- How much time can they devote?
- How will they be paid?

Key questions for CPs
What will I be asked to treat?
- How far will I be able to influence the referral process?
- What structures will there be for me to contribute my knowledge and skills?
- Will I be referred a variety of conditions and levels of illness?
- Will I be asked to work only as a specialist dealing with specific complaints?
- Will I only be sent complex, heartsink patients?
- Will I be able to work to the limits of my practice?
- What will happen when there is an inappropriate referral?
- Will I have a choice about whether I treat everybody sent to me or not?
- How do I give feedback to the GPs?

How will contact with GPs be managed?
Informally:
- Individuals' learning about each other and their therapies.
- Discussing patient care.

Formally:
- For creating and reviewing structures and processes for delivery of the service.
- Reaching agreement.
- Building on the things learnt during informal contact.
- Handling structural problems.

Time limits to treatment:
- How many times will I be allowed to treat each patient?
- What will happen if the patient needs more?
- Are there criteria for extending the treatment period if necessary?

Evaluation:
- How will my work be evaluated?
- Are there any consequences I should know about regarding evaluation?
- Will I receive training to be able to take part in any evaluation procedures?

Practitioner development:
- Can I work as effectively within the NHS as in private practice?
- Do I need to develop any new skills to be able to work effectively within the public health sector?
- What opportunities for learning could working in public health offer me?

Table 5.1 New questions generated and emerging lines of enquiry

Emerging solution to the problems of integrating CTs	Linked processes	Observation/action to be tested
• structured approach to referral: developing guidelines enables increasing clarity about aims/objective of referrals • clear lines of communication shaped by proformas	• professional practice is slow to change • the structures tend to become unwieldy	• re-present guidelines as on-screen computer documents • practical use of a computer-based relational database
• need to collect referral, clinical and outcome data		• continuously adapt system to generate most relevant reporting output
• patient-centred outcome measures built into the referral–treatment cycle	• as far as possible they have to be used consistently	• outcome measures entail particular difficulties for patients with chronic problems and emotional aspects to their illness
• planning high levels of referral of difficult patients and those with chronic health problems	• GPs' expectations of a referral to a CP are not always well articulated • patients' expectations of a CP outcome are not always rational	• review GPs' referrals to CPs in regular clinical meetings
• regular reports produced by the computer system allow tabulated reporting of clinical progress • some patients appear to benefit significantly but some report relapses when CT treatment sessions cease	• is MYMOP always an appropriate way to track clinical change? • e.g. to what extent can the potential benefits of CTs be realized within a resource-limited system?	• use GHHOS to follow samples of patients treated • are referred patients resource hungry, or a special category of need? • would these needs be met cost effectively by greater access to CT? • explore potential cost–benefit of long-term follow-up of chronic high attenders

The future of CTs in integrated mainstream healthcare

When the British Holistic Medical Association was formed in 1986 it put forward its vision of whole person care. Two decades on, its call for seamless holistic approaches and its five founding principles appear less radical than they did then. Perhaps its central proposition now seems almost self-evident—that while health depends on biological influences, and psychological and social factors too, it also has something to do with our humanity and spirituality. Once stated, the other principles follow: that healthcare should involve a wider group of health and social care professionals; that patients need information and resources to ensure appropriate healthcare choices and prevention; that, wherever possible, treatment should encourage the person's innate capacity for health and well-being; and finally that practitioners need education and support in order to maintain their own well-being and capacity to help.

If these five tenets shaped mainstream thinking about healthcare and its delivery, what would public sector medicine look like? An integrated system would have to be pluralistic and centred on primary care, emphasizing prevention and health creation. Treatment would still take place in the context of conventional modern medicine and nursing, but would embrace other physical and psychological treatments—including certain aspects of CT—according to need, appropriateness and patients' beliefs.

Information networks would inform and enhance integrated teamwork; for instance, the internet can make the evidence base highly accessible, it can make information about risks and health promotion available in new ways, and it can improve communication between practitioners. Perhaps most importantly, its potential as a vehicle for the evaluation of outcomes on a large scale is particularly important, because ultimately we have to show that integrating different aspects of healthcare actually improves quality of life and delivers measurable health gain.

In the UK, CTs have been gaining ground in the NHS—a trend driven by public popularity, professional interest and a small but significant amount of research into effectiveness. Yet, although this suggests the integration of certain CTs deserves serious consideration, the case will be unconvincing unless it speaks in terms of identifiable need and cost–benefit. As things stand the lack of cost-effectiveness studies is an obstacle to further integration of CTs. In fact the majority of primary care groups are not planning to commission CTs for this very reason. Perhaps this is no bad thing, because an uncritical acceptance of CT would have been counterproductive. Accepted wisdom—whether orthodox or 'alternative'—deserves to be questioned and wrong expectations of CTs only hinder their appropriate use, perhaps as much as blinkered scepticism. But it appears to many clinicians and patients that some aspects of CT are valuable, and potentially they could be cost effective too. Furthermore, the popularity of CT provides clues about the way health needs and health beliefs are changing. For there is nothing fixed about them, nor are healthcare systems static (some would complain that ours is not static enough!). They evolve as new human and technical capabilities appear and unsuspected needs are recognized. The popularity of CTs might be due to either one or both of these factors. There has been a steady erosion in the 'traditional' GP role, with a significant increase in administrative workload, technical approaches and associated costs. At the same time, global improvements in the basic levels of health and well-being (disease control, public health measures, living conditions) have encouraged a quest for more sophisticated levels of 'holistic' health and lifestyle. Many complementary approaches are effective in this contemporary cultural context and help patients interpret their symptoms—why me? why now? why this?

At a time when 'evidence-based medicine' has such enormous currency, we should remember that some important innovations have in the past been needs driven, developing without a rational base on formal research-derived evidence. Are there parallels between then and now—for instance, between the way CTs have been adopted by the mainstream and how counselling or hospice care were incorporated? Marginal 30 years ago, both have become integral parts of conventional practice. However, these social inventions took root not as a result of clinical trials, but rather because they met previously unspoken needs; in fact, in their early days these new forms of care actually drew attention to the unmet needs of the emotionally distressed and the dying. A few innovators were able to build on the pioneers' experience and create NHS provision. Subsequently, mainstream academic centres for counselling or palliative care arose and became focal points for research and education. They in turn helped to legitimate and spread these new forms of practice.

CTs have had a long journey in from the fringe and the field has reached a point where several UK projects have a similar research and education role. Innovation is under way, alive and well despite the lack of secure funding. However, a research and development effort is overdue, to rectify the lack of quality research and evidence of effectiveness for many complementary medical approaches. Only planned implementation and evaluation will tell us how best to make complementary approaches selectively available, which will be an increasingly important decision as the NHS opens up to these therapies and sensible purchasing policies have to

be developed. Appropriate case selection and 'familiarization' are the keys to successful implementation of complementary medicine, but proof of its efficacy and cost–benefit advantages may not be enough to establish it in the NHS. How the interface between complementary and conventional practice is organized, and how the problems of their interaction are managed, will be crucial. The lack of a common clinical language and theory remains a major obstacle. If the current convergence is to continue, we must face up to the educational task of developing joint learning programmes, as well as the organizational challenge of implementing and evaluating these innovative clinical approaches within the health service.

Thankfully some of the existing projects have survived a major NHS reorganization. Some of the recent pilot schemes are trail blazers for important new models of care. We should be in no doubt that healthcare will change rapidly in the new millennium; an ageing population, new patterns of morbidity and spiralling costs guarantee it. A programme of ongoing action research and evaluation among NHS initiatives would be a step forward. In the medium term, by pooling data and creating information networks, a picture of the problems and benefits of delivering CTs, of learning needs, good practice and outcomes, would unfold. In addition, a proper appraisal of poorly met need, surveying how and why CTs are being used in mainstream practice, is overdue—because, if integrating CTs alongside conventional care mainstream healthcare truly improves outcomes or life quality, then there is an urgent need to know. Eventually the necessary randomized comparative trials could provide the definitive evidence, but meanwhile the test-beds are out there and they deserve our support. To lose them would be to miss a tremendous opportunity.

The history of public provision of complementary therapies has always involved safeguarding the services we have as well as developing them and arguing for further provision. If complementary therapy services are to survive then we need to prove they are cost effective, fulfil unmet needs, provide a high standard of care, are safe and are desired by patients. Services also need to work towards equal access to patients and may be threatened if they can't fulfil on this. When services are closed the expertise of all involved is lost to the public.

It is clear that those who wish to explore the contribution complementary therapies could make to the nation's health need to work together and share their experience. We hope to see a national (even an international) network develop in the coming years, to support best practice and collect outcomes data. We hope that the contents of this workbook will be useful to all those who wish to be involved in the provision of complementary therapies and that it helps consolidate our tenuous position within the mainstream and supports quality care and genuine integration. We welcome comments and criticism from all who use this book and hope to hear how they progress so that we can continue with our learning.

SUMMARY: SOME FINAL POINTERS

In conclusion, we offer some short pointers for would-be integrated teams to bear in mind.

- Don't underestimate the time it takes to change practice. Be prepared for things to take longer than expected.
- Don't expect a consistent level of commitment or enthusiasm over a long period of development.
- Introduce changes in workable chunks.
- Communicate about changes to timetabled events.
- Celebrate small achievements.
- Openly appreciate people's contribution.
- Expect times of confusion, disagreement and a lack of clarity. Articulate these feelings; they are often a kind of group turbulence that precedes a breakthrough!
- Do all you can to engage all concerned in the process: feeding back questions as they emerge, circulating reports, seeking input and aiming for consensus.

REFERENCES

1. Reason R 1991 Power and conflict in multidisciplinary collaboration. Journal of Complementary Medical Research. 5(3): 144–150
2. Balint E, Courtenay M, Elder A et al 1993 The doctor, the patient and the group: Balint revisited. Routledge, London
3. Capra F 1982 The biomedical model. In: The Turning Point. Fontana, New York
4. Gerard T J, Riddell J D 1988 Difficult patients: black holes and secrets. British Medical Journal 297: 530–532
5. Wallcraft J 1998 Healing minds. A report on current research, policy and practice concerning the use of complementary and alternative therapies for a wider range of mental health problems. Mental Health Foundation Complementary Medicine Bulletin on Depression, p. 7
6. Bion W 1959 Attacks on linking. International Journal of Psychoanalysis 30: 308–315, republished in 1967 as Second thoughts. Heinemann, Oxford

Chapter 5 REFLECTIVE LEARNING CYCLE AUDIT

1. **What did you need to know?** *(clarify learning objectives)*

2. **What did you notice?** *(key points)*

3. **What have you learned?** *(learning evaluation)*

4. **How will you apply it to practice?** *(clinical relevance)*

5. **What do I need to do next?** *(reflective educational audit)*

6. **Proceed to next area of interest / section you have identified.**

PART 3

Service documentation and information sheets

6

Information sheets on management of common disorders

The table at the foot of each of the following information sheets assigns a number to the level of research-derived evidence available for using complementary therapies (CTs) to treat the stated condition.

Evidence-linked practice has to include a hierarchy of evidence from clinical case reports through to systematic reviews:

5 = DEFINITELY—good evidence from systematic reviews or meta-analyses

4 = PROBABLY—evidence from one or more sound, randomized and/or controlled trials

3 = POSSIBLY—some evidence from RCTs available: results inconclusive, studies conflicting or methods open to question

2 = OPINION—practitioner conviction, expert opinion or clinical experience, but no reliable research

1 = RUMOUR—'traditional use', but effectiveness doubted or research suggesting that CT is ineffective

The research-derived evidence for using CTs is not always well developed. Consequently, in conditions where practitioners believe they have a useful part to play, even though the RCT-derived evidence is not yet established, a ranking of '2' denotes an area where the particular CT might have a role and where further studies are needed.

The reference numbers in the tables correspond to those in the full evidence table (Table 2.2) and reference details are given in the References to Chapter 2.

ALLERGIES AND INTOLERANCES
an overall multisystem approach

BIOCHEMICAL FACTORS
- ALLERGY = a genetic predisposition to make antibodies to harmless foods and environmental substances. Tiny amounts provoke acute allergic response
- FOOD INTOLERANCE = *not* immune reaction Not sudden. Weak gut enzymes? Deficiencies?

STRUCTURAL FACTORS
- ALLERGIC reactions are acute inflammation, e.g. rashes, fluid retention, swelling, blocked nose, muscle spasm—tightening airways (asthma or gut pain)
- INTOLERANCE: *possible* that intolerances predispose to long-term illness or chronic inflammatory disease

PSYCHOSOCIAL
- build-up of mental, structure or chemical overload?
- allergic symptoms affect feelings and performance
- 'stress' affects gut, respiration, circulation, immunity
- even a true allergy is more a problem when 'stressed'
- possible that unwellness caused by allergy or intolerance exacerbates psychological problems

CONVENTIONAL TREATMENTS
- ALLERGY antihistamines, steroids.
- identify allergens by testing if necessary
- INTOLERANCE? underdiagnosed

NON-CONVENTIONAL
- identify and avoid foodstuffs if suspected; high-quality low-antigen diet (see self-help sheet)
- possible that homeopathy may help to desensitize

REFER TO
- naturopath, homeopath, nutrition counsellor

CONVENTIONAL TREATMENT
- ?stress management and CBT
- hypnotherapy evidence: all allergy

NON-CONVENTIONAL
- relaxation and breathing techniques to relieve stress response and muscle tension

??REFER TO
- meditation programme
- autogenic teacher
- biofeedback relaxation
- hypnotherapist

CONVENTIONAL TREATMENT
- depends on symptoms (see specific conditions: asthma, etc.)

NON-CONVENTIONAL
- depends on symptoms (see specific conditions: IBS, etc.)
- the overall approach aims to increase personal resilience in ways relevant to the individual.
- are structural therapies relevant in this case (e.g. asthma)?

?REFER TO
- osteo/chiropractic, acupuncture

SELF-HELP

Food allergy Common food culprits are cow's milk, eggs, wheat, citrus fruits, soy and nuts. If given in the first year of life—even through breastmilk—they can trigger lifelong allergies in genetically susceptible babies, whose gastrointestinal tracts and immune systems are too immature to process these substances. Avoiding these foods and lowering levels of dust mites, tobacco smoke and animal fur in the home may help prevent infants becoming sensitized. Most people with classic allergic reactions show raised levels of IgE antibodies. IgEs are normal in food intolerance.

Inhalant allergy Commonsense steps to avoid triggers include: special mattress covers to protect against house dust mite droppings; synthetic pillows and duvets; wash bedding every week at 60°C; short-pile synthetic carpets, or none at all; let others vacuum, or use a cleaner that retains most of the dust; no warm-blooded pets; avoid long grass; keep windows closed mid morning and late afternoon/early evening when the pollen count is highest.

Complementary practitioners See allergies and intolerances as a sign of overstrained coping processes—i.e. inadequate diet, environmental pollution and stress are getting the better of the immune system. The overall strategy is to lower the total level of potential irritants—dietary and structural as well as psychological or social—and to maximize resources for wellness and healing, through exercise, relaxation and creativity. Identify allergens *and* irritants and avoid if possible. Strengthen digestion/metabolic processes. Help body systems eliminate toxins and repair damage.

COMMENT

True allergies involve the immune system producing *antibodies*—protein molecules that normally fight bacteria, viruses and other microorganisms—against substances that are normally harmless. These substances may be proteins in food, or be carried on the air we breathe, or come in contact with our skin, or be injected as insect stings (bees, wasps) or ingested as drugs. Allergies are becoming more common in developed countries: already one person in five has some kind of allergy and numbers are increasing, especially among children. Environmental pollutants, food additives and stress have all been blamed. Several different allergens from several different sources may contribute to one disorder. Allergens do not necessarily cause symptoms at the point where they entered the body, but may be carried elsewhere by the bloodstream. Foods can cause asthma in the bronchial tubes (see Asthma card), or house dust mites can trigger eczema on the skin.

	Acupuncture	Homeopathy	Manual therapies	Nutritional therapies	Herbal medicine	Mind–body methods & hypnotherapy
Asthma	3[1] subjectively	3[2]	1 chiro[3] 3 yoga[4]	3 diet strategies[5] 3 Mg, Sn, antiox[6]	3 various herbs[7]	4 hypnotherapy[8] 4 autogenic training[9]
Rhinitis, hay fever	2 prevention?	4[10,11] hay fever		2 exclusion diets?	3[12] urtica	3[13] hypnotherapy
Eczema		2		3 exclusion diets[28] 4 evening prim[29]	3 TCM[30]	4 hypnotherapy[31]

ANXIETY AND ANXIETY ATTACKS (PANIC ATTACKS)

BIOCHEMICAL FACTORS

- persistent 'stress' turns on flight and fight (F&F) response so adrenaline levels rise
- mid brain neurotransmitters disturbed by depressive illness
- anxiety increases if blood sugar level is low (relative hypoglycaemia)

STRUCTURAL FACTORS

- a tense anxious overalert body will cause anxious feelings
- hyperventilation patterns of breathing
- muscle tension
- F&F response causes sweating, rapid heartbeat, gut tension, etc.

PSYCHOSOCIAL

- generalized stresses may push one into overload
- ?anxiety rooted in past experience, family patterns
- a personality tending towards pessimism and neuroticism is susceptible under stress to anxiety, phobias, compulsive/obsessive disorder and panic attacks

CONVENTIONAL TREATMENTS

- short course of tranquillizers
- some antidepressants help panic

NON-CONVENTIONAL

- simple homeopathy (see homeo self-help section)
- avoid alcohol, caffeine
- cut down excess sugar
- try not to miss meals
- supplement with calcium and magnesium (500 mg each daily)

REFER TO

- naturopath, homeopath, nutrition counsellor

CONVENTIONAL TREATMENT

- stress management and CBT
- psychiatry/psychologist if severe

NON-CONVENTIONAL

- relaxation and breathing techniques to relieve stress response and muscle tension

??REFER TO

- meditation programme
- autogenic teacher
- biofeedback relaxation
- hypnotherapist

CONVENTIONAL TREATMENT

- beta blockers reduce symptoms

NON-CONVENTIONAL

- aromatherapy
- yoga

REFER TO

- osteopathy/chiropractic/massage may encourage relaxation, help relieve tension-related symptoms, etc. and indirectly improve circulation and sleep problems
- acupuncture has a reputation for helping with PMS and dysmenorrhoea

SELF-HELP

Anxiety/panic attacks are often linked to hyperventilation patterns of breathing and may improve with breathing retraining. A tendency to anxiety is exacerbated by relative hypoglycaemia. Avoid 'fast-burn' sugar and refined starch, which produce blood sugar dips. Regular high-protein, high-complex carbohydrate, low-fat, low-simple sugar meals.

Biochemical

Avoid alcohol and caffeine. Avoid excessive sugar. Supplement with calcium and magnesium (500 mg of each daily). In an acute anxiety attack rebreathing into a paper bag allows carbon dioxide levels to rise, normalizing blood chemistry.

Structural

Breathing retraining may be difficult if tense short muscles maintain old habits. Careful bodywork (e.g. osteo/chiro) can help. Stretching exercises (see Self-help sheet) and relaxation methods should be encouraged (see Self-help sheet).

Psychosocial

It is essential to realize that though the symptoms of anxiety are real and worrying that they are harmless and transient.

CBT helps change beliefs, expectations and explores coping skills to restore a sense of control.

If anxiety began after a particular traumatic event (PTSD) consider counselling plus CBT. Phobic anxiety and obsessive–compulsive behaviour require expert psychological help.

COMMENT

If anxiety attacks follow a clear traumatic event (PTSD) consider specialist counselling. Phobic anxiety may respond to medication, CBT or hypnotherapy. Hyperventilation is commonly involved in all anxiety attacks. When consciously or unconsciously anxious, breathing becomes rapid, shallow and irregular. The upper chest does the work rather than the diaphragm (see leaflet). Blood acidity changes as too much carbon dioxide is breathed off, and this alters blood chemistry, circulation and nerve conduction. This results in lightheadedness, poor concentration and fainting, tingling and numbness in the face, fingers and feet, muscle pain, cramps and spasms. These feelings become a further source of concern that perpetuates the vicious cycle of symptoms and anxiety. Anxiety is often entangled with depression. Anxiety may link to stress-related disorders such as high blood pressure and irritable bowel syndrome.

	Acupuncture	Homeopathy	Manual therapies	Nutritional therapies	Herbal medicine	Mind–body methods & hypnotherapy
Anxiety		2	3 massage[104] 4 aromatherapy[105]	2 (if hypoglycaemic?)	4 kava[106]	4 relaxation[107] 4 meditation[108]

ASTHMA
(NB ACUTE ASTHMA ATTACKS SHOULD ALWAYS BE TREATED WITH CONVENTIONAL MEDICATION)

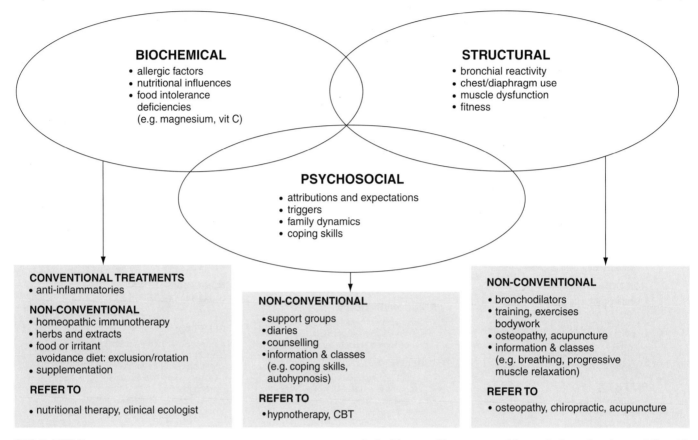

BIOCHEMICAL
- allergic factors
- nutritional influences
- food intolerance deficiencies (e.g. magnesium, vit C)

STRUCTURAL
- bronchial reactivity
- chest/diaphragm use
- muscle dysfunction
- fitness

PSYCHOSOCIAL
- attributions and expectations
- triggers
- family dynamics
- coping skills

CONVENTIONAL TREATMENTS
- anti-inflammatories

NON-CONVENTIONAL
- homeopathic immunotherapy
- herbs and extracts
- food or irritant avoidance diet: exclusion/rotation
- supplementation

REFER TO
- nutritional therapy, clinical ecologist

NON-CONVENTIONAL
- support groups
- diaries
- counselling
- information & classes (e.g. coping skills, autohypnosis)

REFER TO
- hypnotherapy, CBT

NON-CONVENTIONAL
- bronchodilators
- training, exercises bodywork
- osteopathy, acupuncture
- information & classes (e.g. breathing, progressive muscle relaxation)

REFER TO
- osteopathy, chiropractic, acupuncture

SELF-HELP

Biochemical

Dietary factors may contribute to allergy and inflammatory processes. An exclusion diet may help identify the foods involved.

Structural

Exercise and stretching are important ways of making chest muscles work optimally. The skill of diaphragmatic breathing can be helpful. It is more efficient but also more relaxing than upper chest breathing.

Psychosocial

Coping with the uncertainty of when acute attacks happen can be wearing. A diary could help you link the attacks to stresses, environmental and dietary factors. Some people find episodes are triggered by certain emotions.

Commonsense steps to avoid triggers include:

- Use special mattress covers to protect against house-dust mite droppings.
- Use synthetic pillows and duvets and wash bedding every week at 60°C.
- Have short-pile synthetic carpets, or none at all. If possible, let others vacuum, using a cleaner that retains most of the dust.
- Don't keep warm-blooded pets.

- Avoid areas of long grass and keep windows closed, especially mid-morning and late afternoon/early evening when the pollen count is highest.
- Don't smoke and (politely) ask others not to do so near you.
- Avoid exercising on hot summer days when ozone levels are highest. Aerobic exercise, once frowned on for asthmatics, is now recommended to increase lung capacity and strengthen the heart. Some doctors suggest taking medication to open the bronchial tubes at least 20 minutes before exercise, warming up for 10 minutes and carrying an inhaler just in case.
- On cold days, exercise inside and wear a scarf around your face when you go out.
- Avoid hot, centrally heated, atmospheres or use a humidifier and open a small window.
- Check medicines for possible allergens with your pharmacist.
- Stay away from people with colds and ask your doctor about flu injections in winter.
- Occupational allergens are a major problem (paint shops, garages, hairdressers) and consideration should be given to changing the workplace as asthma will worsen and be triggered by more and more irritants as the bronchi become increasingly sensitive.
- Learning techniques to relax and breathe slowly and calmly from the diaphragm helps the sense of control that is so important to people with asthma, and can prevent the panic that may worsen an attack.

	Acupuncture	Homeopathy	Manual therapies	Nutritional therapies	Herbal medicine	Mind–body methods & hypnotherapy
Asthma	3[1] subjectively	3[2]	1 chiro[3] 3 yoga[4]	3 diet strategies[5] 3 Mg, Sn, antiox[6]	3 various herbs[7]	4 hypnotherapy[8] c 4 autogenic training[9]

COMMENT

Recurrent attacks of coughing, shortness of breath and wheezing can be caused by the same inhaled allergens responsible for rhinitis. The condition is becoming increasingly common and can start at any age. Asthma affects 3 million people in the UK, 1 million of whom are children, and more than 200 million people around the world. An incidence of asthma five times higher in developed countries is blamed largely on house-dust mites and car exhaust fumes. Among adults, women are more likely to develop asthma than men. Attempts to identify airborne allergens so that they can be avoided or eliminated do not usually rely on tests. Skin-prick or RAST tests, although not always accurate, may be useful. Most asthmatics have multiple allergies anyway, and desensitization injections—once a common treatment—are now thought to be ineffective. The allergen (or allergens) responsible cannot generally be pinpointed or easily avoided, although avoiding smoke and fumes is always advisable. Mono-diets may help to decrease the overall antigenic load and so indirectly decrease bronchial sensitivity.

CARDIOVASCULAR DISEASE

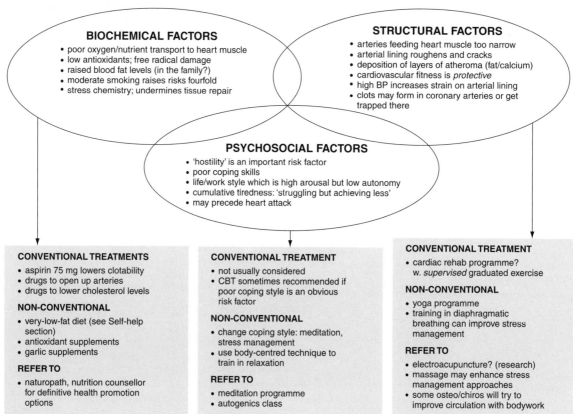

BIOCHEMICAL FACTORS
- poor oxygen/nutrient transport to heart muscle
- low antioxidants; free radical damage
- raised blood fat levels (in the family?)
- moderate smoking raises risks fourfold
- stress chemistry; undermines tissue repair

STRUCTURAL FACTORS
- arteries feeding heart muscle too narrow
- arterial lining roughens and cracks
- deposition of layers of atheroma (fat/calcium)
- cardiovascular fitness is *protective*
- high BP increases strain on arterial lining
- clots may form in coronary arteries or get trapped there

PSYCHOSOCIAL FACTORS
- 'hostility' is an important risk factor
- poor coping skills
- life/work style which is high arousal but low autonomy
- cumulative tiredness: 'struggling but achieving less'
- may precede heart attack

CONVENTIONAL TREATMENTS
- aspirin 75 mg lowers clotability
- drugs to open up arteries
- drugs to lower cholesterol levels

NON-CONVENTIONAL
- very-low-fat diet (see Self-help section)
- antioxidant supplements
- garlic supplements

REFER TO
- naturopath, nutrition counsellor for definitive health promotion options

CONVENTIONAL TREATMENT
- not usually considered
- CBT sometimes recommended if poor coping style is an obvious risk factor

NON-CONVENTIONAL
- change coping style: meditation, stress management
- use body-centred technique to train in relaxation

REFER TO
- meditation programme
- autogenics class

CONVENTIONAL TREATMENT
- cardiac rehab programme? w. *supervised* graduated exercise

NON-CONVENTIONAL
- yoga programme
- training in diaphragmatic breathing can improve stress management

REFER TO
- electroacupuncture? (research)
- massage may enhance stress management approaches
- some osteo/chiros will try to improve circulation with bodywork

SELF-HELP

There is strong evidence that dietary strategies, stress reduction methods (relaxation, meditation, autogenics, etc.) and exercise are helpful.

Biochemical

Diet: Increase fibre, vegetables, complex carbohydrates, cold water fish. Reduce sugar, coffee, excess alcohol and fats—see Self-help skills Supplements? Vitamin E (600 IU daily)—reduces oxidation of low-density lipoproteins (LDL), reduces claudication

Chromium (200 mg daily) regresses atherosclerotic plaques

Magnesium (400 mg elemental daily, orally—enteric coated) reduces LDL and increases high-density lipoproteins (HDL)

Selenium (200 µg daily) can reduce angina

Omega-3 fatty acids. (3 g daily *expensive*) lowers harmful blood fats, clotting, total cholesterol, systolic blood pressure

Omega-6 fatty acids (3 g daily *expensive*) or evening primrose oil (and/or borage oil) lowers LDL and very-low-density lipoprotein (VLDL) cholesterol plasma concentrations

CoQ10 (90 mg daily *very expensive*) reduces anginal episodes, improves cardiac function

Garlic oil (600 mg daily) lowers harmful fats, thins the blood

Ginger (ad lib)—fresh or powdered—inhibits clotting (may be as effective as aspirin)

Gingko biloba—protects against damage from low arterial oxygen

Essential to reduce and stop tobacco

Structural

Aim ultimately for aerobic exercise for 20 minutes 3 × a week. DO NOT EXCEED PULSE RATE GUIDELINES.
Cardiac rehab training needs professional monitoring IF AFTER HEART ATTACK.

Psychosocial

Coping style: are you hostile? See self-assessment section

Lifestyle and work factors. What supports you: what undermines you? See self-assessment section

Stress reduction methods—relaxation, autogenics, meditation—see Self-help skills

	Acupuncture	Homeopathy	Manual therapies	Nutritional therapies	Herbal medicine	Mind–body methods & hypnotherapy
Mild–moderate hypertension			3 tai chi[44]	3 Mg suppl[45] 3 veg diet[46]	3 garlic[47]	3[48] meditation, relaxation biofeedback & exercise
Ischaemic heart disease Intermittent claudication	3[49] reduces pain		3 tai chi[50]	3 CoQ10[51] < 3 gly 3 monascus[52] < 3 gly	3 garlic[53] < 3 gly 3 guar[54] < 3 gly 4 ginkgo[56]	4 Ornish CBT package[55] (< fats, exercise, relaxn)

COMMENT

Susceptibility to heart disease depends on genetic make-up. (Did close relatives get heart disease early? You may have inherited a high cholesterol tendency: get it checked by a medic.) It also depends on your psychological style: do you cope under pressure by getting angry and blaming every one else? You may tend towards 'hostility'. Psychological advice could make you more stress-proof; meditation might be worthwhile and exercise could help you channel some of your agression and burn off your excess stress chemicals. Diet and lifestyle are key factors. Smoking raises your heart disease risk a factor of 4. Eat right and stay slim! Keep an eye on blood pressure and don't work beyond limits of energy and concentration. Get enough sleep. What drains you and what gives you energy? Keep the balance in credit!

HEADACHE AND MIGRAINE

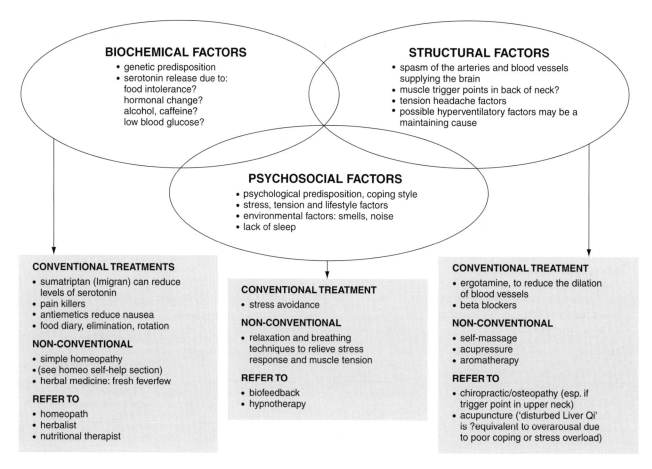

BIOCHEMICAL FACTORS
- genetic predisposition
- serotonin release due to:
  food intolerance?
  hormonal change?
  alcohol, caffeine?
  low blood glucose?

STRUCTURAL FACTORS
- spasm of the arteries and blood vessels supplying the brain
- muscle trigger points in back of neck?
- tension headache factors
- possible hyperventilatory factors may be a maintaining cause

PSYCHOSOCIAL FACTORS
- psychological predisposition, coping style
- stress, tension and lifestyle factors
- environmental factors: smells, noise
- lack of sleep

CONVENTIONAL TREATMENTS
- sumatriptan (Imigran) can reduce levels of serotonin
- pain killers
- antiemetics reduce nausea
- food diary, elimination, rotation

NON-CONVENTIONAL
- simple homeopathy
- (see homeo self-help section)
- herbal medicine: fresh feverfew

REFER TO
- homeopath
- herbalist
- nutritional therapist

CONVENTIONAL TREATMENT
- stress avoidance

NON-CONVENTIONAL
- relaxation and breathing techniques to relieve stress response and muscle tension

REFER TO
- biofeedback
- hypnotherapy

CONVENTIONAL TREATMENT
- ergotamine, to reduce the dilation of blood vessels
- beta blockers

NON-CONVENTIONAL
- self-massage
- acupressure
- aromatherapy

REFER TO
- chiropractic/osteopathy (esp. if trigger point in upper neck)
- acupuncture ('disturbed Liver Qi' is ?equivalent to overarousal due to poor coping or stress overload)

SELF-HELP

Prevention: *Keep a record* of attacks, frequency/possible causes: coincide with certain foods or situations? Read food labels. Get adequate sleep and find time to begin relaxation techniques. If a migraine seems about to start, lie in a dark room and practise relaxation and diaphragmatic breathing.

Structural

Massage to release muscle tension, restore normal blood flow to neck, scalp, face [see section].

Acupressure At the first sign of a headache, squeeze CO-4, LIV-3, GB-14, GB-20 [see section].

Aromatherapy Lavender oil in 5 ml sweet almond oil: circular motion massage to temples and the back of neck, avoiding eyes. Diffuser or warm bath: lavender, peppermint, rosemary, eucalyptus, chamomile or marjoram (for menstrual headaches). Or chamomile, lavender and marjoram.

Yoga Upper back, shoulder and neck exercises.

Biochemical

Food intolerance Some food substances may change the size of blood vessels. *Low-tyramine diet. Food elimination diets. Also rotation diets.*

Herbal medicine Fresh feverfew leaves (*Tanacetum parthenium*) can be effective preventive taken daily (thought to reduce the secretion of serotonin).

Psychosocial

Stress triggers diary

Relaxation/breathing techniques to relieve stress and muscle tension: meditation, yoga and biofeedback may be useful.

COMMENT

High rate of placebo response. Herbal medicine, acupuncture, biofeedback, manipulation, homeopathy and food exclusion all show good results; particularly dietary (inexpensive, reduces dependence on doctor/drugs, and may allow patient to control own problem. No strong comparative evidence to guide treatment choice, but a clear history helps: e.g. if headaches linked to stress or associated with neck pain. Take patient's preference into account. Understand constraints of each approach: e.g. fresh feverfew is preventative only if continued long term; acupuncture is often at least partially effective with approx eight treatments; then suspend treatment until migraines recur.

	Acupuncture	Homeopathy	Manual therapies	Nutritional therapies	Herbal medicine	Mind–body methods & hypnotherapy
Headache	3[14]	2[15]	3 ost/chiro[16]		3[17] apply peppermint oil	3 relaxation[18] 3 hypnotherapy[19]
Migraine	3 prevention[20] 3 treat attacks[21]	3[22]	1 chiropractic[23]	4 exclusion diet[24,25] 2 Mg? B2?	3[26] feverfew prevents	4 biofeedb/relaxn[27]

INFECTIONS
(SEE ALSO INFECTIONS SELF-HELP (RESPIRATORY, URINE, THRUSH, HERPES, AIDS))

BIOCHEMICAL FACTORS
- our natural immunity usually deals with simple infections without antibiotics
- nutritional factors affect immune response
- immunodeficiency rarely inherited
- it occurs after some infection (e.g. HIV) or certain drugs (e.g. cytotoxics)

STRUCTURAL FACTORS
- is it really a repeating infection? diagnosis
- healthy skin/mucus membrane: first line of defence
- rest, nutrition and hygiene assist immune processes
- symptoms are signs that the body is fighting an infection

PSYCHOSOCIAL FACTORS
- occupational and environmental susceptibility?
- chemical immunity is undermined by stress
- 'no time to be ill or get better properly'
- depression can mimic infections

CONVENTIONAL TREATMENTS
- antibiotics for serious infections treat symptoms, e.g paracetamol

NON-CONVENTIONAL
acute   cleanse/plain diet
          simple homeopathy/herbs
prevention basic good diet (see self-help sheet) ± supplements (see relevant sections of repeated infection leaflet)

REFER TO
- naturopath, homeopath, herbalist, nutrition counsellor for definitive prevention options

CONVENTIONAL TREATMENT
Is the problem really 'an infection'? Has diagnosis been confirmed by appropriate tests? Does a symptom diary provide any clues about trigger events? Fear of infection can cause negative expectations & attributions

NON-CONVENTIONAL
- **prevention** ?stress management

REFER TO
- meditation programme
- autogenics teacher

CONVENTIONAL TREATMENT
- support recovery with rest, fluids

NON-CONVENTIONAL
- **acute** support recovery
- **prevention** optimize processes of digestion, circulation, excretion

REFER TO
- acupuncture? experience suggests that it sometimes appears to 'boost immunity'
- massage may enhance stress management approaches
- some osteo/chiros say their approach can improve resistance

SELF-HELP (see Repeating infections leaflet)

Susceptibility possibly increased by A diet high in processed carbohydrates, animal fats, sugars and additives; a low intake of 'antioxidants'; excessive alcohol and caffeine; environmental toxins (industrial pollution and heavy metals, e.g. cadmium, lead and mercury); tobacco smoke; excessive antibiotics and certain drugs; stress, too much or too little exercise; ageing; all put demands on the immune system. If these challenges multiply, the immune system will have difficulty coping and resistance will weaken.

Biochemical
acute Simple homeopathy. Herbs said to fight infections: echinacea, calendula and astragalus. Traditional cleansing: take a laxative at onset, high fluid intake, very plain foods/juices

prevention Diet: low refined carbohydrate, low animal fat, low additive (see Self-help sheet). Antioxidants (vitamins A, C, E, zinc and selenium) help neutralize excess free radicals, produced as part of the body's defence mechanisms but harmful in excess. Herbs said to stimulate the immune system: garlic, ginger, thyme, sage and rosemary.

Structural
acute Rest. Avoid overstimulation. Avoid environmental toxins (including tobacco smoke)

prevention Aerobic exercise for 20 minutes three times a week. Practise stress-reducing technique.

Psychosocial
acute Allow yourself time to recover from 'ordinary illnesses'.

prevention Review lifestyle and work factors. What supports you: what undermines you? Major conflicts or relationships which overburden you? Could you be depressed?

COMMENT

The immune system recognizes our individual chemical signature. It senses anything else in the body as an invader: for instance a cold virus or a bee sting (biochemical immunity). Then defence and repair processes heat up to reject them. The skin and mucous membranes are a physical barrier that keeps most harmful things out and the things we need in. This 'structural resistance' also depends on our internal processes—particularly digestion, circulation and excretion. Heart disease and cancer are neither inflammatory nor infectious conditions; they have little to do with the 'chemical self' kind of immunity though they may reflect a failure of the body to maintain its shape. Psychological resilience is affected by traumatic experiences. And basic personality traits influence how we adapt to psychosocial stress. In turn this can impact on 'biochemical immunity' and structural aspects of resistance.

	Acupuncture	Homeopathy	Osteo/chiro	Nutritional therapies	Herbal medicine	Mind–body therapies & hypnotherapy
some acute and repeated infections	2	3 oscillo-coccinum (flu)	2	3 e.g. Zn	5 echinacea for colds	4 evidence that 'stress' decreases mucosal resistance

IRRITABLE BOWEL SYNDROME

BIOCHEMICAL
- ?disturbed 'chemical messengers' in gut can disrupt normal rhythm of peristalsis
- food intolerance? (lactose not uncommon)
- 'dysbiosis': disturbance of normal gut flora
- increased mucosal permeability? ('leaky gut') after parasitic (NB giardiasis) gastro-enteritis, or yeast infection or antibiotics

STRUCTURAL FACTORS
- spasm of the intestinal wall
- bloating due to excess gas produced by fermentation
- habitual 'air swallowing'
- muscle trigger points in abdominal wall?

PSYCHOSOCIAL CHANGES
- stress, tension and lifestyle factors
- some people with IBS have tendency to anxiety
- depression may present as abdominal pain
- eating habits: ?junk food, low fibre, high sugar

CONVENTIONAL TREATMENTS
- if recent onset consider role of infection and intolerance

NON-CONVENTIONAL
- simple homeopathy (see homeo self-help section)
- herbal: peppermint oil caps
- food diary, elimination, rotation: especially wheat and/or dairy

REFER TO
- nutritional therapist/naturopath
- ?homeopath
- ?herbalist

CONVENTIONAL TREATMENT
- stress avoidance

NON-CONVENTIONAL
- stress management
- relaxation and breathing techniques to relieve stress response and muscle tension

REFER TO
- biofeedback or autogenic training
- hypnotherapy
- brief counselling if possibility of underlying psychological issues

CONVENTIONAL TREATMENT
- antispasmodics reduce pain

NON-CONVENTIONAL
- self-massage
- acupressure
- aromatherapy

REFER TO
- possibly acupuncture: 'stagnant Liver Qi'? = overarousal due to poor coping or stress overload
- 'deficient Kidney/Spleen' = poor digestion/absorption
- ?Damp Heat = gut flora disturbance

SELF-HELP

A multifactorial condition: often interacting—causes.* Did it began after acute diarrhoea or antibiotics? IBS does not usually begin in middle age or later. Check with GP if persistent change in bowel habit.*

Keep a record of episodes, frequency/possible causes: do they coincide with certain foods or situations? Read food labels. Take exercise, get enough sleep and start relaxation techniques.

Structural

Acupressure At the first sign of a pain, squeeze CO-4, LIV-3 (see leaflet).

Yoga as aid to relaxation.

Biochemical

Reduce fat intake. Avoid refined carbohydrate (encourages smooth-muscle spasm). Increase soluble fibre if general tendency to constipation. Rule out food sensitivities. Foods most implicated in studies: dairy produce and grains (wheat, barley, oats, rye, millet). *Food elimination diets* (see leaflet); *rotation diets* (see leaflet).

Herbal medicine Enteric-coated peppermint oil capsules reduce abdominal symptoms—1 to 2 (0.2 ml/cap) 3 × daily between meals.

Psychosocial

Stress triggers diary (see leaflet). *Relaxation/breathing techniques* (see leaflet) to relieve stress and muscle tension: meditation, yoga and biofeedback may be useful.

COMMENT TO PRACTITIONERS (see stress and the gut section)

Precise causes not known. Stress appears to trigger and aggravate symptoms but diet may be the key factor.

If IBS interferes with normal life and does not respond to simple treatment then psychological or nutritional therapies will usually help. *Clues.* Sometimes infection (e.g. parasite, bacterial or yeast overgrowth) possibly producing 'leaky gut mucosa' or a food intolerance may precede the onset of IBS (e.g. began after acute diarrhoea or after antibiotics). Is there evidence of emotional stress, poor coping, high anxiety, depression? Coping skills relevant (relaxation, breathing: evidence ++ for hypnotherapy). If emotional triggers or distress despite reassurance ? counselling or CBT.

Concern about underlying disease is common. GPs may opt to arrange colonoscopy and stool tests for blood to reassure about cancer. Change of bowel habit in middle age should not be attributed to IBS.

	Acupuncture	Homeopathy	Manual therapies	Nutritional therapies	Herbal medicine	Mind–body methods & hypnotherapy
IBS	3[36]	2		3 exclusion diet[37]	3 p'mint oil[38] 3 TCM herbs[39]	4 hypnotherapy[40]

MECHANICAL BACK, NECK AND HEAD PAIN

BIOCHEMICAL FACTORS
- a familial (?genetic) component may render family members susceptible
- injured tissue releases inflammatory chemicals
- inflammatory chemicals cause swelling, and stimulation of pain nerves

STRUCTURAL FACTORS
- strains even without injury or inflammation cause protective muscle tension (stiffness)
- local muscle tension restricts circulation in joints and muscle (therefore painful waste products accumulate) causing tenderness
- stiff areas soon weaken so that other muscles must compensate

PSYCHOSOCIAL FACTORS
- occupational and environmental susceptibility
- trigger events tend to happen when tense or hurried
- exercise and rehab needs info, motivation, support
- long-term pain avoidance leads to inactivity, loss of fitness and confidence: anxiety and pain behaviour

CONVENTIONAL TREATMENTS
- pain killers, anti-inflammatories
- short-term rest

NON-CONVENTIONAL
- **acute** arnica 30 4×D
- **inflammatory** bromelaine 500 mg 4 ×D
- **persistent** (if joint or disc pain) chondroitin sulphate or glucosamine 500 mg 3×D + diet (if joint or disc pain) reduce arachidonic acid (low animal fat, high fish oil) (see self-help sheet)

REFER TO
- naturopath, nutrition counsellor if persistent

CONVENTIONAL TREATMENT
- **persistent** stress management, CBT and rehab exercises

NON-CONVENTIONAL
- **persistent** relaxation and breathing techniques relieve stress response & muscle tension

REFER TO
- meditation programme
- autogenic teacher
- biofeedback relaxation
- hypnotherapist

CONVENTIONAL TREATMENT
- early mobilization, physiotherapy

NON-CONVENTIONAL
- **acute** acupressure, osteo/chiro
- **persistent** yoga, Alexander tech

REFER TO
- osteopathy/chiropractic; shorten acute episodes and may prevent recurrences; experience suggests early intervention worthwhile
- acupuncture experience suggests especially useful in combo with manipulation

Role of CTs unclear in persistent pain

SELF-HELP (see Back pain leaflet)

Susceptibility	Poor posture, working in a fixed position for long periods; poorly designed and oversoft chairs and sagging mattresses;
increased by	Excess weight; pregnancy; tense areas remaining long after an acute backache seems to have got better; ageing joints; stress and anxiety (causes muscle tension): depression.
Triggers	Lifting heavy objects incorrectly; twisting while bending; unaccustomed spells of manual work; carrying overloaded shoulder bags and cases.
Resilience	Improving back strength and flexibility; bodywork to relax and stretch particular tight and tender areas
increased by	Improved posture; good working position (esp workstations); a bed that supports the back.
Biochemical *acute*	Arnica 30 4× daily, plus bromelain enzymes (500 mg 4× daily away from food) if inflamed.
persistent	If inflamed joints or disc bulge ?try chondroitin sulphate or glucosamine 500 mg 3 × daily. Diet: reduce arachidonic acid (low animal fat and high fish oil intake (see self-help sheet)
Structural *acute*	Use acupressure or ice massage to Co4 (see acupressure self-help sheet.)

persistent	Acute back pain exercises (see self-help sheet). Rehab exercises (see self-help sheet).
Psychosocial *acute*	Allow yourself time out. If pain is bad REST and DO NOTHING WHICH INCREASES PAIN during the recovery phase—for 2–3 days. THEN START GENTLE MOBILIZATION EXERCISES AS SOON AS POSSIBLE. Long spells of immobility will mean patient takes longer to recover.
persistent	Requires expert rehabilitation as pain avoidance habits lead to a loss of fitness, confidence, strength and mobility. A mind–body approach is essential. Consider depression.

COMMENT

Acute back pain commonly recurs; possibly in the majority of complainants. Most backache is not due to a prolapsed ('slipped') disc even where there is leg pain ('sciatica'). More commonly the pain is due to muscle or ligament strain and the build-up of painful tension and stiffness—often around one of the small spinal (facet) joints, or the sacroiliac joint or in the big back and buttock muscles. Occasionally the cause is inflammatory disease or an infection so a correct diagnosis is important. Long-term persistent back pain has psychological elements which need to be dealt with. Exercise programmes are best long-term therapy. Job satisfaction is the best correlator with good recovery.

	Acupuncture	Homeopathy	Manual therapies	Nutritional therapies	Herbal medicine	Mind–body methods & hypnotherapy
Back pain	4 (chronic)[58]		4 ost/chiro (acute)[59]		4 devil's claw[60]	4 exercise progs[61] 4 yoga[62]
Neck pain	3[63]		3[64]			

OSTEOARTHRITIS

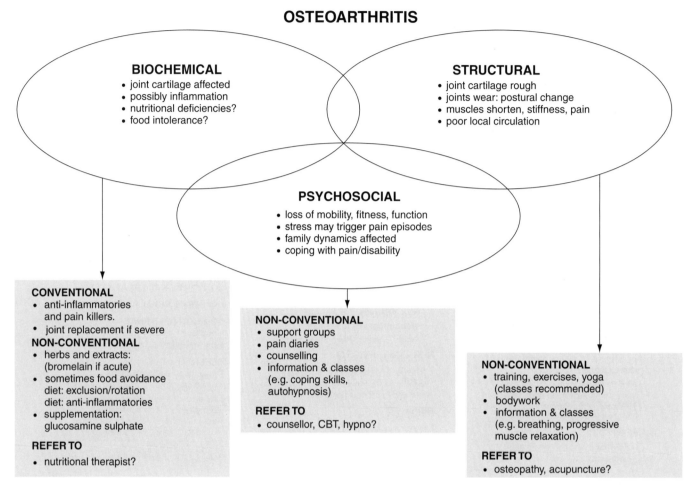

BIOCHEMICAL
- joint cartilage affected
- possibly inflammation
- nutritional deficiencies?
- food intolerance?

STRUCTURAL
- joint cartilage rough
- joints wear: postural change
- muscles shorten, stiffness, pain
- poor local circulation

PSYCHOSOCIAL
- loss of mobility, fitness, function
- stress may trigger pain episodes
- family dynamics affected
- coping with pain/disability

CONVENTIONAL
- anti-inflammatories and pain killers.
- joint replacement if severe

NON-CONVENTIONAL
- herbs and extracts: (bromelain if acute)
- sometimes food avoidance diet: exclusion/rotation diet: anti-inflammatories
- supplementation: glucosamine sulphate

REFER TO
- nutritional therapist?

NON-CONVENTIONAL
- support groups
- pain diaries
- counselling
- information & classes (e.g. coping skills, autohypnosis)

REFER TO
- counsellor, CBT, hypno?

NON-CONVENTIONAL
- training, exercises, yoga (classes recommended)
- bodywork
- information & classes (e.g. breathing, progressive muscle relaxation)

REFER TO
- osteopathy, acupuncture?

SELF-HELP

Biochemical

Dietary factors may contribute to pain and inflammation. A diet low in fats and arachidonic acid can help.

Structural

Exercise and stretching are important ways of making muscles work more normally. They also improve circulation. Tense muscles become painful. OA pain is often muscular and not due to sore joints.

Psychosocial

Coping with pain and disability may become important if the OA is severe.

COMMENT

Osteoarthritis is a degeneration of the joint cartilage, ultimately interfering with movement. About one-third of adults have radiographic evidence of OA in the hand, foot, knee or hip by the age of 65 years. OA is considered to be a natural result of the ageing process, as nearly everyone over the age of 60 shows some signs of the disease. Age, excess weight, general wear and tear, previous fracture near a joint, and a lifetime of inadequate diet and exercise are probably the main causes of OA. Skeletal defects, genetic factors and hormone deficiencies (e.g. many women have OA after the menopause) are other important factors. Many people with OA never suffer from aches, pains or the stiffness associated with the disease. Much can be done to restore function and well-being even when the disease has been treated conventionally. Many CTs are effective in OA.

Complementary therapies for osteoarthritis avoid the side-effects associated with NSAIDs. Generally they can alleviate pain and stiffness to the same degree as paracetamol. Physical therapies like acupuncture need to be repeated every few months as maintenance. Exercise programmes are an essential part of the integrated package.

If—as sometimes happens—the OA responds well to biochemical/nutritional/exercise approaches, self-help may be enough on its own.

	Acupuncture	Homeopathy	Manual therapies	Nutritional therapies	Herbal medicine	Mind–body methods & hypnotherapy
OA	**4** knee[65] **2** hip	**3**[66]	**4** ost/chiro (back/neck)[67] **3** yoga (hands)[68]	**4** glucosamine[69] **4** chondroitin[70] **4** avocado unsap[71]	**4** devil's claw[72] **4** phytodolor[73]	

PAINFUL PERIODS (DYSMENORRHOEA)

BIOCHEMICAL FACTORS
- uterus sensitive to prostaglandins?
- build-up of waste products in tense muscles due to poor circulation (cramp)

STRUCTURAL FACTORS
- unusually heavy period?
- tense painful uterus muscles
- tense muscles, pelvis, diaphragm muscles restrict circulation
- muscle trigger points in back/abdominal wall

PSYCHOSOCIAL CHANGES
- stress, emotional and lifestyle factors influence local muscle tension and pain perception
- is dysmen part of a widespread lack of well-being?
- dysmen/PMS is associated with CFS, IBS, FMG

CONVENTIONAL TREATMENTS

primary dysmen
- pain killers, e.g. paracetamol anti-inflammatories, e.g. ibuprofen
- antispasmodics
secondary dysmen
- depends on cause

NON-CONVENTIONAL
- simple homeopathy [see homeo self-help section]
- herbal: phyto-oestrogens, *Vitex agnus castus*
- ?supplements: vitamin E, OEP

REFER TO
- herbalist/naturopath

CONVENTIONAL TREATMENT
- stress management;
- gynaecologist if severe

NON-CONVENTIONAL
- relaxation and breathing techniques to relieve stress response and muscle tension

REFER TO
- biofeedback or autogenic training
- hypnotherapy if severe, persistent
- rarely counselling if possibility of underlying psychological issues

CONVENTIONAL TREATMENT
- physiotherapy exercises to improve mobility and circulation

NON-CONVENTIONAL
'pelvic congestion'
- local heat helps circulation
- aromatherapy
- yoga

REFER TO
- osteo/chiropractic to low back and pelvis can prevent/relieve dysmen
- acupuncture shown to relieve cramp and pain

SELF-HELP

Dietary and herbal measures help restore normal menstrual function. Exercise, heat, massage improve local circulation. Relaxation methods can reduce sensitivity to pain/cramp.

Structural

Acupressure To SP-6, CO-4, LIV-3. *Self-stretching* For pain from low-back and abdominal muscles (see self-help sheet).

Yoga as aid to general relaxation and to stretch widespread tense muscles.

Biochemical

Herbal extract of *Vitex agnus castus* [Agnolyt] 20 drops in water on rising for 2 months *or* 1 to 2 g of powdered root or 1 ml of fluid extract three times daily of dong quai (*Angelica sinensis*) may help dysmen or heavy periods.

Vitamin E 150 mg daily for 10 days premenstrually and for the next 4 days may help dysmenorrhoea.

Diet: reduce arachidonic acid by cutting animal fats (dairy, meat); increase fish oil (see self-help sheet). Increase natural phytoestrogens from fennel, celery, parsley, any of the cabbage family, soy-based foods.

Psychosocial

Stress triggers diary (see section) to check whether these factors make pain worse. *Relaxation/breathing techniques* to relieve stress and muscle tension: meditation, yoga, hypnotherapy and biofeedback may be useful.

COMMENT

Primary dysmenorrhoea is due to uterine contractions caused by an excess of—or sensitivity to—inflammatory prostaglandins (hormone-like fatty acids) when progesterone levels decline at the onset of a period. Contributing factors may include stress and anxiety, poor circulation, muscle tension and lack of exercise. Secondary dysmenorrhoea is due to uterine congestion. Possible underlying causes should be discussed with your doctor (fibroids, endometriosis, pelvic infection, an intrauterine contraceptive device or constipation).

Some dysmen/PMS seems to be related to a more widespread lack of well-being. This 'unwellness' could be mediated by biochemical (e.g. food intolerance, poor nutritional status), structural (lack of fitness, poor posture/breathing, fibromyalgia syndrome) and/or psychosocial factors (emotional or work overload, poor coping skills, anxiety, depression).

	Acupuncture	Homeopathy	Manual therapies	Nutritional therapies	Herbal medicine	Mind–body methods & hypnotherapy
Period pain	3[93]	2	3 chiropractic[94]	2	2	2

PERSISTENTLY ACHING JOINTS AND MUSCLES
INCLUDING 'FIBROMYALGIA'

BIOCHEMICAL FACTORS
- inflammation after *recent* injury or strain
- inflammation due to immune processes (virus infection, arthritis)
- build-up of waste products in muscles due to poor circulation (e.g. cramp)
- long-term muscle pain not usually inflammatory

STRUCTURAL FACTORS
- inflamed or injured tissues are hot, swollen
- tense painful muscles produce pain/stiffness
- tense muscles restrict circulation
- muscle trigger points can produce referred pain some distance away
- 'fibromyalgia syndrome': multiple tender points (esp. neck/back) and sleep disturbance

PSYCHOSOCIAL
- persistent pain is depressing, frightening, exhausting
- 70% of depression initially presents as pain
- stress, tension, postural and lifestyle factors relevant
- sleep disturbance: important factor in FMS
  (**NB:** FMS is closely associated with CFS, PMS, IBS)

CONVENTIONAL TREATMENTS
- pain killers, e.g. paracetamol
- anti-inflammatories, e.g. ibuprofen if evidence of ongoing inflammation.
- low-dose amitriptyline at night

NON-CONVENTIONAL
- simple homeopathy [see homeo self-help section]
- herbal: oils and ointments
- food diary, elimination, rotation diet if clues that it is relevant
- ?supplements*

REFER TO
- nutritional therapist/naturopath

CONVENTIONAL TREATMENT
- stress management
- ?sleep disturbance in FMG

NON-CONVENTIONAL
- relaxation and breathing techniques to relieve stress response and muscle tension

REFER TO
- biofeedback or autogenic training
- hypnotherapy
- brief counselling if possibility of underlying psychological issues

CONVENTIONAL TREATMENT
- physiotherapy exercises to improve mobility and circulation

NON-CONVENTIONAL
- self-massage
- acupressure
- aromatherapy
- yoga

REFER TO
- osteo/chiropractic
- acupuncture if *single* or *few* trigger points

SELF-HELP

Persistent muscular pain in the absence of ongoing injury or inflammation is not uncommon. Pain and muscle irritability produce a sequence of self-perpetuating pain—spasm—pain, which needs to be interrupted. Pain avoidance can lead to immobility, a loss of strength and fitness and poor morale. Therefore exercise, stretching and careful rehabilitation with adequate encouragement and support are essential. In addition, if any inflammation is involved it can be reduced in several ways.

Structural

Acupressure To trigger points within reach. Self-stretching for trigger-point pain involving specific areas (see self-help sheet). **Yoga** as aid to general relaxation and to stretch widespread tense muscles.

Biochemical

*Chondroitin sulphate or glucosamine 500 mg three times daily if active ongoing inflammation.

Diet: reduce arachidonic acid by cutting animal fats (dairy, meat); increase fish oil (see self-help sheet).

Food intolerance sometimes produces persistent muscular aching or joint pain (see self-help sheet).

Psychosocial

Stress triggers diary (see self-help leaflet) if these factors make pain worse. *Relaxation/breathing techniques* to relieve stress and muscle tension: meditation, yoga, hypnotherapy and biofeedback may be useful.

COMMENT

It is important to know whether pain is due to active inflammation or injury. If not then can trigger points be detected? If they are *widespread* consider fibromyalgia syndrome. FMS is associated with and is made worse by lack of sleep.

The pain from trigger points usually spreads and may generate secondary tender points.

Anxiety about the cause of pain is understandable. Pain avoidance may become counterproductive: rehabilitation will be essential. Depression often presents as pain or results from persistent pain. Antidepressants or CBT can help. FMS is closely associated with several painful conditions: dysmenorrhoea, PMS, IBS, chronic fatigue syndrome. Hyperventilation may be a connecting factor.

	Acupuncture	Homeopathy	Manual therapies	Nutritional therapies	Herbal medicine	Mind–body methods & hypnotherapy
Fibromyalgia	3[62]	3[83]	3 massage[84]	2	3 capsaicin oint > grip[85]	3 hypnotherapy[86] 3 meditation[87] 4 exercise[88]
Persistent pain	3[125]					4 meditation prog[126]

PREMENSTRUAL SYNDROME

BIOCHEMICAL FACTORS
- poor nutrition and too much strenuous exercise may disturb hormone cycle
- serotonin and adrenaline affect mood
- hormone prolactin regulates oestrogen and progesterone
- four types of PMS may link to different nutritional needs

STRUCTURAL FACTORS
- see dysmen if this is relevant
- moderate exercise, increased 1 or 2 weeks before a period, improves blood flow, affects fluid retention, relieves stress and stimulates production of endorphins

PSYCHOSOCIAL CHANGES
- hormone cycle controlled by the areas of the brain affected by stress
- is PMS part of a widespread lack of well-being?
- dysmen/PMS is associated with CFS, IBS, FMG

CONVENTIONAL TREATMENTS
- hormonal (including 'the pill')
- antihormonal (bromocriptine suppresses prolactin),
- diuretics, lithium, tranquillizers, antidepressants and pain killers

NON-CONVENTIONAL
- simple homeopathy (see homeo self-help section)
- herbal: phyto-oestrogens *Vitex agnus castus*
- ?supplements: 'Optivite', B6, OEP

REFER TO
- herbalist/naturopath, homeopath

CONVENTIONAL TREATMENT
- stress management

NON-CONVENTIONAL
- relaxation and breathing techniques to relieve stress response and muscle tension

REFER TO
- severe prolonged PMS can strain a relationship and family stability. ?CBT, couples or family therapy if significant psychological causes or results of PMS

CONVENTIONAL TREATMENT
- exercises

NON-CONVENTIONAL
- aromatherapy
- yoga

REFER TO
- osteopathy/chiropractic; soft tissue manipulation may help relaxation, headaches, etc. and indirectly improve circulation and tensions within the pelvis
- acupuncture helps PMS and dysmenorrhoea

SELF-HELP

Dietary strategies can help modify PMS severity.

Different types of PMS have been identified (see opposite), each requiring slightly different supplementation.

Structural

Yoga as aid to general relaxation.

Aromatherapy: daily bath with essential oils of lavender, clary sage and geranium for 2 weeks before period.

Biochemical

Herbal extract of *Vitex agnus castus* [Agnolyt] 20 drops in water on rising for 2 months.

Some nutritional *supplements* thought to regulate hormonal production include vitamin B6 and B complex, vit E, zinc, magnesium, calcium and essential fatty acids found in evening primrose oil and fish oils. 'Optivite' is an OTC supplement.

Diet: Craving can be due to low blood sugar and carbohydrates intolerance. Reduce salt, sugar, saturated fats.

Psychosocial

Hormonal and nutritional factors are only one way of looking at PMS. Clearly anxiety and depression types of PMS are also a psychological state involving altered moods and disturbances in relationships. Some practitioners say PMS is not an illness and should be 'reframed' as a cyclical hypersensitivity that has potential benefits of assertiveness, creativity and female empowerment.

COMMENT

Most women experience cyclical changes in mood and sensitivity during the cycle. Sometimes these can be extreme and debilitating. Over 150 symptoms have been reported, which disappear with the onset of menstruation. There are four clinical types of PMS: *anxiety* (irritability, mood swings, insomnia and depression before a period); *craving* (increased appetite, headache, palpitations, fatigue and fainting); *depression* (forgetfulness, confusion and lethargy) and *fluid retention* (weight gain over 3 1b, breast congestion, abdominal bloating, swelling of the face, hands and feet). Each type seems to have a particular cause, possibly different kinds of hormonal and nutritional imbalances.

Complementary approaches offer significant advantages over the use of conventional hormonal methods in view of their reported efficacy and lack of significant side-effects.

	Acupuncture	Homeopathy	Manual therapies	Nutritional therapies	Herbal medicine	Mind–body methods & hypnotherapy
PMS	2	2	3 reflexology[89]	3 B6[90] 4 calcium[91]	2	4 aerobic exercise[92]

PROBLEMS AROUND THE MENOPAUSE

BIOCHEMICAL FACTORS
- less progesterone & oestrogen produced
- fluctuating levels of oestrogen disturb the circulation
- reduced oestrogen slowly reduces bone mass
- if heavy periods precede menopause they may cause anaemia

STRUCTURAL FACTORS
- circulatory disturbances (sweats, flushes, itching)
- dryness and loss of skin elasticity (vaginal dryness, hair loss, skin changes)
- muscular tension (aches and pains)
- gradual loss of calcium from bones which can result in osteoporosis: risk of bone fractures

PSYCHOSOCIAL
- time of major change in a woman's sense of self- and body image; plus unstable hormonally
- mental, emotional difficulties (concentration, memory, libido, depression, low energy) partly hormonal
- women who are busy in paid or voluntary work seem to suffer fewer menopausal problems
- clinical depression??

CONVENTIONAL TREATMENTS
- hormone replacement therapy (HRT) prevents osteoporosis, treats hormone-related symptoms (flushes, dryness)

NON-CONVENTIONAL
- herbal: dong quai (*Chin angelica*) 3 × day for hot flushes or heavy periods
- phyto-oestrogen cream (wild yam), nutritional support may be relevant

REFER TO
- naturopath, nutrition counsellor herbalist, ?homeopath

CONVENTIONAL TREATMENT
- antidepressants have a place
- stress management, counselling, relaxation techniques: improve coping with periods of transition

NON-CONVENTIONAL
- consider imagery, meditation

??REFER TO
- meditation programme?
- support for lifestyle, nutritional change; support groups available? (Stress, Relaxation self-help leaflets)

CONVENTIONAL TREATMENT
- beta blockers may help flushes
- regular exercise of any sort helps muscle tension and bone loss (see self-help sheet)

NON-CONVENTIONAL
- work on body/self image through yoga, tai chi? massage?
- acupuncture apparently helpful with flushes

?REFER TO
- massage therapist? acupuncturist? yoga therapist?

SELF-HELP

Most discomforts of menopause may be relieved by lifestyle, nutritional and herbal influences.

Biochemical

After menopause, women not taking HRT need an intake of 1500 mg calcium a day; 1000 mg if on HRT. Limit salt/sugar, caffeine, alcohol. Eat low-fat, high-fibre wholefood diet with plenty of fruit and vegetables. Lacto-ovo-vegetarian diet (very low in meat) reduces bone density loss (see self-help sheet).

Biomechanical

Aerobic exercise lowers frequency/severity of hot flushes; helps maintain bone density (see self-help sheet). Artificial lubricants (KY jelly or cocoa butter) can counteract vaginal dryness during intercourse.

Psychosocial

A time of major life-change: issues about loss, self-image, body image, sexuality, spirituality. Midlife crisis demands a changed perspective. The culture does not support women in this. Previous emotional problems may seem worse at menopause, a reminder of increasing age, loss of fertility and a sense of transition from 'mother' to 'elder'. Hormonal changes often coincide with the 'empty nest' syndrome, a mother's perceived loss of identity as children grow up and leave home. How to raise self-esteem? improve self/body image? increase overall well-being? Make regular time for oneself every day. Stress management, counselling and relaxation techniques may all improve coping with periods of transition. ?Role of support groups.

COMMENT

Average age 51. Any time from 45—or earlier—to 55. Hormonal changes take place over several years and may be accompanied by a number of symptoms—although many women sail through with no problems. Many symptoms (e.g. depression, insomnia, flushes) are treated symptomatically. Most settle down once menopause passes. Osteoporosis (OP) is exception. (Risk factors for OP: history of low Ca diet, excessive exercise, close relatives with OP.) Short-term HRT effective with body symptoms and helps prevent OP, but long-term HRT possibly linked with uterine/breast cancer but risks minimal if HRT < 10 years. HRT *may* lower risk of heart disease/strokes and protect against Alzheimer's disease.

CT systems attribute symptoms around menopause to poor detoxification and elimination, food intolerance, lack of stress management and exercise skills. The ovaries stop producing oestrogen during the menopause, but the adrenal glands continue to manufacture small amounts and it is also made in fatty parts of the body. But when the adrenal glands are strained by poor diet, low blood sugar levels and stress of rapid bodily/psychological change this back-up system fails. If hypoglycaemic (low blood sugar) tendency avoid refined carbohydrates, sugar, caffeine; learn to manage stress to take the load off the adrenals. (See hypoglycaemia self-help leaflet.)

	Acupuncture	Homeopathy	Manual therapies	Nutritional therapies	Herbal medicine	Mind–body methods & hypnotherapy
Perimenopausal problems	**4**[95]	**2**		**3** dietary phyto-oestrogens[96]	**3** St J wort[97] **3** bl cohosh[98]	**3** exercise > bone mass[99]

RHEUMATOID ARTHRITIS

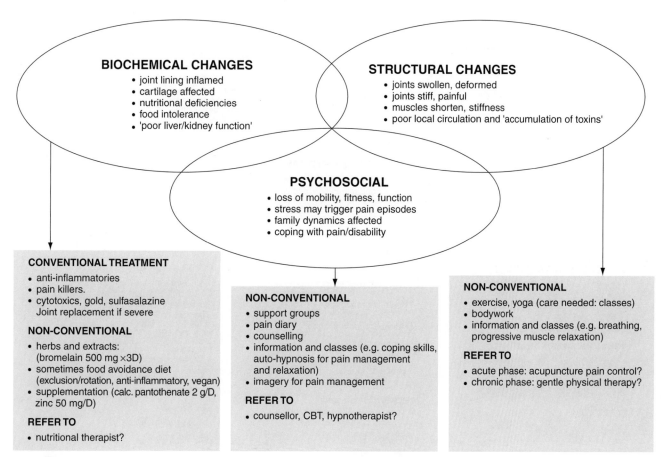

BIOCHEMICAL CHANGES
- joint lining inflamed
- cartilage affected
- nutritional deficiencies
- food intolerance
- 'poor liver/kidney function'

STRUCTURAL CHANGES
- joints swollen, deformed
- joints stiff, painful
- muscles shorten, stiffness
- poor local circulation and 'accumulation of toxins'

PSYCHOSOCIAL
- loss of mobility, fitness, function
- stress may trigger pain episodes
- family dynamics affected
- coping with pain/disability

CONVENTIONAL TREATMENT
- anti-inflammatories
- pain killers.
- cytotoxics, gold, sulfasalazine
  Joint replacement if severe

NON-CONVENTIONAL
- herbs and extracts:
  (bromelain 500 mg ×3D)
- sometimes food avoidance diet
  (exclusion/rotation, anti-inflammatory, vegan)
- supplementation (calc. pantothenate 2 g/D,
  zinc 50 mg/D)

REFER TO
- nutritional therapist?

NON-CONVENTIONAL
- support groups
- pain diary
- counselling
- information and classes (e.g. coping skills,
  auto-hypnosis for pain management
  and relaxation)
- imagery for pain management

REFER TO
- counsellor, CBT, hypnotherapist?

NON-CONVENTIONAL
- exercise, yoga (care needed: classes)
- bodywork
- information and classes (e.g. breathing,
  progressive muscle relaxation)

REFER TO
- acute phase: acupuncture pain control?
- chronic phase: gentle physical therapy?

SELF-HELP

Biochemical

In complex chronic inflammatory disease, dietary factors may contribute to pain and inflammation. In 'traditional' terms they are due to poor digestive ('liver') and excretion ('kidney') function leading to 'accumulation of toxins'. Research suggests that diet may help.

Structural

In active RA, care is needed with exercise and stretching. They are important ways of making muscles work more normally and also improve circulation. Taught muscles become painful in themselves. Exercise in warm water is safer.

Psychosocial

Coping with pain and disability are important if the RA is severe. Stress may trigger flare-ups. Studies suggest a range of mind–body approaches may be useful.

COMMENT

Complementary therapies for RA avoid the side-effects associated with NSAIDs. Acupuncture may help for pain control (evidence supports its use as an analgesic only and not as an anti-inflammatory) but needs repeating every few months. Exercise and physical therapy programmes are an essential part of the integrated package as they help maintain function, but they need to be supervised expertly. Good evidence for homeopathy, and for dietary change in acute or chronic phase of RA. Check diet recommended is nutritionally adequate. Very few adverse reactions to homeopathy reported, compared with conventional medicines.

	Acupuncture	Homeopathy	Manual therapies	Nutritional therapies	Herbal medicine	Mind–body methods & hypnotherapy
RA	3[74]	3[75]	2 massage	4 veg diet[76] 4 fasting[77] 4 fish oil suppls[78]	4 devil's claw[79] 4 phytodolor[80]	4 relaxation < pain[81]

TIREDNESS AND FATIGUE
A MULTISYSTEM APPROACH

BIOCHEMICAL
- TREATABLE DISEASES esp. anaemia, cancer, autoimmune disorders, TB, sarcoid
- NUTRITIONAL DEFICIENCIES iron? magnes?
- FOOD INTOLERANCE and HYPOGLYCAEMIA
- POSTVIRAL FATIGUE (sudden onset)
- 'BIOCHEMICAL DEPRESSION' midbrain serotonin deficit

STRUCTURAL
- strong link between CFS with fibromyalgia and hyperventilation: why?
- hyperventilation is a common finding
- fibromyalgia includes sleep- deficit-related muscle pain and tiredness
- loss of fitness contributes to exhaustion

PSYCHOSOCIAL
- build-up of mental, structural or chemical overload?
- 'stress' affects gut, respiration, circulation, immunity
- affects disproportionate number of young professional women; the majority are clinically depressed
- 'CFS personality'—perfectionist, takes on too much, finds it hard to relax, tends to get depressed, introverted

CONVENTIONAL TREATMENTS
- diagnose cause: is it depression? are there indicators of disease?
- basic blood tests are worthwhile
- viral trigger relevant in some cases (but no treatment available)

NON-CONVENTIONAL
- once pathology ruled out consider deficiencies and intolerances
- herbs: hypericum extract?
- homeopathy has CFS reputation

REFER TO
- naturopath, nutrition counsellor
- homeopath? herbalist?

CONVENTIONAL TREATMENT
- ?stress management
- CBT with carefully supervised graduated exersise

NON-CONVENTIONAL
- relaxation and breathing techniques to relieve stress response and muscle tension

??REFER TO
- cognitive behaviour modification, stress counselling
- meditation programme?

CONVENTIONAL TREATMENT
- non-specific; ongoing rest risks loss of fitness, low morale, phobic avoidance, isolation, illness behaviour

NON-CONVENTIONAL
- is yoga, tai chi feasible?
- massage for sore muscles?
- bodywork to support breath retraining?
- acupuncture theoretically helpful

REFER TO
- massage therapist? acupuncturist? yoga therapist?

SELF-HELP

Biochemical

Consider whether nutritionally compromised (iron?); likelihood of food intolerances? endocrine imbalances (thyroid?) or viral/other infection.

Exclusion diet for food intolerances (see self-help sheet).
Hypoglycaemic-rebalancing diet (high protein, low sugar, grazing pattern) (see self-help sheet).
Anticandida diet—if history is appropriate (see questionnaire and self-help sheet).

Biomechanical

Evaluate breathing. Is there a tendency to upper chest pattern? Consider hyperventilation (see self-help sheet). Is there an obvious element of physical tension (posture, body language, clenching teeth, rapid heart, etc.)—encourage relaxation methods (see self-help notes)?

Psychosocial

Enough sleep? Under real or imagined 'stress'? Other symptoms of depression? (up to 75% of CFS patients are clinically depressed—whether as a cause or consequence of their fatigue).

Stress management (see self-help sheet). Relaxation methods (see self-help sheet). Graduated exercise programme.

COMMENT

Rule out treatable or serious diseases. If persistent check for cancer, autoimmune problems, TB, etc. If intermittent consider possibility of food intolerance.

If worse a.m., prelunch and late afternoon: ?hypoglycaemic trait.

If constant consider depression, significant nutritional deficiency, hypothyroid, etc.

If thrush and/or IBS are associated: ?candida overgrowth, especially if history of antibiotic use++ (see self-help sheet).

CFS defined as physical and mental fatigue that reduces daily activity by at least 50%; illness lasting more than 6 months and associated symptoms in the muscles, nerves and cardiovascular systems despite all examinations and investigations being normal. CFS may be a complex interaction between trigger factors (stress, viral infection), psychological factors, brain chemistry and social attitudes. Severe persistent fatigue sometimes responds to antidepressants, and supportive psychotherapy with graduated exercise programme. Not all persistent fatigue is the same: there may be diverse syndromes but as yet hard to distinguish causes and best treatments. However, a 'mind–body approach' supporting recovery biochemically, structurally and psychosocially is always relevant.

	Acupuncture	Homeopathy	Manual therapies	Nutritional therapies	Herbal medicine	Mind–body methods & hypnotherapy
Chronic fatigue syndrome	2	3[101]	2 (if hyperventilation?)	2 (if food intolerance?)	3 St J wort [102] (depression?)	4 CBT and exercise progs[103]

7

Patient advice and self-help sheets

INTRODUCTION

The patient advice and self-help sheets may be photocopied for personal use. Some are intended to be folded once only, while others need to be folded twice. They have been printed in such a way that when both sides of each leaflet are copied onto one sheet of A4 paper, the leaflet is ready to fold.

We have included leaflets covering therapies that are most commonly integrated into NHS practice. marylebone Health Centre has integrated the use of acupuncture, homeopathy, massage, naturopathy and osteopathy but we have also included leaflets about chiropractic, herbal medicine, hypnotherapy and nutritional therapy as a guide for other centres.

© Harcourt Publishers Ltd 2002 Peters D, Chaitow L, Harris G, Morrison S Integrating Complementary Therapies in Primary Care: A Practical Guide for Health Professionals

ACUPUNCTURE

What you need to know about

WHAT IS ACUPUNCTURE?

Acupuncture is a form of medicine which developed in China. Very fine needles are inserted into the body at specific points according to your complaint where they stimulate the body's ability to heal and create well-being.

WHAT DOES IT TREAT?

Acupuncture is used to treat many common conditions. In this practice it is used to treat migraine headaches, irritable bowel syndrome, recurrent infections, musculoskeletal pain and tiredness.

VISITING THE ACUPUNCTURIST?

The acupuncturist will want to find out all about you and your health. The first visit will take about an hour and following visits about 40 minutes. You will need to see the acupuncturist once a week for about 6 weeks.

WILL I STILL BE ABLE TO SEE MY DOCTOR?

Yes, your doctor will want to know how you are progressing and will discuss this with your acupuncturist.

WILL I STILL BE ABLE TO TAKE MY MEDICINE?

In most cases yes. There are a few medicines which do not mix well with acupuncture but if

your doctor has suggested that you will be able to continue taking your medicine the acupuncturist will want to know all about the medicine you are taking. If the medicine you take needs to be changed during the time that you see the acupuncturist this can be discussed with both your doctor and the acupuncturist.

IS THERE ANYTHING ELSE I NEED TO KNOW?

Acupuncturists use only sterile needles which are used once and thrown away. Many people ask whether it is painful. You may feel a pinprick followed by a dull ache which the majority of people find acceptable.

SERVICES OUTSIDE THE NHS

The London School of Acupuncture and Traditional Chinese Medicine at the Poly Clinic at the University of Westminster, 115 New Cavendish Street, W1 (call 020 7-911 5041)

HOW TO MAKE AN APPOINTMENT WITH THE ACUPUNCTURIST

- You have been given a form called 'The Measure Yourself Medical Outcome Profile' known as the MYMOP form. Please read the information on this page and fill it in.
- Take the completed form to reception where you will be given an appointment with the acupuncturist at the earliest opportunity.

- Sometimes there is a short waiting list for treatment. We like to make the maximum use of the service and so you will be asked if you are able to come for treatment at short notice so that if an appointment becomes available you could be offered it.

CANCELLATION POLICY

This service is popular. If you cannot attend for your appointment please give reception as much notice as you can so that someone else can be given it.

ACUPUNCTURE—COSTS

No charge is made for this service.

CHIROPRACTIC

What you need to know about

WHAT IS CHIROPRACTIC?

Chiropractic is a 'hands-on' therapy, using manual techniques to diagnose and treat disorders of the spine, joints and muscles. It views the body as a mechanism, with the spine as the key support that protects the nervous system and links the brain to body. The underlying principle is that any strain, damage or distortion of the spine can lead to problems in the internal organs, glands and blood vessels, so the aim of treatment is to bring the body's systems back into harmony, and allow its self-healing processes to function efficiently, by realigning the spine.

WHAT DOES IT TREAT?

Chiropractic is used to treat many conditions, including spine and neck disorders; muscle, joint and postural problems; sciatica; headaches, migraine; gastrointestinal disorders; tinnitus, vertigo; menstrual pain; and asthma. A number of studies have shown it can relieve lower back pain.

VISITING THE CHIROPRACTOR

The chiropractor will want to find out all about you and your health and will take a detailed medical history, asks questions about lifestyle and may carry out standard diagnostic tests, including X-rays (unless the practitioner uses the McTimoney method). Tell your practitioner if you have osteoporosis or inflammation, infections or tumours, circulatory problems (particularly aneurysms) or a

recent fracture. During treatment you may need to undress to your underwear. Treatment of stiff or 'locked' joints usually takes place on a specially adjustable chiropractic couch, and consists of precise and well-controlled techniques known as 'adjustments'. The practitioner begins by moving the joint as far as it will go (mobilization) then giving a rapid, measured thrust to move it slightly further. With any adjustment, there may be an audible painless 'click' in the joint. This is caused by a tiny gas bubble created by the change in pressure when the joint is suddenly stretched.

After an initial 30–60-minute diagnostic session, subsequent sessions may be brief and the number depends on the condition and how quickly you respond to treatment.

WILL I STILL BE ABLE TO SEE MY DOCTOR?

Yes, your doctor will want to know how you are progressing and will discuss this with your chiropractor.

WILL I STILL BE ABLE TO TAKE MY MEDICINE?

In most cases, yes. The chiropractor will want to know all about the medicine you are taking. If the medicine you take needs to be changed during the time that you see the chiropractor this can be discussed both with your doctor and the chiropractor.

IS THERE ANYTHING ELSE I NEED TO KNOW?

Your chiropractor may give you exercises to do at home to help you improve quicker.

CHIROPRACTIC – COSTS

No charge is made for this service.

SERVICES OUTSIDE THE NHS

British Chiropractic Association 01734 757557

McTimoney Chiropractic Association 01865 880974

Scottish Chiropractic Association, 30 Raeburn Place, Edinburgh EH12 5NX

HOW TO MAKE AN APPOINTMENT WITH YOUR CHIROPRACTOR

- You have been given a form called 'The Measure Yourself Medical Outcome Profile', known as the MYMOP form. Please read the information on this page and fill it in.
- Take the completed form to reception where you will be given an appointment with the chiropractor at the earliest opportunity.
- Sometimes there is a short waiting list for treatment. We like to make maximum use of the service and so you will be asked whether you are able to come for treatment at short notice so that if an appointment becomes available you could be offered it.

CANCELLATION POLICY

This service is popular. If you cannot attend for your appointment please give reception as much notice as you can so that someone else can be given it.

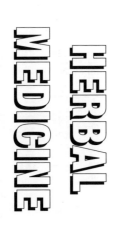

What you need to know about

HERBAL MEDICINE

WHAT IS HERBAL MEDICINE?

Herbal remedies are made from leaves, flowers and other plant parts. Many laboratory-produced drugs are derived from plants but, whereas these contain isolated and synthesized single active chemical ingredients, herbalists make use of the whole plant. Its components, they believe, have greater therapeutic power together than separately (they work in 'synergy'). Like other traditional systems, herbalism seeks to restore the body's self-healing processes. Practitioners look for the cause of illness, such as poor diet, an unhealthy lifestyle or excessive stress, which may have disrupted the body's natural state of harmony, and will prescribe herbal formulae, and possibly diets, for different body systems—for example, to stimulate the circulation or the liver, or calm the digestive system. The remedies prescribed are tailored to the patient, not the symptoms.

WHAT DOES IT TREAT?

Herbal medicine is used to treat many conditions, including persistent conditions such as migraine and arthritis; respiratory, digestive and circulatory problems; skin conditions; mild depression; insomnia; benign prostatic disease, cystitis, PMS and menopausal problems.

VISITING THE HERBALIST

The medical herbalist will want to find out all about you and your health. A herbalist will take a detailed medical history and may give you a physical examination or carry out simple tests. You should also tell your herbalist if you are taking prescribed medication, are pregnant, or have heart disease, high blood pressure, diabetes or glaucoma. You will be prescribed one or more herbal remedies tailored to your individual condition, which will normally be made up on the spot. Remember that herbal remedies take longer to work than conventional medicine.

WILL I BE ABLE TO SEE MY DOCTOR?

Yes, your doctor will want to know how you are progressing and will discuss this with your herbalist.

WILL I STILL BE ABLE TO TAKE MY MEDICINE?

In most cases, yes. There are a few herbal remedies may interfere with some conventional drugs but if your doctor has suggested that you will be able to continue taking your medicine the herbalist will want to know all about the medicine you are taking. If the medicine you take needs to be changed during the time that you see the herbalist this can be discussed both with your doctor and the herbalist.

IS THERE ANYTHING ELSE I NEED TO KNOW?

Your herbalist may suggest changes to your diet to help you improve quicker.

HERBALISM—COSTS

No charge is made for this service.

SERVICES OUTSIDE THE NHS

National Institute of Medical Herbalists 01392 426022

Register of Chinese Herbal Medicine 07000 790332

European Herbal Practitioners Association 01993 830419

HOW TO MAKE AN APPOINTMENT WITH YOUR HERBALIST

• You have been given a form called 'The Measure Yourself Medical Outcome Profile', known as the MYMOP form. Please read the information on this page and fill it in.

• Take the completed form to reception where you will be given an appointment with the herbalist at the earliest opportunity.

• Sometimes there is a short waiting list for treatment. We like to make maximum use of the service and so you will be asked if you are able to come for treatment at short notice so that if an appointment becomes available you could be offered it.

CANCELLATION POLICY

This service is popular. If you cannot attend for your appointment please give reception as much notice as you can so that someone else can be given it.

© Harcourt Publishers Ltd 2002 Peters D, Chaitow L, Harris G, Morrison S Integrating Complementary Therapies in Primary Care: A Practical Guide for Health Professionals

HOMEOPATHY

What you need to know about

WHAT IS HOMEOPATHY?

Homeopathy is a form of natural medicine developed in Europe over the last 200 years. It uses dilute amounts of naturally occurring substances to stimulate the body's healing processes.

WHAT DOES IT TREAT?

Homeopathy is used to treat a wide range of disease. In this practice it is used for treating, for example, migraine headaches, irritable bowel syndrome, recurrent infections, musculoskeletal pain and tiredness, etc.

VISITING THE HOMEOPATH

The homeopath will want to find out all about you and your health. The first visit will take about half an hour. You will need to see the homeopath every month or two.

WILL I STILL BE ABLE TO SEE THE DOCTOR?

Yes, your doctor will want to know how you are progressing and will work with your homeopath. Your doctor will talk to you about when you need to see them.

WILL I STILL BE ABLE TO TAKE MY MEDICINE?

In most cases yes. There are a few medicines which do not mix well with homeopathy but if your doctor has suggested that you have homeopathy you will be able to continue taking your medicine. The homeopath will want to know all about the medicine you are taking. If the medicine you take needs to be changed during the time that you see the homeopath this can be discussed with both your doctor and the homeopath.

IS THERE ANYTHING ELSE I NEED TO KNOW?

Homeopathy does not just treat the symptoms you come with. So the homeopath will want to know about any changes to your health including changes in your general well-being. Homeopathy usually takes time to work.

HOMEOPATHY – COSTS

No charge is made for this service.

HOW TO MAKE AN APPOINTMENT WITH THE HOMEOPATH

- You have been given a form called 'The Measure Yourself Medical Outcome Profile', known as the MYMOP form. Please read the information on this page and fill it in.

- Take the completed form to reception where you will be given an appointment with the homeopath at the earliest opportunity.

- Sometimes there is a short waiting list for treatment. We like to make the maximum use of the service and so you will be asked if you are able to come for treatment at short notice so that if an appointment becomes available you could be offered it.

CANCELLATION POLICY

This service is popular. If you cannot attend for your appointment please give reception as much notice as you can so that someone else can be given it.

HYPNOTHERAPY

What you need to know about

WHAT IS HYPNOTHERAPY?

When profoundly relaxed, most people become more open to suggestion. Modern hypnotherapy uses this, and also the way the mind tends to drift in and out of daydream-like states in the course of normal waking life. During this 'everyday trance', the conscious, rational part of the brain is temporarily bypassed, making the subconscious, which influences mental and physical functions, extremely receptive to suggestion. You will, however, remain aware of your surroundings and are unlikely to accept unreasonable suggestions. A related technique known as 'guided imagery' harnesses the imagination to help people visualize positive images and desired outcomes to help cope with stress, achieve their potential and stimulate the body's self-healing processes.

WHAT DOES IT TREAT?

Hypnotherapy is used to treat many conditions including fear and phobias, addictions, pain, stress, anxiety, depression; insomnia; digestive disorders; weight problems; menstrual problems; bedwetting, asthma, allergies; and skin conditions. Guided imagery also is used in heart conditions; cancer; autoimmune disease; and stress-related gastrointestinal and reproductive disorders.

VISITING THE HYPNOTHERAPIST

The hypnotherapist will want to find out all about you and your health. Tell your practitioner if you have suffered from severe depression, psych-

osis or another serious psychiatric condition, or epilepsy. The hypnotherapist will begin by getting you to relax and then giving you suggestions to help you drift off into a trance-like state. Once in this state the hypnotherapist will make specific suggestions related to your problem—for example, to help you overcome fears, phobias, or pain, or to wean you off an addiction. You may also be given a posthypnotic suggestion; this enables you to undergo self-hypnosis in between treatments or after the course is completed. There is usually a long initial consultation, followed by a course of shorter appointments.

WILL I STILL BE ABLE TO SEE MY DOCTOR?

Yes, your doctor will want to know how you are progressing and will discuss this with your hypnotherapist.

WILL I STILL BE ABLE TO TAKE MY MEDICINE?

In most cases, yes. If your doctor has suggested that you will be able to continue taking your medicine the hypnotherapist will want to know all about the medicine you are taking. If the medicine you take needs to be changed during the time that you see the hypnotherapist this can be discussed both with your doctor and the hypnotherapist.

IS THERE ANYTHING ELSE I NEED TO KNOW?

You may also be taught various methods that need to be practised daily. These may include visualization and imagery techniques, in which a relaxed state is induced and then suggestions for visualization are given, or relaxation techniques that encourage the removal of unconscious muscle tension in the body, by encouraging you to become aware of and release tension.

HYPNOTHERAPY–COSTS

No charge is made for this service.

SERVICES OUTSIDE THE NHS

Association of Professional Therapists 01989 764905
British Council of Hypnotist Examiners 01723 585960

Central Register of Advanced Hypnotherapists 0207 354 9938
National Association of Counsellors, Hypnotherapists and Psychotherapists 01974 241 376

HOW TO MAKE AN APPOINTMENT WITH YOUR HYPNOTHERAPIST

* You have been given a form called 'The Measure Yourself Medical Outcome Profile', known as the MYMOP form. Please read the information on this page and fill it in.

* Take the completed form to reception where you will be given an appointment with the hypnotherapist at the earliest opportunity.

* Sometimes there is a short waiting list for treatment. We like to make maximum use of the service and so you will be asked whether you are able to come for treatment at short notice so that if an appointment becomes available you could be offered it.

CANCELLATION POLICY

This service is popular. If you cannot attend for your appointment please give reception as much notice as you can so that someone else can be given it.

© Harcourt Publishers Ltd 2002 Peters D, Chaitow L, Harris G, Morrison S Integrating Complementary Therapies in Primary Care: A Practical Guide for Health Professionals

What you need to know about

MASSAGE

WHAT IS MASSAGE?

Therapeutic massage is a 'hands on' therapy and has been used for hundreds of years to treat aches and pains in muscles and stiff joints, to keep people mobile and active and to bring about a feeling of well-being.

WHAT DOES IT TREAT?

Massage, as well as treating pain and stiffness, can also help with the treatment of stress and for stress-related conditions such as sleeplessness anxiety, depression and digestive disorders. In this practice massage will be suggested for a wide variety of complaints.

VISITING THE MASSAGE THERAPIST

Each treatment will last for 45 minutes and the therapist will ask you about your general health and where in your body you are currently experiencing any tension or pain. You may need between one and four treatments initially. You will need to undress to your underwear to receive massage.

WILL I STILL BE ABLE TO SEE THE DOCTOR?

Yes. Your doctor will want to know how you are progressing and will discuss this with your massage therapist.

WILL I CONTINUE TO TAKE MY MEDICINE?

Yes. It is safe for you to continue taking any tablets or medicine that the doctor has asked you to take.

IS THERE ANYTHING ELSE I NEED TO KNOW?

You may feel tired but more relaxed after treatment and perhaps a little sore, especially if your therapist has been working on a specific area. This feeling will pass very quickly. Each person responds differently and your therapist will want to know about these changes. If it is possible please do not have a large meal before a massage and you may want to make sure that you do not have to rush about afterwards. Your practitioner may also suggest some exercises for you to do at home.

MASSAGE—COSTS

No charge is made for this service.

For services outside the NHS consult your practitioner.

HOW TO MAKE AN APPOINTMENT WITH THE MASSAGE THERAPIST

- You have been given a form called 'The Measure Yourself Medical Outcome Profile', known as the MYMOP form. Please read the information on this page and fill it in.

- Take the completed form to reception where you will be given an appointment with the massage therapist at the earliest opportunity.

- Sometimes there is a short waiting list for treatment. We like to make the maximum use of the service and so you will be asked whether you are able to come for treatment at short notice so that if an appointment becomes available you could be offered it.

CANCELLATION POLICY

This service is popular. If you cannot attend your appointment please give reception as much notice as you can so that it can be given to someone else.

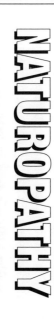

What you need to know about

NATUROPATHY

WHAT IS NATUROPATHY?

Naturopathy means 'natural cure'. By using a combination of healthy diet, simple self-help techniques, for example, breathing and relaxation exercises, beneficial herbs and general exercise, naturopathy seeks to promote the body's own ability to heal itself.

WHAT DOES IT TREAT?

Naturopaths treat most long-term conditions. In this practice it is used to treat recurrent infections, long-term fatigue, anxiety and irritable bowel syndrome. It is also useful for allergic conditions, chronic muscle pain and chronic disease in general.

VISITING THE NATUROPATH

The naturopath will want to find out all about you and what you do. The 'treatment' will often involve the practitioner suggesting you either change your diet or the type of exercise you take. This means that you will be able to experiment with what works for you so that you can learn about how to stay well. Some changes are harder to make than others especially when you don't feel well. Your naturopath understands this and is there to help you make the changes. You will need to see the naturopath at least twice. Each appointment will take about 30 minutes.

WILL I STILL BE ABLE TO SEE THE DOCTOR?

Yes. Your doctor will want to know how you are progressing and will discuss this with your naturopath.

WILL I STILL BE ABLE TO TAKE MY MEDICINE?

In most cases yes. If your doctor has suggested that you have naturopathy you will be able to continue taking your medicine. Your naturopath will want to know about the medicines you are taking. If the medicine you take needs changing during the time that you see the naturopath this can be discussed with both your doctor and the naturopath.

IS THERE ANYTHING ELSE I NEED TO KNOW?

Naturopathy may require that you supplement your diet with vitamins and minerals so there may be some extra costs.

NATUROPATHY–COSTS

No charge is made for this service.

SERVICES OUTSIDE THE NHS

British College of Naturopathy and Osteopathy, Netherhall Gardens, London NW3

HOW TO MAKE AN APPOINTMENT WITH THE NATUROPATH

- You have been given a form called 'The Measure Yourself Medical Outcome Profile', known as the MYMOP form. Please read the information on this page and fill it in.

- Take the completed form to reception where you will be given an appointment with the naturopath at the earliest opportunity.

- Sometimes there is a short waiting list for treatment. We like to make the maximum use of the service and so you will be asked whether you are able to come for treatment at short notice so that if an appointment becomes available you could be offered it.

CANCELLATION POLICY

This service is popular. If you cannot attend for your appointment please give reception as much notice as you can so that someone else can be given it.

NUTRITIONAL THERAPY

What you need to know about

WHAT IS NUTRITIONAL THERAPY?

Nutritional therapists use diet and food supplements to treat as well as prevent disease. They look for nutritional deficiencies, allergies or intolerance to food and for environmental factors that could cause poor digestion or absorption of food in the gut, preventing nutrients reaching the bloodstream. All nutritional practitioners believe that good health is directly related to the quality of food eaten, and that an inadequate diet affects mood, fitness and well-being, and hastens ageing.

WHAT DOES IT TREAT?

Nutritional therapy is used to treat many conditions, including headache and migraine; fatigue, chronic fatigue syndrome; irritable bowel syndrome; digestive disorders; arthritis; high blood pressure; circulatory disorders; menstrual problems; asthma, eczema; allergies and food sensitivities.

VISITING THE NUTRITIONAL THERAPIST

The nutritional therapist will want to find out all about you and your health. The first consultation lasts about an hour and covers details of your medical history and questions about your diet and lifestyle. The practitioner may also look at your skin, eyes, tongue, nails and reflexes for clues that suggest deficiencies, imbalances or toxicity. If a food allergy or intolerance is suspected you may be asked to follow an exclusion or elimination diet. A range of standard testing procedures, including blood, stool, urine, sweat and hair analysis, may be used as well. Other tests include muscle testing, or kinesiology, which uses lack of muscle strength to confirm a suspected food sensitivity, and the Vega test, in which you are connected to an electrical device designed to detect the presence of deficiencies and sensitivities. Supplements, including vitamin and mineral supplements, herbal products, enzymes, and 'live' bacteria to normalize gut bacteria, may be suggested, as well as lifestyle changes or other complementary therapies. The practitioner may recommend and monitor one of various diets. You will probably be advised to minimize the effect of toxins by eating plenty of fibre and organically grown fruit and vegetables.

WILL I STILL BE ABLE TO SEE MY DOCTOR?

Yes, your doctor will want to know how you are progressing and will discuss this with your nutritional therapist.

WILL I STILL BE ABLE TO TAKE MY MEDICINE?

In most cases, yes. There are a few medicines that do not mix well with nutritional therapy but if your doctor has suggested that you will be able to continue taking your medicine the nutritional therapist will want to know all about the medicine you are taking. If the medicine you take needs to be changed during the time that you see the nutritional therapist this can be discussed both with your doctor and the nutritional therapist.

IS THERE ANYTHING ELSE I NEED TO KNOW?

Nutritional therapy may require that you supplement your diet with vitamins and minerals so there may be some extra costs. Nutritional advice may also include following specialized diets, such as a detoxification diet, gluten-free, dairy-free or wheat-free diet, for which you may need to buy special 'replacement' foods.

NUTRITIONAL THERAPY—COSTS

No charge is made for this service.

SERVICES OUTSIDE THE NHS

British Association of Nutritional Therapists
0870 606 1284

Institute for Optimum Nutrition 020 8877 9993

HOW TO MAKE AN APPOINTMENT WITH YOUR NUTRITIONAL THERAPIST

• You have been given a form called 'The Measure Yourself Medical Outcome Profile', known as the MYMOP form. Please read the information on this page and fill it in.

• Take the completed form to reception where you will be given an appointment with the nutritional therapist at the earliest opportunity.

• Sometimes there is a short waiting list for treatment. We like to make maximum use of the service and so you will be asked whether you are able to come for treatment at short notice so that if an appointment becomes available you could be offered it.

CANCELLATION POLICY

This service is popular. If you cannot attend for your appointment please give reception as much notice as you can so that someone else can be given it.

OSTEOPATHY

What you need to know about

WHAT IS OSTEOPATHY?

Osteopathy is known as a 'hands on' therapy. It uses manual methods to stretch muscles and joints. Sometimes the treatment involves skilful manipulation of the spine and may produce a sudden 'popping' feeling as the joint stretches and relaxes. Muscles sometimes feel sore but treatment is not painful. Your treatment might also involve medical acupuncture—a technique whereby very fine needles are inserted into the skin. You might feel a brief pinprick and a dull ache during the acupuncture.

WHAT DOES IT TREAT?

Osteopathy is well known for treating pain in the back, neck and joints but can also treat other conditions. In this practice it is also used to treat asthma, digestive disorders and headaches.

VISITING THE OSTEOPATH

To receive treatment from an osteopath you may need to undress to your underwear. Each treatment will last 15–30 minutes and you are likely to require at least two treatments.

WILL I STILL BE ABLE TO SEE THE DOCTOR?

Yes, your doctor will want to know how you are progressing and will discuss this with your osteopath.

WILL I CONTINUE TO TAKE MY MEDICINE?

In most cases yes. The osteopath will want to know all about the medicine you are taking. If the medicine you take needs to be changed during the time that you see the osteopath this can be discussed with both your doctor and the osteopath.

IS THERE ANYTHING ELSE I NEED TO KNOW?

Your osteopath may give you exercises to do at home to help you improve quicker.

OSTEOPATHY—COSTS

No charge is made for this service.

SERVICES OUTSIDE THE NHS

British School of Osteopathy 0207 930 9254
London College of Osteopathy 0207 262 5250
London School of Osteopathy 0207 538 8334

HOW TO MAKE AN APPOINTMENT WITH THE OSTEOPATH

• You have been given a form called 'The Measure Yourself Medical Outcome Profile', known as the MYMOP form. Please read the information on this page and fill it in.
• Take the completed form to reception where you will be given an appointment with the osteopath at the earliest opportunity.

- Sometimes there is a short waiting list for treatment. We like to make the maximum use of the service and so you will be asked whether you are able to come for treatment at short notice so that if an appointment becomes available you could be offered it.

CANCELLATION POLICY

This service is popular. If you cannot attend for your appointment please give reception as much notice as you can so that someone else can be given it.

HOUSE DUST MITE—ALLERGEN AVOIDANCE MEASURES

Allergen removal

- Vacuum thoroughly and regularly with a medical vacuum cleaner; conventional vacuum cleaners are counterproductive and will actually increase airborne levels of house dust mite allergen following use.
- Vacuum mattresses when changing bedding for laundering.
- Remove your bedroom carpet. Replace with hard wood, cork or linoleum. Keep the floor totally dust free.
- Damp dust rather than using a dry cloth.

Allergen deactivation

- Neutralize the house dust mite allergen in carpets, upholstery and bedding with an antiallergy spray such as 'Banamite' (a non-toxic product consisting of aqueous solution of tannins). This must be repeated at regular intervals (3- to 6-monthly).
- Do not use mite-killing chemicals (acaricides) as these are also toxic to humans!

Allergen exclusion

- Use antiallergy barrier covers on mattresses, duvets and pillows.
- Use antiallergy synthetic duvets and pillows to discourage the colonization of mites.
- Pillow cases, duvet covers and sheets should be laundered weekly, and the pillows and duvets themselves washed every 3 months (60° centigrade or the maximum the fabric will allow).

Dehumidification

- Use a special antiallergy dehumidifier fitted with an electrostatic air filter.

Other measures

- Increase ventilation—open bedroom windows.
- Mites can be destroyed by putting pillows and soft toys in a polythene bag and leaving in the freezer for 6 hours, followed by machine wash in hot water.
- Wash curtains every 2 or 3 months; avoid venetian blinds as these collect a lot of dust.
- Put clothes and toys away; avoid having books in the bedrooms.
- Clean tops of wardrobes and other tall furniture.

Allergies

Patient Advice

ALLERGIES

True allergies—as opposed to food intolerances—involve the immune system, the body's defence against infection. In this case, antibodies—protein molecules that fight bacteria, viruses and other microorganisms—are produced against substances which are normally harmless. These substances, called allergens, may be proteins in the food we eat or be carried on the air we breathe, that come in contact with our skin or are injected as insect stings (bees, wasps) or ingested as drugs. Allergies are becoming more common in developed countries: already one person in five has some kind of allergy and numbers are increasing, especially among children. Nobody knows for sure why this is so, although environmental pollutants, food additives and stress have all been blamed.

WHAT IS AN ALLERGIC REACTION?

Allergic reactions follow quickly after exposure to the allergens (anything from a few minutes to a few hours), and take the form of several classic allergic disorders—hay fever, perennial rhinitis (constant runny or congested nose), asthma, urticaria (hives), atopic eczema and food allergies. Most common symptoms include rashes, fluid retention, swelling, blocked nose and headaches, muscle spasm leading to tightening of the airways and gut spasms, increased mucus secretions causing streaming eyes and nose and asthmatic coughs.

WHY DO PEOPLE GET ALLERGIES?

The allergen sparks production of particular antibodies known as immunoglobin E (IgE), which are attached to special immune cells, called mast cells, throughout body tissues. Antibodies latch on to a target (the antigen) on the invading cell, flagging its presence so that killer cells from the immune system can attack. When IgE antibodies bind to an invading antigen, they prod their mast cells into action, releasing histamine and so precipitating the allergic response.

A general predisposition to producing IgE, known as 'atopy', tends to run in families; so a parent might suffer from hay fever, her son from eczema and her daughter from asthma. It is now thought that a single gene may lie behind this sensitivity. Everyone who carries this gene reacts positively to tests for allergens, but about 15% show no symptoms of allergies, and sensitivity varies among the rest from very weak to extreme. Some people are allergic to just one substance; others are susceptible to a whole range and may even develop new allergies as time goes by. Other possible contributing factors include environmental pollutants such as industrial chemicals and car exhausts, diet, infections and even anxiety and stress. Several different allergens from several different sources may contribute to one disorder. Nor do allergens necessarily cause symptoms at the point where they entered the body, but may be carried elsewhere by the bloodstream. Foods, therefore, can cause asthma in the bronchial tubes, or house dust mites trigger eczema on the skin.

CONVENTIONAL TREATMENT

One of the main chemicals released in an allergic reaction is histamine, which triggers certain body changes to repel invaders. In urticaria and hay fever it causes the itching and swelling. A mainstay in treating allergies are drugs that combat its effects, known as antihistamines.

DIAGNOSIS

There are two main diagnostic methods to identify an allergen:

The skin prick test   A purified extract of the suspected allergen is inserted under a scratch in the skin. If the area develops a red itchy bump, known as the 'wheal-and-flare' response, then immune system activity is indicated. These tests often work better with inhaled allergens than those in food, where antibodies can remain in the gut rather than entering the bloodstream and reaching the skin.

Radioallergosorbent test (RAST)   This is more reliable for true food allergies. Most people with classic allergic reactions show raised levels of IgE antibodies. A sample of the patient's blood serum is added to an extract of the suspect substance. If the blood contains IgE antibodies, they will bind to antigens in the substance. These are revealed by a liquid carrying a radioactive or coloured marker and containing special antibodies (anti-IgE) that bind to IgE antibodies. Measuring the amount of radioactivity or colour given off can indicate the amount of IgE present.

COMPLEMENTARY THERAPY

Practitioners tend to see allergies and intolerances as a sign of overstrained coping processes—a sign that inadequate diet, environmental pollution and stress are getting the better of the immune system. The overall strategy is to lower the total level of potential irritants—dietary as well as psychological or social—and to maximize resources for wellness and healing, through exercise, relaxation and creativity. To aid healing, the allergen must be identified if possible and avoided. Complementary practitioners aim to restore and strengthen digestion and metabolic processes and help body systems to eliminate toxins and repair any damage.

SELF-HELP

'True' food allergy   Causes sudden acute, severe illness. Common food culprits are cow's milk, eggs, wheat, citrus fruits, soy and nuts. If given in the first year of life—even through breastmilk—they can trigger lifelong allergies in genetically susceptible babies, whose gastrointestinal tracts and immune systems are too immature to process these substances. Avoiding these foods and lowering levels of dust mites, tobacco smoke and animal fur in the home may help prevent infants becoming sensitized.

Food intolerance   Most people with classic allergic reactions show raised levels of IgE antibodies. IgEs are normal in 'food intolerance', which is sometimes confused with true food allergy. Food intolerance is sometimes implicated in migraine, irritable bowel syndrome and rheumatoid arthritis. It is possible too that food intolerance can undermine well-being in susceptible individuals and contribute to long-term ill health (see Oligoantigenic diet and exclusion rotation diet self-help sheets).

Inhalant allergy   Commonsense steps to avoid triggers include: house dust and pollen avoidance (see below): no warm-blooded pets; avoid long grass; keep windows closed mid-morning and late afternoon/early evening when the pollen count is highest.

coltsfoot and hyssop to loosen phlegm and relax the bronchial muscles. Liquorice may be suggested as an anti-inflammatory and to support the adrenals, chamomile (also an anti-inflammatory), and vervain and skullcap (antispasmodics) to reduce tension.

Osteopathy/chiropractic   Practitioners would try to relax the chest muscles and rib joints to improve mobility by treating the neck, back of the chest and the rib cage. Some practitioners think the manipulative work also calms oversensitivity of the breathing passages.

Yoga   Yoga breathing and stretching postures can help increase respiratory stamina, relax chest and diaphragm muscles, improve energy levels and relieve tension. During an attack, controlled abdominal breathing may help control panic. Several studies show yoga may be helpful for asthma. At City Hospital, Nottingham, yoga exercises that focused on deep breathing twice a day for 2 weeks helped strengthen breath flow in asthmatics, who then found they depended less on inhalers and showed less reaction to histamines. In India, yoga training that included internal cleansing techniques (including 'purging' by induced vomiting and diarrhoea) had reduced symptoms and the need for medication at a 2-year follow-up [Jain et al, Journal of Asthma 1991].

Diet and nutrition

Naturopathy   Practitioners advise a low-allergy diet (milk, eggs, nuts—especially peanuts, seafood, yeast and foods containing mould—see Oligoantigenic self-help sheet). Take care with processed foods, food preservatives and additives and colouring. Sulphites may still be found in low levels in some sausages, burgers, jams, processed vegetables, cider and wine—care should be taken where labels are not always accessible, such as in restaurants. Oily fish and fish oil supplements are a rich source of omega-3 fatty acids, thought to have an anti-inflammatory effect. Foods containing B vitamins—in particular vitamin B6 and niacin, sometimes deficient in asthmatics—may help stress-provoked attacks. Antioxidant foods could strengthen the lungs against free radicals, generated as part of the asthmatic response to allergens. Low levels of magnesium make asthma attacks worse, and foods rich in magnesium (fish, green vegetables, sunflower seeds and dried figs) may help relax the airways. Caffeine is a bronchodilator and in emergencies two cups of strong coffee may bring relief—but should not be used by those whose medication contains the chemically similar substance theophylline.

During attacks, warm compresses to chest and back or steam inhalations may ease lung congestion and help breathing. Daily breathing and mobility exercises are recommended.

Homeopathy   Constitutional treatment is recommended and is compatible with conventional treatment. Specific allergens should be identified and can be given as a remedy at homeopathic potency.

Feelings and lifestyle

Relaxation and breathing   Learning to relax muscle tension, especially in the shoulder and stomach muscles, and to breathe calmly with the diaphragm helps improve breathing efficiency. Being able to use these skills during an attack is particularly helpful. A simple technique to help slow breathing: some practitioners advise breathing as if actively sucking air slowly into the nose; hold the breath for about half the length of time it took to inhale, then just as slowly exhale (see Anti-arousal breathing self-help leaflet).

Psychotherapy and counselling   Might be useful if emotional triggers seem to be important.

Hypnotherapy   Several studies have found that hypnosis can significantly reduce the need for medication and improve symptoms.

For house dust mite—allergen avoidance measures—SEE Allergies patient advice sheet.

Asthma [also see Allergies]

Patient Advice

ASTHMA

Recurrent attacks of coughing, shortness of breath and wheezing can be caused by the same inhaled allergens responsible for rhinitis. The condition is becoming increasingly common and can start at any age; it affects three million people in the UK, one million of whom are children, and more than 200 million people around the world. An incidence of asthma five times higher in developed countries is largely blamed on house dust mites and car exhaust fumes. Among adults, women are more likely to develop asthma than men. There are varying degrees of severity but about a quarter of people with asthma feel that the disease totally controls their life or has a major effect on it. Severe attacks when the patient's heart races and the person sweats and gasps for breath feel very frightening and if untreated can be dangerous—even fatal. Fortunately conventional treatment is almost always effective.

CAUSES

Airborne allergens and irritants stimulate special cells called 'mast cells' in the bronchi, the airways to the lungs. In response, the small breathing passages tense up (called bronchospasm) and the membranes lining the passages become inflamed, thickening and eventually producing a sticky white mucus. Air flow is restricted, causing breathlessness and a sense of tightening of the chest. For some people, symptoms get no worse, but others progress to a full asthma attack. As the smooth muscles of the bronchi contract and narrow, the struggle to breath out through the constricted tubes causes the characteristic wheezing and whistling sound.

Asthma triggers vary from one individual to another, but may include allergens in the form of animal hairs, feathers, dust, house dust mites, latex rubber, cockroaches, pollen, moulds or foods such as dairy products, alcohol, seafood, yeast and nuts (see Allergies patient advice leaflet); viral infections; and environmental pollutants such as car fumes, tobacco smoke, industrial fumes and other chemicals, especially when air quality is poor. The following are not usually primary causes of asthma, but can trigger an attack when the bronchi are already sensitized: changes in weather conditions, such as cold, damp, dry or stormy weather; aspirin-based medicines, anti-inflammatories and some other drugs; times of hormonal transition, as before a period; and physical and emotional stress. Too much salt and monosodium glutamate in the diet also seems to make the bronchial tubes more reactive to histamine and increase the risk of an attack. Electromagnetic radiation from mobile telephones, televisions and computers are also suspected of triggering reactions [Centre for Immunology and Cancer Research, St Vincent's Hospital, Sydney—reported in Journal of Alternative and Complementary Medicine]. Recent research suggests that a diet high in polyunsaturated oils, found in many margarines, may predispose some people to asthma.

CONVENTIONAL TREATMENT

It is essential to see a doctor and to have emergency medicines available, as asthma can be fatal and conventional medication is life saving. Attempts to identify airborne allergens so that they can be avoided or eliminated do not usually rely on tests. But skin-prick or RAST tests, though not always accurate, can be useful. Most asthmatics have multiple allergies anyway and desensitization injections—once a common treatment—are now thought to be ineffective. The allergen (or allergens) responsible cannot generally be pinpointed or easily avoided, although avoiding smoke and fumes is always advisable. Medication includes sodium cromo-

glycate and corticosteroid taken continuously to build up 'resistance' and prevent unexpected attacks, bronchodilator drugs inhaled through inhalers, or nebulizers to prevent bronchospasm in the air tubes during attacks.

PREVENTION AND SELF-HELP

Commonsense steps to *avoid triggers* include:

- Use special mattress covers to protect against house dust mite droppings.
- Use synthetic pillows and duvets and wash bedding every week at 60°C.
- Have short pile synthetic carpets or none at all. If possible, let others vacuum, using a cleaner that retains most of the dust.
- Don't keep warm-blooded pets.
- Avoid areas of long grass and keep windows closed, especially mid morning and late afternoon/early evening when the pollen count is highest.
- Don't smoke and (politely) ask others not to do so near you.
- Avoid exercising on hot summer days when ozone levels are highest. Aerobic exercise, once frowned on for asthmatics, is now recommended to increase lung capacity and strengthen the heart. Some doctors suggest taking medication to open the bronchial tubes at least 20 minutes before exercise, warming up for 10 minutes and carrying an inhaler just in case.
- On cold days, exercise inside and wear a scarf around your face when you go out.
- Avoid hot, centrally heated atmospheres or use a humidifier and open a small window.
- Check medicines for possible allergens with your pharmacist.
- Stay away from people with colds and ask your doctor about flu injections in winter.
- Occupational allergens are a major problem (paint shops, garages, hairdressers) and consideration should be given to changing one's workplace as asthma will worsen and be triggered by more irritants as the bronchi become increasingly sensitive.

Learning techniques to relax and breathe slowly and calmly from the diaphragm helps the sense of control that is so important to people with asthma, and can prevent the panic that may worsen an attack.

COMPLEMENTARY TREATMENT (see also Allergies patient advice leaflet)

Alexander technique   Some asthma patients make their problem worse by hunching their shoulders and sinking their neck into their chest. Better posture allows the chest to relax and improves breathing.

Acupuncture   There is some evidence that needling appropriate acupoints may relieve asthma symptoms, but benefits seem to be modest and short lived. [Jobst et al, Lancet 1986; Kleijnen et al, Thorax 1991; Tashkin et al, Annals of Allergy 1977, Journal of Allergy and Clinical Immunology 1985].

Aromatherapy   Eucalyptus inhaled on a tissue (not in a steam inhalation) or massaged on the chest in a carrier oil may ease breathing.

Herbal medicine   It is essential to consult a properly trained practitioner if herbal medicine is wanted. The practitioner would try to reduce the sensitivity and reaction of the bronchial tubes to allergens and irritants. Relaxants and antispasmodics may help ease symptoms but herbalists would seek an underlying cause. Ephedra, lobelia and jimson weed relax bronchial muscle but must be used only by qualified herbalists because of the risk of side-effects (ephedra and lobelia are listed by the US Food and Drug Administration as causing serious problems). Other remedies include euphorbia, thyme, grindelia, blood root, skunk cabbage, down an arm or leg. For occasional backache, a friend could help: firm stroking movements up either side of the spine, fanning across the shoulders, and circular thumb movements over the small muscles either side of the spine may ease discomfort.

Osteopathy   Techniques for treating acute and chronic back pain range from gentle massage to ease muscle tension, to pressure and stretching movements for joint mobility, and manipulation of stiff joints. Several studies have shown that osteopathy can speed recovery from low back pain.

Acupuncture   Practitioners in Chinese medicine focus on 'removing blockages and enhancing the flow of Qi', stimulating points on appropriate meridians according to the type and locality of pain.

Acupressure   Firm pressure for 1 minute on Bladder points BL-31, BL-25 (points between vertebrae on the lower back), BL-40 (knee joint, front of leg) and Gall Bladder point 30 (hip joint, front of leg) may relieve low back pain.

Alexander technique   If you are prone to repeated episodes of back pain becoming aware of how you move helps you realign and correct your posture, easing areas of muscle tension.

Yoga   Most yoga postures help stretch and release tense muscles and encourage suppleness and flexibility. Breathing exercises gently work the muscles of the upper back. Check first with your doctor and avoid positions that hurt. Better still, ask a qualified teacher to tailor a yoga programme to your individual requirements. The corpse position (lying flat on your back) is good for releasing tension and relieving pain; shoulder rotations ease tension in the upper back; back rolls massage the spine. (Contact Yoga Biomedical Trust 020 7833 7267).

Hydrotherapy   Alternate hot and cold compresses to the painful area, 3 minutes with the hot compress, 1 minute for the cold, repeating every 20 minutes.

Relaxation and breathing   Learning to breathe well and relax reduces anxiety that causes muscle tension and exacerbates pain. Progressive muscle relaxation or a relaxation tape may be very effective.

Back and Neck Pain

Patient Advice

BACKACHE

Backache is the most frequent complaint that people take to complementary therapists and the leading cause of disability for people under 45. Even severe episodes of back pain usually get better after a few weeks with little treatment, but repeat episodes commonly follow.

Most backache is not due to a prolapsed ('slipped') disc even when there is leg pain ('sciatica'). More commonly the pain is due to muscle or ligament strain and the build-up of painful tension and stiffness—often around one of the small spinal (facet) joints, or the sacroiliac joint or in the big back and buttock muscles. Occasionally the cause is inflammatory disease or an infection so a correct diagnosis is important. Long-term persistent back pain has psychological elements which need to be explored.

Susceptibility increased by: poor posture, working in a fixed position for long periods; poorly designed and oversoft chairs and sagging mattresses; excess weight; pregnancy; tense areas remaining long after an acute backache seems to have got better; ageing joints; stress and anxiety (causes muscle tension); and depression.

Triggers: lifting heavy objects incorrectly; twisting while bending; unaccustomed spells of manual work; or carrying overloaded shoulder bags and cases.

Resilience is increased by: improving back strength and flexibility; bodywork to relax and stretch particular tight and tender areas; improved posture; good working position (esp. workstations); and a bed that supports the back.

CONVENTIONAL TREATMENT

Acute Take rest and pain killers; never more than 2–3 days in bed; active exercise for rehabilitation as soon as bearable. Use manipulation if not improving within 6 weeks: physiotherapist/osteopath or chiropractor for mobilization (not if disc pain). If pain still continues and is severe your practitioner will consider specialist diagnostic tests (early on if loss of power suggest persisting disc prolapse or other cause).

Persistent Depending on symptoms, treatment options include anti-inflammatory and muscle relaxant drugs, traction, a collar or surgical corset, epidural anaesthetic injections, antidepressants, TENS (transcutaneous nerve stimulators) and in extreme cases surgery to relieve pressure on a disc/spinal nerve root. In a number of cases of chronic back pain, no obvious orthopaedic or neurosurgical abnormality can be found.

PREVENTION

- Improve posture—avoid rounding your back or slumping. Imagine you are being lifted up from the top of your head.
- Keep fit and supple—walking and swimming (especially backstroke) are excellent exercise for the back. Stop if a movement hurts. To avoid morning stiffness, lie on your back, clasp your knees, slowly pull them towards your chest and hold for 10 seconds. To help stretch and strengthen the back, sit on the floor with legs bent and arms wrapped around the knees. Rock slowly backwards and forwards until the whole spine touches the floor. For an ache that is worse when standing still or sitting, sit on the edge of a chair with legs apart. Starting at the top of the neck, slowly bend your spine until your head and arms are between your legs. Hold for five seconds than slowly return upright, feeling a gentle stretch along your back.
- Make sure your chair correctly supports the small of your back and allows a wide thigh to trunk angle. Buy special back rests for car seats if driving long distances.

- Avoid heavy lifting, but, if it is unavoidable, keep your back straight, bend your hips and knees and grip the load with elbows close to the body. Don't carry loads on one hip but in front of you.
- Wear comfortable low-heeled shoes.
- Invest in a good supportive mattress for your bed (not necessarily 'orthopaedic').
- Arrange cupboards and furniture to avoid bending, stooping and reaching.

SELF-HELP

For sudden, acute back pain:

- Stop what you are doing and lie face down on the floor, hands by your sides, to take pressure off the back.
- Go to bed for 1 or 2 days and rest completely. Take paracetamol (two 500-mg tablets every 6 hours, up to eight a day).
- Apply an ice pack (or bag of frozen vegetables) if it brings relief—but not directly on the skin. If this doesn't work, try a warm covered hot water bottle.
- See the doctor after 1 or 2 days if the pain is still bad.

Pain and inflammation produce a self-perpetuating cycle of pain—spasm—pain, which needs to be calmed down. Inflammation is a key repair function but it can be resolved in ways which reduce discomfort.

Diet and nutrition

Acute inflammation Bromelain enzymes 500 mg 4 × daily outside meal-times. Arnica 30 two tablets 4 × daily outside meal-times.

Chronic inflammation Chondroitin sulphate or glucosamine (if joint or disc involvement) 500 mg three times daily.

Diet Reduce arachidonic acid by cutting animal fats and increasing fish oil intake (see Anti-inflammatory self-help sheet).

Bodywork

Acute Use acupressure or ice massage to CO-4. Acute back pain exercises (see Back and Neck exercise self-help sheets).

Persistent, recurring Consider yoga, Alexander technique or graduated exercise programme.

Back rehabilitation exercises (see self-help sheet).

Feelings and lifestyle

Acute Take time out, rest and *do nothing which increases pain* during the recovery phase—for at least 3 days. *Start gentle mobilization exercises as soon as possible.* Long spells of immobility will mean you take longer to recover.

Chronic Persistent back pain may require expert rehabilitation as pain avoidance habits lead to a loss of fitness, confidence, strength and mobility. A mind-body approach is essential.

Bodywork and exercise

Massage Massage can help relax tense muscles and alleviate aches and pains, provided you are sure the problem is muscular. See a doctor, chiropractor or osteopath if pain runs

Dysmenorrhoea

Patient Advice

DYSMENORRHOEA (painful periods)

Dull aches in the lower back, cramping pains, headaches are common during the first 2 or 3 days of a period. But they can be severe. There are two kinds of dysmenorrhoea. Primary dysmenorrhoea starts soon after puberty but tends to disappear between 25 and 30 or after childbirth. In secondary dysmenorrhoea, periods start to become painful after a number of years without problems.

CAUSES

Primary dysmenorrhoea may be due to uterine contractions caused by an excess of—or sensitivity to—prostaglandins (hormone-like fatty acids) as progesterone levels decline with the onset of a period. Contributing factors include stress and anxiety, poor circulation, muscle tension and lack of exercise. Secondary dysmenorrhoea usually has an underlying cause that should be discussed with your doctor, such as fibroids, endometriosis, pelvic infection, an IUD (intrauterine contraceptive device) or constipation.

CONVENTIONAL TREATMENT

Primary dysmenorrhoea may be treated with pain killers, drugs to relax the muscles, anti-inflammatory tablets (e.g., ibuprofen), drugs to inhibit uterine contractions, or the contraceptive pill. Danazol, a drug that stops the secretion of the pituitary hormones which regulate periods, is used only if dysmenorrhoea is very severe. Treatment for secondary dysmenorrhoea depends on the cause.

PREVENTION AND SELF-HELP

Exercise to improve circulation and tone muscles may relieve pain.

Bodywork and exercise

Massage   Massaging the lower abdomen, sacrum, lower back and legs can relieve pain. Massage the uterus to relieve spasm and promote blood flow by lying on your back with knees bent and making circular motions over the lower abdomen with the palm of your hand.

Chiropractic / osteopathy   Manipulation of the spine and pelvis and soft tissue manipulation of the abdominal muscles may improve uterine circulation and relieve muscle tension. Controlled trials have shown that chiropractic can be effective in relieving period pain. Poor posture and muscle tone, tight clothing and shallow breathing can influence blood supply to the uterus.

Diet and nutrition

Acupuncture / acupressure   In a clinical trial, 91% of patients improved with acupuncture, compared with 36% with sham acupuncture and 10% with no treatment. Pressure on the acupoint Bladder 23 may ease pain.

Yoga   Yoga is said to relieve stress, normalize hormone balance, relax muscles and tone the pelvis. Postures that open and release tension in the lower abdomen may be helpful, especially the shoulder stand, triangle, forward stretch and the corpse pose for relaxation.

Naturopathy   A healthy diet with plenty of fruit and vegetables. Essential fatty acids, found in oily fish and evening primrose oil, seem to inhibit prostaglandins. Some practitioners recommend avoiding meat, dairy products and eggs as these contain arachidonic acid, which promotes prostaglandin manufacture. In one small study, bilberry flavonoids seemed to relax uterine muscle.

Hydrotherapy   Alternating hot and bathing may improve uterine blood circulation.

Nutritional therapy   Supplements that encourage normal hormonal production include vitamin B6 and B complex, vitamin E, zinc, magnesium, calcium and essential fatty acids found in evening primrose oil and fish oils.

Herbal medicine   Herbs used to relieve cramp and muscle spasm include cramp bark, black haw and blue cohosh. False unicorn root (helonias root) lady's mantle, calendula and raspberry leaves are frequently prescribed to relieve uterine congestion and agnus castus (chaste tree), shatavari and false unicorn root to help balance female reproductive hormones. Cayenne and ginger may improve circulation.

Homeopathy   Take one of the following remedies every 2 hours as needed:

Colocynth 6C—for cramping pain, better from hard pressure and bending double.
Chamomilla 6C—for waves of labour-like pains.
Sepia 6C—for heavy bearing-down pains with tiredness and irritability.
Sabina 6C—bright blood with dark clots and pain stretching from sacrum to pubes.
Mag. Phos—two tablets dissolved in warm water and sipped frequently.

Feelings and lifestyle

Relaxation and breathing   Stress-management techniques can reduce pain and relieve muscle tension (see self-help sheet). Diaphragmatic breathing improves blood circulation.

© Harcourt Publishers Ltd 2002 Peters D, Chaitow L, Harris G, Morrison S Integrating Complementary Therapies in Primary Care: A Practical Guide for Health Professionals

in salami). Food elimination and rotation diets have had good results (see Exclusion rotation diet self-help sheet).

Herbal medicine Fresh feverfew leaves (*Tanacetum parthenium*) can be an effective preventive if taken daily (thought to reduce secretion of serotonin).

Feelings and lifestyle

Try keeping stress triggers diary (see Stress management self-help sheet). Use relaxation/breathing techniques to relieve stress and muscle tension: progressive muscle relaxation (see Relaxation and breathing self-help sheets), diaphragmatic breathing (see Anti-arousal breathing self-help sheet); meditation, yoga and biofeedback may also be useful.

COMPLEMENTARY THERAPIES

Herbal medicine, acupuncture, biofeedback, manipulation, homeopathy and food exclusion all show good results; particularly dietary (inexpensive, reduces dependence on doctor/drugs, and may allow patient to control own problem). There is no strong comparative evidence to guide treatment choice, but a clear history helps (e.g. if your headaches are linked to stress or associated with neck pain). Take your own preference into account understanding the constraints of each approach, e.g. feverfew is preventative only if continued long term; acupuncture is often at least partially effective with approx. eight treatments, then have more treatment if migraines come back eventually.

Headache & Migraine

Patient Advice

HEADACHE

Headache is a common complaint. Stress/anxiety that stiffens neck and shoulder muscles is probably the most usual reason for tension headache, but there are a number of possible triggers, acting either alone or in combination. These can range from simple lifestyle factors to psychological problems or musculoskeletal disorders, so it's important to find and deal with any underlying causes.

CAUSES AND SYMPTOMS

Stress, anxiety and tiredness account for most headaches, especially those in the back of the head or behind the forehead. Tension in the muscles connecting the shoulders and neck to the base of the skull is the usual cause. Other frequent lifestyle reasons are lack of sleep; eye strain and neck strain (especially if working too long at a computer screen); lack of exercise; constipation; drinking too much caffeine, as in tea and coffee, and sudden withdrawal from caffeine; skipping meals, which can result in low blood sugar (*hypoglycaemia*). External triggers include bright sunlight, wind and changes in atmospheric pressure.

Poor posture or arthritis in the neck vertebrae (*cervical spondylosis*) can trap the nerves to the muscles of the scalp and forehead. Physiological causes include fever; premenstrual tension and other hormonal swings; sinusitis, when thick catarrh blocks sinus cavities after a cold; and high blood pressure.

See a doctor if you have:

- a headache, drowsiness, nausea, vomiting, intolerance of light, especially following a head injury
- a headache, fever, stiff neck, nausea, vomiting, drowsiness, intolerance of light (possible meningitis)
- a headache that is worse in the mornings, lasts several days, with nausea or vomiting, especially if accompanied by altered vision or drowsiness (possible high blood pressure or brain tumour)
- a headache and self-help remedies haven't worked in 3–7 days
- a persistent one-sided headache.

CONVENTIONAL TREATMENT

This includes pain killers such as paracetamol, aspirin, or ibuprofen. If persistent, the doctor will do a physical examination and arrange blood tests, X-rays and a brain scan if necessary. You may be referred to a specialist for a sinus examination.

PREVENTION AND SELF-HELP

Make sure you get plenty of fresh air, exercise and sleep. Eat sensibly and regularly, and avoid too much caffeine in tea, coffee, cocoa and cola. Look at the causes of stress in your lifestyle and be prepared to make changes. Use stress-management techniques (see Stress self-help leaflet). Avoid a combination of known trigger factors.

MIGRAINE

This is an intense, often one-sided headache attack frequently preceded or accompanied by hallucinatory auras, visual disturbances such as flashing lights, odours, pins and needles in the arms and hands, intolerance of light or noise, nausea and vomiting. Lasting anything from

2 to 72 hours, the condition affects about one person in ten (though some say the figure is as high as one in five), three times as many women as men, and tends to diminish after middle age.

CAUSES AND SYMPTOMS

The pain is caused by a spasm of the arteries and blood vessels supplying the brain. In a 'classic' migraine, the initial constriction of the blood vessels restricts blood flow to the brain, causing the aura. The dilation that follows is responsible for the throbbing head and light intolerance. With a 'common' migraine, there is no aura. A 'cluster' migraine (which tends to be more common in men) occurs daily for as long as 3 months; symptoms include watery eyes.

Triggers are usually the same as for headaches: stress, tension, hormonal cycles (in women), low blood sugar and lifestyle factors. Migraines may also be due to the contraceptive pill and food intolerance.

CONVENTIONAL TREATMENT

After a prescription from your GP to control the nausea, simple dispersable pain killers can be very effective (e.g. Aspro Clear or soluble paracetamol). In severe cases, other drug approaches may be used. These include ergotamine, to reduce the dilation of blood vessels, beta blockers and drugs such as sumatriptan (Imigran) that reduce levels of the hormone serotonin, which is believed to be involved in migraine attacks. Pain killers and antinauseants are also effective in the short term.

If migraines are due to the contraceptive pill, the doctor will probably recommend another form of contraception.

PREVENTION

Keep a record of your attacks, their frequency and possible causes. Notice if they coincide with certain foods or situations. Read food labels carefully for possible links. Get plenty of exercise and start relaxation techniques. If a migraine seems about to start, lie in a dark room and practise relaxation and deep diaphragmatic breathing.

SELF-HELP

Bodywork and exercise

Massage   to release muscle tension and restore normal blood flow to vessels in the neck, scalp and face. Hot or cold packs may be useful, try both.

Acupressure   At the first sign of a headache, squeeze CO-4, LIV-3, GB-14, GB-20.

Aromatherapy   Mix 5 drops lavender oil in 5 ml sweet almond oil and using a circular motion massage your temples and the back of your neck, avoiding the area around your eyes. Put 6 drops of the following essential oils in a diffuser or warm bath: lavender, peppermint, rosemary, eucalyptus, chamomile or marjoram (for menstrual headaches). Or try a mixture of 3 drops each of chamomile, lavender and marjoram.

Yoga   Upper back, shoulder and neck exercises may help to prevent attacks.

Diet and nutrition

Migraine has been linked to food intolerance (some food substances cause arteries in the head to expand, e.g. amines found in aged cheese, pickled herrings, red wine, and preservative nitrites

SELF-HELP FOR CIRCULATORY DISEASE

There is strong evidence for lifestyle changes including dietary, stress reduction and exercise.

Diet

Eat more high-fibre vegetable and complex carbohydrate and cold-water fish. Reduce sugars, saturated fats and alcohol. Smoking *must* be stopped.

Supplement with antioxidants, vitamins A, C and E and selenium (200 μg).

Body work and exercise

Take aerobic exercise 20 minutes three times weekly—avoiding exceeding pulse rate guidelines.

Relaxation, breathing exercises, or meditation can also be helpful.

Heart & Circulation Problems

Patient Advice

HEART DISEASE

Coronary heart disease starves the heart muscle of nourishment. The thick muscle of the heart has to do. Risk factors include smoking, diabetes, high levels of blood fats, 'type A' (hostile, hurried) personality, sedentary lifestyle, poor diet and a family history of coronary artery disease. Correct diagnosis is essential and examination might include blood tests, X-rays of the coronary arteries and an exercise electrocardiogram.

Coronary heart disease starves the heart muscle of nourishment. The thick muscle of the heart wall has its own blood supply from the two coronary arteries, which get narrowed in two ways: the inner lining furs up with a fatty chalky deposit (*atheroma*) and the muscular artery wall hardens (*arteriosclerosis*). These tend to occur at the same time (*atherosclerosis*). If they are very narrowed the heart muscle will get cramp (angina) or even die off (a heart attack). Narrow arteries are more likely to close up entirely if a blood clot blocks them up (a *coronary thrombosis*). Damage to the heart muscle can be fatal but, if not, then the depth, extent and quality of the scar tissue determine the length and quality of life after an attack.

CAUSES, RISK FACTORS AND TREATMENT

Genetic make-up influences likelihood of atherosclerosis and therefore of heart disease. Psychological and lifestyle factors (diet, smoking, exercise, adequate rest and sleep) are the other key factors. How hostility is handled is important and learning to channel aggressive tendencies is probably helpful.

CONVENTIONAL TREATMENT

Conventional treatment uses drugs to improve blood flow, lower cholesterol and reduce the work of the heart. Aspirin, 75 mg daily in those who can tolerate it, reduces the risk of heart attack and stroke. Beta blockers reduce the risk of heart attack in susceptible people. Surgical options are a heart bypass and angioplasty.

HIGH BLOOD PRESSURE

High blood pressure (*hypertension*) is diagnosed when the lowest blood pressure (called the diastolic BP) reading is above 90 mmHg; when this is above 100 it increases the risk of heart attack and stroke—which is why doctors try to spot it and treat it even though there are usually no symptoms until late in the disease. Hypertension is generally discovered only during routine physical examination. Untreated high BP probably decreases lifespan by 10–20 years, principally by increasing atherosclerosis. Death is usually from heart disease, stroke or kidney failure. Each 1 mmHg reduction of diastolic BP below the potential danger level of 90 lowers your risk by 2–3%. Regular checks should give advance warning of potential problems.

CONVENTIONAL TREATMENT

Conventional treatment consists of stress management, dietary modification (decreased salt intake, decreased calorie intake if overweight, decreased cholesterol and saturated fats), regular exercise, control of risk factors for atherosclerosis (see above) and drug therapy.

ANGINA

This is attacks of aches or pain at the front of the chest, similar to a heart attack but generally less severe and relieved by rest. In a more serious form, called 'unstable angina,' pain is prolonged or occurs while resting. *See a doctor immediately as you could be at risk of a heart attack.* The cause is usually atherosclerosis.

Angina mostly affects men. The average age of a patient with angina is between 50 and 60 years. The pain is caused by cramp from chemical build-up in the heart wall because the

CONVENTIONAL TREATMENT

Nitroglycerine tablets temporarily increase blood supply to the heart, limiting damage to the heart muscle. Other drugs used include beta blockers, calcium channel blockers and various antihypertensives to reduce blood pressure. If the narrowing is severe and attacks worsen, angioplasty (a balloon inserted into the artery to reopen it) or coronary artery bypass surgery may be advised. Gentle exercise such as walking can benefit angina but needs medical supervision.

STROKE

Areas of the brain are damaged when their blood supply is blocked. This can result in sudden loss of speech or movement on one side of the body, affecting the face, arm, leg, or all three. The attack is often accompanied by numbness and heaviness in the limbs, blurred vision, loss of bladder or bowel control, dizziness, confusion or loss of consciousness for hours or even weeks. About 30% of cases are rapidly fatal, 30% cause permanent paralysis or loss of function to some degree and 30% make a complete recovery. The eventual amount of damage depends on the patient's age, state of health and size and location of the stroke. It is unusual for total recovery to occur but the sooner improvement is seen the better are the chances. Any deficit present after 6 months is likely to be permanent, but retraining programmes appear to be having some success. Further attacks are common.

CAUSES

A stroke is usually due to a blood clot or haemorrhage in the brain. The cerebral artery is usually so narrowed or damaged by atherosclerosis (plaques of cholesterol and fats that build up on artery walls) that flow is sluggish, blood becomes sticky and a clot (or thrombus) forms, blocking the supply of blood to the brain.

In a *transient ischaemic attack* (TIA), or 'stuttering stroke', the blood flow is briefly interrupted, causing minor episodes of dizziness or vertigo. Any paralysis is usually temporary. The risk of a full-blown stroke is higher in someone who gets TIAs. It is often advisable to take aspirin 75 mg daily after such an episode.

CONVENTIONAL TREATMENT

Call the doctor as soon as possible. Damaged brain cells never recover, but other cells can take over their job, so the emphasis in both conventional and complementary treatment is on rehabilitation. Physiotherapy, occupational and complementary treatment can help restore movement and speech. Anticoagulants may be prescribed to prevent further clots forming. Steroids will reduce brain swelling. Treatment should include correcting any risk factors for atherosclerosis: lowering cholesterol or reducing hypertension.

Patient Advice

Infections that Keep Coming Back

RECURRING CYSTITIS (bladder infections) SELF-HELP MEASURES

Avoid habitual retention of urine—'too busy to go'. Maintain high water intake—2 litres daily minimum.

Maintain scrupulous hygiene. Wipe from front to back only. Wear cotton underwear. Empty bladder before and after sex. Avoid tampons. Avoid bubble baths and soap in the genital area.

Diet and nutrition

Cranberry juice (unsweetened) or freeze-dried cranberry powder (any health store) contains hippuric acid, which cuts down bacteria sticking to the bladder lining. Plus drinking not less than 2 litres water daily eases cystitis symptoms rapidly.

Dissolve two high-quality acidophilus capsules in 1 litre of warm water and apply vaginally as a douche several times daily.

Bodywork and exercise

During acute attacks take hot Sitz baths twice daily for up to 20 minutes to ease pain.

Osteopathic/manipulative methods and/or Alexander technique training and/or yoga therapy may be useful it structural factors are involved, e.g. poor posture, slumped standing position, abdominal weakness.

Toning exercises (see Abdominal toning self-help sheet).

Feelings and lifestyle

Stress probably increases likelihood of outbreaks. Try keeping a trigger event diary, and meditation, (see self-help sheet) or stress management (see self-help sheet).

THRUSH (a common yeast infection: candidiasis) SELF-HELP MEASURES

Patients with multiple problems, especially if there is antibiotic overuse, 'the pill', steroids by mouth, or high sugar/fat intake, may have candida hypersensitivity related to overgrowth of candida in the gut. Symptoms apart from constant or recurrent thrush may include IBS, skin problems, mood changes, 'foggy' brain, PMS, etc. Currently the concept is unproven but widely accepted based on clinical experience.

Some common medications encourage yeast overgrowth. Evidence suggests that local treatment sometimes leads to short-lived benefits unless the intestinal yeast reservoir is also treated. A dietary strategy can usually help.

Diet and nutrition

Probiotic (*Lactobacillus acidophilus & Bifidobacteria*) supplementation helps (BioCare brand—1 capsule each meal) (see Probiotics self-help sheet).

Antifungal medication If non-conventional is preferred choose from caprylic acid (three to six capsules daily with meals) and/or garlic capsules (3 × daily with meals). Follow a low-sugar, low-caffeine, low-yeast ('anticandida') bifidogenic diet (see self-help sheet). Use local antifungal applications for symptomatic relief.

Feelings and lifestyle

Many people who have been told they have 'candida' probably do not. A blood test detecting fasting alcohol levels in response to a loading dose of glucose is suggestive. (This is called a gut fermentation product test and it is available from Biolab, Weymouth St, London W1).

Stress probably increases likelihood of outbreaks. Again try keeping a trigger event diary (see Meditation self-help sheet and Stress management self-help sheet).

© Harcourt Publishers Ltd 2002 Peters D, Chaitow L, Harris G, Morrison S Integrating Complementary Therapies in Primary Care: A Practical Guide for Health Professionals

THE IMMUNE SYSTEM AND RECURRING INFECTIONS

RESISTANCE IS NOT THE SAME AS IMMUNITY

Strictly speaking the immune system's task is to recognize our individual chemical signature: the 'chemical self'. It senses anything entering the body as an invader: for instance a cold virus or a bee sting. When this happens, defence and repair processes heat up to reject the intruder. Resistance is more than just immunity though: the skin and mucous membranes present a physical barrier which keeps most harmful things out and the things we need in. These boundaries and the moving forms the body contains, like our muscles, gut and blood vessels, for example, form a kind of 'structural self'. So some diseases (like heart disease or cancer) are not inflammatory or infectious conditions. They have little to do with the 'chemical self', though they do reflect a failure of the body to keep its shape. The 'psychological self' is our personal sense of 'I'. Traumatic experiences—not all of them remembered—and basic personality traits—some learned, some inherited—will influence how we adapt to psychosocial stress. This can undermine the chemical and structural aspect of resistance.

CAN RESISTANCE BE WEAKENED?

A diet high in processed carbohydrates, animal fats, sugars and additives; a low intake of 'antioxidants'; excessive alcohol and caffeine; environmental toxins (industrial pollution and heavy metals, e.g. cadmium, lead and mercury); tobacco smoke; excessive antibiotics and certain drugs; stress, too much exercise and ageing: all these put demands on us which are chemical, structural and psychological. If these challenges multiply, the system will have difficulty in coping.

RESISTANCE-BOOSTING SELF-HELP

Diet and nutrition

Eat a balanced diet, relatively free from chemicals, with plenty of vegetables and fruit, nuts, seeds and wholegrains, low in saturated animal fats, sugars, processed carbohydrates and chemical additives. Avoid caffeine and excessive alcohol. Essential nutrients for the immune system include the following.

Antioxidants (vitamins A, C and E, zinc and selenium) and bioflavonoids (natural protective chemicals found in plants) help neutralize superfluous free radicals, produced as part of the body's defence processes but harmful in excess.

Betacarotene (the natural form of vitamin A), found in spinach, sweet potatoes, carrots and other yellow, red and orange vegetables, strengthens immune barriers such as the skin and mucous membranes.

Vitamin C (high in oranges and other citrus fruits, blackcurrants, strawberries and kiwi fruit) helps increase antibody levels.

Vitamin E (wholegrain cereals, nuts, olive oil, avocados) protects body cells and tissues. Oily fish contain vitamin D (vital to the immune system), selenium (which helps maintain the immune system) and essential fatty acids, (involved in inflammation—white cell activity to fight infection).

B vitamins—especially B6, involved in antibody production, and B12—maintain body tissues and mucous membranes.

Minerals Deficiencies of zinc (in pumpkin seeds, seafoods, oysters, lean beef), magnesium (in soy beans, nuts, brewers' yeast), manganese (in tea, leafy green vegetables) and calcium (in dairy foods, tinned fish) affect the immune system. Iron (in red meat, egg yolks, parsley) nourishes white blood cells.

Ageing depletes immunity and studies of elderly people show that a multivitamin and mineral supplement improves their immune responses. Anyone who suspects their immune system may be compromised—after a viral infection, encountering environmental pollution or under stress—might consider similar supplementation.

Herbs Herbs said to stimulate the immune system include garlic, ginger, thyme, sage and rosemary.

Herbs said to fight infections include echinacea, calendula (marigold) and astragalus.

Bodywork and exercise

Take aerobic exercise for at least 20 minutes three times a week.

Practise stress-reducing techniques, such as meditation and relaxation. Avoid environmental toxins as far as possible.

The stress connection

The structural self is obviously responsive to feelings: we blush, we blanch, we become tense or relaxed; blood pressure goes up or down. But mind and body are also linked by chemicals involved in the 'chemical self' which affect the immune system. Examples include: emotions release chemical messengers (neurotransmitters) that can deplete or enhance immune responses. Laughter, for example, seems to increase cytokines that boost production of white cells called lymphocytes. Persistent loneliness, fear, anger and sadness can trigger the pituitary gland to activate the adrenal glands whose stress hormones (cortisol, adrenaline and noradrenaline) change the way certain white cells divide and multiply.

REPEATED BOUTS OF INFECTION

HERPES SIMPLEX (cold blisters on lips or genital sores) SELF-HELP MEASURES

Diet and nutrition

Eat a high lysine/low arginine diet to control viral activity. Take L-lysine (500 mg 4 to 8 times daily away from meals with carbohydrate snack) during acute herpes attacks until symptoms ease, twice daily prophylactically.

Echinacea purpurea (500 mg powdered root 6× daily) immediately on experiencing first signs of herpes activity, and every 3 hours can abort outbreak and decrease likelihood of further attacks.

Glycyrrhizin (500 mg 3 × daily) controls herpes virus activity.

Topical application Extract of liquorice root (3% glycyrrhizinic acid) reduces healing time and pain in recurrent genital and oral herpes. Rub ointment on to site several times daily until symptoms ease.

Feelings and lifestyle

Stress increases likelihood of outbreaks. Keep a stress review, and trigger diary. Practise meditation, autogenics or relaxation (see self-help sheets).

RECURRENT RESPIRATORY TRACT INFECTIONS SELF-HELP MEASURES

Immune-enhancing methods involving nutrition, herbs and hydrotherapy can reduce the number and severity of infectious episodes.

Diet and nutrition

Echinacea purpurea (900 mg daily) for upper respiratory infections (antiviral, antifungal, antibacterial).

Bromelain (500 mg 4 × daily away from mealtimes) for sinusitis.

Pollen extracts for upper respiratory infections.

Garlic capsules for all respiratory tract infections.

A well-formulated antioxidant combination (vitamins A, C and E, selenium and zinc).

Zinc gluconate lozenges sucked for at least 10 minutes at onset of a cold may abort it.

Bodywork and exercise

Daily cool baths (5 minutes) taken in a warm bathroom have an immune-enhancing effect over a period of 3–6 months.

Feelings and lifestyle

Stress probably increases likelihood of outbreaks. Use a stress review, trigger event diary, or try meditation.

Mind and emotions

Although rheumatoid disease is often quite mild, for some it becomes severely disabling. Pain and stiffness vary, possibly triggered or made worse by stress—including emotional stresses as well as bodily stresses (like weather change, diet, or physical overexertion). Self-help approaches can make a big difference: good stress management and relaxation skills will help you cope with pain (see Stress management self-help leaflet). Studies suggest that visualization and biofeedback help some people. Having a complex long-term painful and potentially disabling disease will have an impact on your partner, colleagues and family. It can also undermine your morale and self-esteem. Consider whether a short course of counselling might help. Support from a group of people who have experienced what it is like to have RA may be important for you. Depression should not be ignored, whether it is a result of the painfull condition or exists with it. If you experience mood swings, sleep disturbance, low energy and negative ideas about yourself then see your doctor.

Inflammatory Joint Disorders

Patient Advice

INFLAMMATORY JOINT DISORDERS

Potentially severe, painful and disabling chronic diseases sometimes begin in childhood or young adulthood. These conditions are actually widespread diseases which happen to affect joints as well as other organs (e.g. rheumatoid arthritis, psoriatic arthritis). The synovial membrane which lines the joint space becomes painfully swollen and there is destruction of bone and cartilage within the joint.

RHEUMATOID ARTHRITIS

Inflammation of the joint lining (synovial membranes) can spread to the joint itself and, in severe cases, the bones resulting in deformity and disability. Small joints, such as the knuckles and toes, are most susceptible, but the wrists, ankles, knees and neck can also be affected. Rheumatoid arthritis is less common in the spine and hips, which are more prone to osteoarthritis. Young adults and the early middle aged (between 40 and 50) are most at risk, and women three times more than men.

SYMPTOMS

First indications may be a vague aching and morning stiffness and feeling generally unwell, with joint pain and swelling coming later. In other instances the onset is sudden and severe. However the disease starts, the joints become swollen, painful and stiff, particularly first thing in the morning. Occasionally the lungs, eyes and other organs may be affected and the condition is also associated with low-grade anaemia.

CAUSES

The specific trigger for this autoimmune disease is unknown but various factors may be involved. Postviral infection, stress, diet, food intolerance and bacterial overgrowth in the gut have all been implicated.

CONVENTIONAL TREATMENT

Diagnosis involves careful examination and blood tests to establish the presence of a substance called rheumatoid factor and X-rays to determine joint damage. Exercises, physiotherapy, heat treatment, pain killers and non-steroidal anti-inflammatory drugs are treatment options. In serious cases, steroid or gold injections and immunosuppressors may be used but need careful medical supervision. Joint replacement surgery may be indicated if joint destruction is disabling.

COMPLEMENTARY TREATMENT

Massage Using a light cream or oil to massage the tissues around a joint with gentle strokes towards the heart may improve circulation, and promote lymphatic draining that reduces swelling and eases pain. An experienced practitioner will be needed.

Aromatherapy Massaging painful joints with essential oils of rosemary, benzoin, chamomile, camphor, juniper or lavender may be soothing. Cypress, fennel and lemon oils are said to be detoxifying and may help inflammation.

Chiropractic / osteopathy There is no place for joint manipulation, but soft tissue stretching and careful trigger-point treatment may improve mobility.

Acupuncture Chronic inflammatory diseases are a deep-seated problem so practitioners consider the individual's overall pattern of disharmony. Stimulation of appropriate acupoints, depending on the location of the joint, may relieve pain.

Diet and nutrition

Naturopathy / nutritional therapy See Anti-inflammatory diet self-help sheet. Flaxseed, evening primrose oil and fish oil supplements may help directly decrease inflammation.

A diet high in wholegrains, vegetable and fibre and low in sugar, animal produce and refined carbohydrates is generally recommended. There is strong evidence that food intolerance sometimes plays a role in the inflammatory process in rheumatoid arthritis. Common suspects include dairy products, eggs and cereals. Scientific evidence also shows that omega-3 fatty acids have an anti-inflammatory effect on the joints of some rheumatoid arthritis patients. Oily fish (salmon, trout, herring, mackerel and sardines) and fish oils (cod liver oil) are good sources of these. So are soy beans and tofu (useful for vegetarians). There is evidence that evening primrose oil also has anti-inflammatory effects. In fact, according to several studies, a long-term vegetarian diet can relieve some of the symptoms of rheumatoid arthritis.

Supplements Vitamins C and E, selenium, zinc and magnesium are recommended as antioxidant levels are often low in rheumatoid arthritis patients. Flavonoids, pancreatic enzymes and bromelain, a digestive enzyme found in fresh pineapple that breaks down protein, are all natural anti-inflammatories sometimes recommended for this condition. Tryptophan the precursor to the mood hormone serotonin may reduce pain. In one study, patients taking zinc supplements reported less swelling and discomfort.

Copper bracelets are said to allow the absorption of copper into the body through the skin. There is some evidence that patients with rheumatoid arthritis may be deficient in copper, which is necessary for muscle function and repair, and an Australian study found copper bracelets effective in relieving pain and stiffness in arthritis. Claims for their benefits are controversial, however, although there seems little harm in wearing them.

Herbal medicine Traditionally, feverfew is said to be anti-inflammatory though this is unconfirmed by modern research, and devil's claw may be recommended as an analgesic, an anti-inflammatory and to reduce uric acid. Anti-inflammatory herbs include Bupleuri root, licorice, turmeric (curcumin) and Chinese skullcap, which also has a high flavonoid content. Oil of wintergreen, a traditional anti-inflammatory remedy, may be applied as a liniment.

Hydrotherapy If arthritis is in the hands, exercise them in hot soapy water first thing in the morning and throughout the day. Hot or cold compresses over any painful area may be soothing. Frequent hot baths and showers help relax tense muscles and relieve joint pain. Ice packs (a pack of frozen peas wrapped in a towel) may also prove beneficial.

Exercise

It is important to try to maintain strength and mobility. But exercise is likely to be painful, especially if weight-bearing joints are inflamed. So water exercises are an important way of keeping fit and flexible. Many public pools organize 'aqua-aerobic' sessions or make time available for arthritis sufferers.

Homeopathy A Scottish trial found that homeopathic treatment of rheumatoid arthritis compared favourably with aspirin or a placebo. Practitioners would treat constitutionally and prescribe individually suited remedies.

Most long-term IBS sufferers experience anxiety, fatigue, hostility, depression and sleep disturbances. Stressful events provoke contractions of the colon in everyone. Possibly some IBS sufferers have particular difficulty in adjusting to life events and experience more stress. The fact that other 'non-organic' syndromes—fibromyalgia syndrome, chronic fatigue syndrome, hyperventilation syndrome, pelvic pain—are more common in IBS raises important questions about common causes. A history of childhood problems and emotional conflicts has been identified in more than 50% of people with IBS—a surprisingly high proportion. Cognitive behavioural therapy may help change ways of thinking and behaving.

Some people find it difficult to relax on their own and hypnotherapy helps them achieve a deeply relaxed state. Hypnotherapy can be successful in relieving symptoms of IBS when medical treatment has failed.

Biofeedback   can help especially when combined with other behavioural and psychological methods.

Irritable Bowel Syndrome

Patient Advice

IRRITABLE BOWEL SYNDROME

IBS—formerly known as spastic colon, mucus colitis, or functional bowel disorder—is one of the commonest of all gastrointestinal complaints. The gut is sheathed in a thin muscle wall that constantly contracts and relaxes, a regular wave-like motion (known as peristalsis) that pushes digested food and waste products gently towards the rectum. In IBS this rhythm appears to be disturbed as a result of sensitivity of the muscle in the gut wall. About 10% of the population are affected, particularly those between 20 and 45. Although IBS is one of the most frequent reasons for hospital referral, many people apparently put up with symptoms and never consult a doctor about their IBS.

SYMPTOMS

IBS sufferers have a highly variable bowel habit and symptoms, and may have pain and bloating. It tends to be made worse by stress. If symptoms are severe and persistent or distressing your doctor might suggest an investigation. However, if three or more of the following symptoms are present then irritable bowel syndrome is the most likely diagnosis: recurrent griping stomach pains relieved by bowel movements, more frequent and looser stools after onset of pain, a swollen abdomen, slimy mucus in the faeces, and a feeling of incomplete evacuation. Blood in the stool is not a symptom and should always be discussed with the doctor. IBS usually ceases in middle age, so an onset of symptoms after age 40 should always be checked medically.

CAUSES

If the bowel muscle propels contents too quickly, diarrhoea results; if too slowly, then constipation. Overactivity or spasm causes colicky cramping pain, which may be uncomfortable. However, the exact causes are unknown. There is no evidence of damage in the bowel, nor is it linked to any serious illness. Stress and anxiety appear to trigger and aggravate symptoms and a diet low in roughage or fibre is sometimes associated with the condition. Psychological factors are clearly important. Sometimes IBS is triggered after gastroenteritis.

CONVENTIONAL TREATMENT

Diagnosis is usually straightforward but it is important to rule out any serious complaint. A full history and physical examination is made and a colonoscopy (a tube inserted through the rectum to view the bowel) or barium enema (X-ray of the intestines) may be carried out. Stools may be examined to exclude infections. Treatment depends on the kind of symptoms and includes high-fibre diets, bulking agents such as ispaghula to soften stools, sometimes antidiarrhoeal (like codeine or imodium) and antispasmodic drugs (like mebeverine).

PREVENTION AND SELF-HELP

If you tend to be constipated, eat a high-fibre diet, aiming for 18 grams of soluble fibre a day from ordinary foods.

Avoid stressful situations at meal times, eat slowly and calmly and chew food thoroughly. Practise stress management techniques (see self-help sheet).

Take plenty of exercise; as well as reducing stress, it is good for all muscles, especially the abdominals and low back muscles.

Most IBS symptoms respond to simple treatments. If not, then dietary change may be the next step. Sometimes simple psychological techniques are necessary too.

© Harcourt Publishers Ltd 2002 Peters D, Chaitow L, Harris G, Morrison S Integrating Complementary Therapies in Primary Care: A Practical Guide for Health Professionals

COMPLEMENTARY TREATMENT

IBS responds to many kinds of simple treatment, suggesting that once psychological, nutritional, stress-related and musculoskeletal elements are dealt with it is not difficult to recover well-being. It seems that dietary factors are relevant in at least 50% of cases. Perhaps a continual low level of stress response interferes with digestive processes: the flight and fright reaction will slow up the bowel, and reduce digestive enzymes, as well as tightening up blood vessels in the gut and leading to poor absorption.

Bodywork and exercise

Acupuncture Practitioners will treat according to the individual, aiming to restore balance in the autonomic nervous system.

Diet and nutrition

Naturopathy / nutritional therapy Practitioners attribute IBS to a number of factors, including food intolerance (especially wheat, corn and dairy products) and bowel bacteria overgrowth. Increasing dietary fibre is almost universally recommended, but be careful how you take it. Fresh and dried fruit, green leafy vegetables, oat bran, psyllium and guar gum are good sources of easily digested water-soluble fibre. Drinking at least 3 pints of water a day helps progress through the bowel. Insoluble fibre—wheat bran, beans and lentils—may irritate the gut and produce wind; nor is bran a good idea if diarrhoea is a predominant symptom.

Approximately half the mass of stools is made up of microbes, so any disruption of bacteria in the colon is likely to affect bowel movements. Normally they help protect the gastrointestinal tract from toxin-producing organisms and aid digestion. But they may have been disturbed by stress or medication. If so 'live' yoghurt or tablets containing gut-friendly *Lactobacillus acidophilus*, *Lactobacillus bulgaricus* and *Bifidobacteria* supplements may help (probiotics—see self-help sheet). Some practitioners claim that two-thirds of IBS sufferers have at least one food intolerance and maybe more, so would try to identify the foods involved by exclusion diets (see self-help sheets). Reaction to different foods and combinations varies between individuals. Exclusion of cow's milk products improves symptoms in about 50% of IBS sufferers; wheat exclusion helps a further 25%. Citrus fruits, coffee and alcohol may also be implicated. Tea, coffee and alcohol affect gastrointestinal function. Practitioners will also take measures to reduce yeast overgrowth if they see it as a complicating factor.

Herbal medicine Peppermint is traditionally used to relieve intestinal spasm and gas. Specially coated capsules which release peppermint on reaching the colon help reduce contractions of the intestinal muscle. Peppermint tea and infusions are also recommended. Ginger relieves nausea. Other herbal preparations which relieve intestinal cramps, expel gas, tone and strengthen the stomach and relieve pain include chamomile, valerian, rosemary and lemon balm.

Homeopathy Practitioners would treat according to the individual's constitution, but the following remedies may be tried: *Argentum nit* for wind and constipation or diarrhoea, triggered by apprehension or nervousness; *Nux vomica* for flatulence and spasms with an ineffectual urge to move the bowels; *Colocynth* for griping pains and an attack associated with anger; *Arsenicum alb* for diarrhoea with colic and anxiety.

Feelings and lifestyle

Relaxation and breathing Techniques that induce relaxation and release muscle tension can help manage stress and relieve anxiety.

Menopause

Patient Advice

MENOPAUSE

The menopause describes the 'change of life' surrounding a woman's last period. Although the average age is 51, it can happen anytime from 45—or even earlier—to 55. Hormonal changes leading up to, and beyond, this event take place over several years and may be accompanied by a number of symptoms—although many women sail through with no problems at all.

SYMPTOMS

These may include circulatory disturbances (flushes, sweats, itching), mental and emotional difficulties (concentration, memory, loss of self-esteem, identity, sex drive, depression, low energy, anxiety), hormonal changes (vaginal dryness, hair loss, skin changes) and muscular disorders (aches and pains).

CAUSES

Some time during the 40s, levels of oestrogen produced by the ovaries begin to decrease. As a result, eggs mature less regularly, which means less progesterone is produced. The lining of the womb thickens less and periods become increasingly erratic and eventually stop. Sometimes they get highly irregular and very heavy. Fluctuating blood levels of oestrogen disturb the circulation. Reduced oestrogen slowly reduces bone mass and can result in osteoporosis and an increased risk of bone fractures. Many psychological symptoms such as depression may link more with a woman's changing sense of who she is rather than with just hormones (for instance those busy in paid or voluntary work seem to suffer fewer menopausal problems).

CONVENTIONAL TREATMENT

Many symptoms, such as depression, insomnia and bladder infections, are treated specifically, although most settle down once the menopause is past. The exception to this is osteoporosis. Hormone replacement therapy (HRT) is most commonly prescribed in the form of pills, skin implants, slow-release skin patches and vaginal creams. It does exactly as the name suggests—replaces oestrogen and progesterone, the hormones lost during menopause—so that hot flushes and vaginal dryness are relieved and brittle bones can be prevented. They prevent calcium loss from the bones. In the short term HRT is very effective for women whose symptoms are causing problems, but long-term use is still being researched. A link with breast cancer is not ruled out—although risks are minimal if taken for less than 10 years. HRT undoubtedly helps prevent osteoporosis, though only for as long as it is taken, and there is increasing evidence that it may reduce the risk of heart disease and strokes and protect against Alzheimer's disease.

PREVENTION AND SELF-HELP

The earlier a woman can begin protecting herself against the effects of declining oestrogen production the better.

- Help prevent osteoporosis with a diet rich in calcium and vitamin D (necessary for calcium absorption). After menopause, women not taking HRT should have an intake of 1500 mg a day, or 1000 mg for those on oestrogen replacement.
- The most important factor is not to smoke.

- Weight-bearing exercise (walking, dancing, weight training and lifting, tennis and hiking) strengthens bones.
- Regular exercise of any sort helps relaxation and relieves stress.
- Limit intake of sodium and sugar, caffeine and alcohol and eat a healthy low-fat, high-fibre wholefood diet with plenty of fruit and vegetables.
- Plants containing natural oestrogens (phyto-oestrogens) could protect against osteoporosis, heart disease and breast cancer. These include carrots, corn, apples and oats, but soy beans and soy bean-based products such as tofu, soy milk and miso soup are thought to be particularly effective at increasing oestrogen production in the body.
- Make regular time for yourself every day and allow yourself treats, such as a meal out with friends or a beauty treatment.
- Artificial lubricants (KY jelly or cocoa butter) may counteract vaginal dryness during intercourse.

Diet and nutrition

Naturopathy   Naturopaths attribute many of the symptoms of unwellness around menopause to poor detoxification and elimination, food intolerance, lack of stress management and exercise skills. Avoiding refined carbohydrates, sugar, caffeine and stress may help. If you get easily exhausted when you miss a meal it might be due to hypoglycaemia (low blood sugar). For this reason, eat a number of small meals throughout the day rather than three large ones.

Homeopathy   Practitioners would prefer to treat constitutionally as menopausal problems are thought to represent long-standing imbalances, and there are hormonal homeopathic remedies. The following general remedies may be useful: *Sepia*: poor memory, mood changes, anxiety, irritability, vaginal dryness, night sweats; *Sulphur*: hot flushes worse in a warm room, poor memory and depression; *Lachesis*: difficulty in concentrating, hot flushes and sweats, overexcitement, feeling faint; *Natrum mur.*: depression, weepiness, vaginal dryness, weariness, faintness; *Calcarea*: irritability, panic attacks, mood changes, anxiety, hot flushes, tendency to put on weight; *Graphites*: overexcitement and for difficulty in concentrating, irritability, weepiness, fearfulness and faintness in a warm room.

Traditional Chinese medicine   There is some scientific evidence to support the use of TCM herbs including dong quai (Chinese angelica).

Feelings and lifestyle

Relaxation and breathing   Stress, whether from overwork or emotional problems, can make menopausal symptoms worse. Stress management techniques that relieve tension and promote relaxation may help (see self-help sheet).

Psychotherapy and counselling   Previous emotional problems may seem worse at menopause, a reminder of increasing age, loss of fertility and a sense of transition from 'mother' to 'elder'. Hormonal changes often coincide with the 'empty nest' syndrome, a mother's perceived loss of identity as children grow up and leave home. Therapy and counselling can help resolve these issues with bitter taste, drowsiness after eating, dry cough, stiff back from moving, sensitivity to cold, everything worse for cold, wet, damp, sleep and rest, better for warmth, dryness, movement, rubbing and stretching.

Feelings and lifestyle

Psychotherapy and counselling   Cognitive behavioural therapy helps people break cycles of depression, inactivity and pain that may have developed.

Hypnotherapy   In one trial, FMS patients who had not responded to physical therapies reported less pain, fatigue and stiffness and greater well-being after hypnotherapy [Haanen, Journal of Rheumatology 1991].

Muscular Pain [trigger point pain: fibromyalgia syndrome]

Patient Advice

MYOFASCIAL (TRIGGER POINT) PAIN AND DYSFUNCTION (MFP & D)

At one time muscular pain and tension might have been attributed to 'muscular rheumatism' or 'fibrositis' (a term now medically obsolete). All three terms suggest symptoms of muscular pain, tenderness and possibly weakness. Often the cause is likely to be myofascial trigger points. Myofascial pain and dysfunction is a term not yet widely recognized outside osteopathic circles. It can affect any muscle group in the body, including the back, and it is probably the commonest cause of simple back pain of the kind given vague labels like lumbago, recurrent back strain and even 'arthritis' of the spine'. Muscles with trigger points often hurt when they contract, as in moving or lifting, and subsequently never fully relax, even at rest. Many people have trigger points around their necks and shoulders owing to postural stress from poorly designed desks and chairs.

CAUSES

There are a variety of causes, but usually it will be a minor injury, overuse, tension, viral illness or repetitive use that causes a muscle to become irritable.

CONVENTIONAL TREATMENT

Anti-inflammatory drugs, pain killers, physiotherapy and pain-relieving injections into the trigger points may be prescribed and attempts made to diagnose the factors which keep the trigger points active.

COMPLEMENTARY TREATMENT

Bodywork and exercise

Exercise and bodywork (osteopathy, chiropractic, yoga, rolfing) that stretches the muscle can help reduce the vicious circle of pain and tension.

Acupuncture Needling of trigger points—80% of which appear to be in exactly the same position as acupoints—can relieve pain.

Massage / aromatherapy Massage with a vegetable oil helps relieve muscle tension and pain. The addition of aromatherapy essential oils, particularly lavender and rosemary, is soothing.

Diet and nutrition

Nutritional therapy If it is a long-term problem, a raw food or fruit diet may be recommended.

Hydrotherapy Ice packs, hot and cold compresses and Epsom salt baths may relieve stiffness and discomfort.

FIBROMYALGIA SYNDROME (FIBROSITIS) (see also sheets on pain, chronic fatigue syndrome)

Formerly known as fibrositis, fibromyalgia syndrome (FMS), unlike MFP & D, is a generalized muscle pain that affects several areas, often with vague aches, stiffness, fatigue, sleep disturbance and poor concentration. (Myofascial pain, in comparison, is usually limited to a well-defined area although the two conditions are often confused.) The American College of Rheumatology considers a diagnosis of FMS when there is a history of widespread pain involving whole regions of the body and pain in 11 out of 18 accepted trigger points. It is probably significant that 75% of people with diagnosed chronic fatigue syndrome (also known as ME) have the same symptoms. As many as two-thirds of FMS sufferers also have irritable bowel syndrome. In one American survey, more than 35% of patients with FMS were unable to work. FMS is an important cause of chronic pain and it requires holistic management.

CAUSES

Causes are unknown or inconclusive, although trigger point pain is probably an important aspect. Factors that appear to affect trigger FMS include low thyroid hormone, premenstrual syndrome, menopause, poor tissue circulation made worse by tension and stress, food intolerance (especially wheat and dairy), infections (bacterial, viral or yeast), nutritional deficiencies (vitamins B, C and iron), faulty breathing patterns and lack of exercise.

PREVENTION AND SELF-HELP

Aerobic exercise for at least 20 minutes three times a week helps the body release its own pain killers (endorphins), enhances self-esteem and feelings of well-being and is as effective in mild to moderate depression as antidepressant medication. Cycling or swimming are probably the best kinds of exercise if you are prone to FMS.

CONVENTIONAL TREATMENTS

Small doses of antidepressants appear to be beneficial, but anti-inflammatories are not helpful.

COMPLEMENTARY TREATMENT

Acupuncture In general, needling trigger points is not as successful in treating FMS as it is in myofascial pain, although in a Swiss study three-quarters of FMS patients improved with acupuncture.

Bodywork and exercise

Massage, osteopathy Soft tissue treatment focusing on muscle stretching and lengthening appears to achieve better results than joint manipulation. In a small study at the Touch Research Institute, Miami, a group receiving massage to painful areas reported less pain, fatigue and stiffness than one receiving TENS (transcutaneous electrical nerve stimulation). Patients have reported that osteopathic soft tissue treatment reduced pain and tender trigger points and improved sleep patterns.

Diet and nutrition

Nutritional therapy Both FMS and chronic fatigue syndrome have been linked to a deficiency in the brain chemical serotonin, which may explain why antidepressant medication helps both conditions. Supplements of B vitamins, magnesium and the amino acid tryptophan may help manufacture serotonin. Supplements said to help sleep patterns include calcium, zinc and melatonin, and vitamin B complex, Vitamin C. Essential fatty acids are advised to support general nutritional well-being. Practitioners would also consider exclusion diets to identify any food intolerances.

Homeopathy Constitutional treatment is preferred. Rhus tox is worth trying if you fit this constitutional profile: restlessness, apprehension especially at night, heavy head, coated tongue

Osteoarthritis & Cervical Spondylosis

Patient Advice

OSTEOARTHRITIS

Arthritis is a blanket term for inflammation of one or several joints. There is actually little inflammation in osteoarthritis, which is mainly the result of wear and tear and injury to joint cartilage. The most common form of joint disease, particularly women after the menopause—and largely affects the lower back, hip, knee, neck, hands and fingers. Pain, stiffness and swelling—worse in the morning or after rest—can come and go for months and even years. Some joints may become quite knobbly and creak when roughened surfaces move together; in other cases inflammation is scarcely visible.

CAUSES

Whether from age degeneration, overuse or injury, the cartilage that lines bones at their point of contact thins, flakes and cracks from overuse and the bone can become thickened and distorted. Movement of the joint becomes painful and difficult and the muscles that move it gradually weaken so that function is lost.

CONVENTIONAL TREATMENT

Pain killers, non-steroidal anti-inflammatory drugs (such as aspirin or ibuprofen), heat treatment, exercise to maintain activity and physiotherapy to prevent muscle wasting are the usual treatments. Severe cartilage loss may require joint replacement surgery (hips, knees).

PREVENTION AND SELF-HELP

Keep weight down, as obesity increases pressure on weight-bearing joints. Take gentle exercise (swimming, cycling, walking) to strengthen the muscles responsible for protecting the joints, but avoid activities that put pressure on affected joints, for example, walking over rough terrain could exacerbate osteoarthritis of the knees.

Wear comfortable, well-fitting shoes that reduce stress on weight-bearing joints. Avoid carrying or lifting heavy loads if your neck or shoulders are vulnerable. If possible use the palm of the hand or forearm instead of arthritic fingers.

If you already suffer from arthritis, avoid prolonged periods in one position or you may stiffen up.

Find a system of exercise that suits you and do it regularly. Swimming is particularly good.

COMPLEMENTARY THERAPIES

Bodywork and exercise

Massage   Massage will improve circulation to the tissues, promote lymphatic drainage that reduces swelling and ease pain. Stretching and trigger-point work will help relax painful tension.

Acupuncture   According to the World Health Organisation, osteoarthritis is one of 104 conditions that acupuncture can treat effectively.

Acupressure   See Acupressure self-help sheet.

Diet and nutrition

Naturopathy / nutritional therapy   General dietary measures are designed to improve overall nutrition, digestion and elimination. Cutting down on highly refined processed foods, saturated animal fats, sugar and salt and eating more wholegrain cereals, fresh fruit and vegetables helps keep weight down. According to some researchers, supplements of methionine, an essential amino acid, may be more effective than the anti-inflammatory drug ibuprofen. Some studies indicate that taking glucosamine sulphate, one of the major ingredients of the synovial fluids that cushion joints, may be helpful. Vitamins E and C (often deficient in the elderly) and pantothenic acid have been shown to have positive effects on cartilage. Supplements of vitamin A, vitamin B6, zinc and magnesium (involved in the production of the structural protein collagen) may also be recommended. (See Anti-inflammatory diet self-help sheet.)

Herbal medicine   Herbal remedies to reduce joint inflammation include juniper and devil's claw. Circulatory stimulants such as angelica root and cinnamon may also be suggested. In one study, capsaicin cream from chili peppers reduced tenderness and pain by 40%.

Hydrotherapy   Alternate hot and cold compresses on the joint are used to stimulate circulation and ease stiffness. Swimming strengthens muscles and loosens stiff joints. Osteoarthritis of the fingers is helped by alternate hot and cold bathing.

Yoga   Stretching postures help strengthen muscles that protect joints. They also increase flexibility and improve circulation. (Contact the Yoga Biomedical Trust on 020 7833 7267.)

CERVICAL SPONDYLOSIS

In this form of osteoarthritis, degenerating joints in the neck region of the spine press on adjacent nerves. This may cause a painful or stiff neck, sometimes associated with arm pain, tingling, numbness, pins and needles, pain in the hands and legs and sometimes headache, double vision, dizziness or unsteadiness when the neck is turned. Pain and tingling are often worse in bed.

CONVENTIONAL TREATMENT

Physiotherapy   Neck exercises, anti-inflammatories (like Nurofen) and a soft neck collar worn at night may help speed recovery.

Touch and movement therapies

Aromatherapy   Massage with lavender oil and warm baths with essential oils of rosemary, cedarwood and benzoin may relieve symptoms.

Massage   Firm stroking movements down the neck and back may alleviate muscle tension associated with pain and enhance blood supply and lymphatic drainage in the area, but consult a qualified practitioner.

Exercises   See Chronic neck pain exercises self-help sheet.

Chiropractic / osteopathy   Gentle soft tissue manipulation and trigger point work can help, but manipulation of the elderly neck has to be very carefully done.

Acupuncture   Needling of local trigger points can be very helpful.

Acupressure   Firm stimulation of Gall Bladder points GB-20 and GB-21 and Large Intestine point 4 may help alleviate pain.

Patient Advice

Premenstrual Syndrome

Homoeopathic self-help

Dysmenorrhea, every 2 hours as needed:

Colocynth 6C—for cramping pain, better from hard pressure and bending double

Chamomilla 6C—for waves of labour-like pains

Sabina 6C—bright blood with dark clots and pain stretching from sacrum to pubes

Sepia 6C—for heavy bearing-down pains with tiredness and irritability.

PMS Possible remedies include Pulsatilla, Calcarea, Sepia, Lycopodium, Sulphur, Natrum Mur, Nux Vom and Phosphorus. Sepia is likely to be most effective if you experience premenstrual headaches, irritability, confusion and depression. A combination of irritability, anxiety, anger, hot flushes and cravings for sugar may be more suited to Sulphur. It is likely that symptoms will get worse before they get better (aggravation reaction), so be patient as this shows the treatment is working.

COMPLEMENTARY THERAPIES

Consider naturopathy, homeopathy, acupuncture if after trying self-help approaches your PMS is still a problem. Ask your GP for advice on what to do next.

PREMENSTRUAL SYNDROME (PMS)

Most women experience cyclical changes in mood and sensitivity during the month. Sometimes these can be extreme, however. Over 150 symptoms have been reported, but PMS can be divided into four types: *anxiety* (including irritability, mood swings, insomnia and depression before a period); *craving* (including increased appetite, headache, palpitations, fatigue and fainting); *depression* (including forgetfulness, confusion and lethargy) and *fluid retention*.

CAUSES

Each type seems to have a particular cause, possibly different kinds of hormonal and nutritional imbalances. The female hormone cycle is controlled by the same areas of the brain that are affected by factors such as stress. Worry, poor nutrition and too much strenuous exercise all have a strong effect on women's periods. Anxiety is linked to the most common type of PMS and may be due to high oestrogen levels, which can disturb levels of brain chemicals such as serotonin and adrenaline that affect mood. The pituitary hormone prolactin regulates oestrogen and progesterone, but deficiencies in vitamin B complex and essential fatty acids (EFAs) may alter prolactin levels. Craving can be due to low blood sugar and an intolerance of carbohydrates. Depression is sometimes linked to high progesterone and low oestrogen. Fluid retention is attributed to elevated aldosterone, the adrenal hormone responsible for salt and water balance.

Biochemical

PMT-A ('anxiety') Symptoms include anxiety, irritability, insomnia and depression.
Dietary strategies: reduce or eliminate dairy produce; avoid caffeine.
Supplementation:
pyridoxine (B6)—200 mg daily
calcium—1 g daily

PMT-D ('depression') Symptoms include depression, forgetfulness, confusion, lethargy
Dietary strategies: cut refined carbohydrate drastically, increase complex carbohydrates—vegetables, pulses, wholegrains, fruit. Reduce salt to 1 g daily.
Animal fat should be reduced and vegetable oils increased—especially safflower oil (cis-linoleic acid).
Supplementation:
magnesium—400 mg daily
vitamin E—300 iu daily
omega-6 fatty acids (either as borage oil, flaxseed oil, evening primrose oil) in doses of 1 to 2 g daily.

PMT-C ('craving') Symptoms include cravings for sweet foods/drinks, increased appetite, headaches, fatigue and palpitations.
Dietary strategies: low fat, low refined carbohydrates, increased complex carbohydrates.
Supplementation:
magnesium supplementation—400 mg daily
pyridoxine (B6) supplementation—200 mg daily.

PMT-H ('hyperhydration') Main symptoms include weight gain, breast congestion and tenderness, abdominal bloating, oedema of face and extremities.
Dietary strategies: low-fat diet.

Supplementation:
pyridoxine (B6)—200 mg daily
vitamin E—300 iu daily
magnesium—400 mg daily.

The PMS personality?

Hormonal and nutritional factors are only one way of looking at PMS. Clearly anxiety and depression types of PMS are also psychological states involving altered moods and potentially disturbances in relationships. Some practitioners say PMS is not an illness at all and should be 'reframed' as a cyclical hypersensitivity. Ninety-five per cent of women notice some changes before a period, but many are not bothered by them, only about 5% being sufficiently disturbed to seek medical help. Of those complaining of PMS, only one in four has 'true PMS'. In the rest, mild to moderate premenstrual symptoms are exacerbated by factors such as depression, anxiety, relationship problems and heavy, irregular or painful periods. It seems that perfectionists, pessimists and those who never say no and take on too much are most prone to symptoms. It may be useful to keep a daily of daily events and moods.

CONVENTIONAL TREATMENT

There are a variety of treatments, ranging from supplements of vitamin B6 to progestogen treatment, oestrogen implants, the contraceptive pill, diuretics, bromocriptine (a powerful antihormonal drug which suppresses prolactin), lithium, tranquillizers, antidepressants and pain killers.

PREVENTION AND SELF-HELP

Moderate exercise, increased 1 or 2 weeks before a period, improves blood flow, prevents fluid retention, relieves stress and stimulates the production of endorphins.

For all forms of PMS supplement with Optivite (multivitamin/mineral) 1 to 2 × daily and oil of evening primrose 1000 mg daily. Some nutritional supplements thought to regulate hormonal production include vitamin B6 and B complex, vitamin E, zinc, magnesium and calcium. It may be worth trying a herbal extract of Vitex agnus castus [Agnolyt] 20 drops in water on rising for 2 months.

Bodywork and exercise

Yoga is an aid to general relaxation. Regular practice is advised to control circulatory surges. Helpful postures are the triangle, bow, half shoulderstand and butterfly. If breasts are painful, avoid the plough and shoulderstand.

Aromatherapy Practitioners recommend a daily bath with essential oils of lavender, clary sage and geranium for 2 weeks before your period is due (take care if you are pregnant). Massage with these oils can relieve tension and reduce fluid retention. A chamomile steam inhalation may help associated headaches.

Relaxation and breathing Stress management techniques are strongly advised to relieve anxiety and tension and encourage the relaxation response (see Stress management self-help sheet). Other therapies to relieve stress include meditation (see self-help sheet), visualization, autogenic training and hypnotherapy.

Feelings and lifestyle

Poor sleep, anxiety and depression are common causes of tiredness. Do you get enough sleep? Are you under real or imagined 'stress'? Do you have other symptoms of depression (mood swings, early-morning waking, loss of appetite/libido, negative self-image)?

Stress management and relaxation methods (see self-help sheets) plus graduated exercise programmes can be discussed with your practitioner.

Tiredness & [Postviral] Fatigue

Patient Advice

© Harcourt Publishers Ltd 2002 Peters D, Chaitow L, Harris G, Morrison S Integrating Complementary Therapies in Primary Care: A Practical Guide for Health Professionals

CHRONIC (AND POSTVIRAL) FATIGUE SYNDROME

Fatigue is a symptom of a number of diseases—anaemia, depression, chronic infection, cancer, autoimmune disorders and thyroid disorders among them. But no apparent cause can be found for a state of extreme and disabling exhaustion that has acquired a number of names, the most generally accepted worldwide being chronic fatigue syndrome (CFS). In the UK, where it is (often incorrectly) known as ME (myalgic encephalomyelitis), 150 000 people are said to be affected. Other terms used for the condition are postviral fatigue syndrome (PVFS) and chronic fatigue and immune dysfunction syndrome (CFIDS). Symptoms may begin suddenly, sometimes after an acute viral infection, and commonly include incapacitating and persistent fatigue, muscle aches, joint pains, weakness after exercise, headaches, swollen glands, digestive disorders, inability to concentrate, memory loss, recurring minor infections or low-grade fevers, depression, an increasing sense of being unable to function, sleep disturbance, light sensitivity, food intolerance and environmental allergies. Diagnosis is controversial and, with the lack of an obvious cause, conventional medical opinion is divided over whether CFS is a disease in its own right or a form of depression. None the less, the symptoms are very real, can last for years and are severe enough to ruin people's lives. In the US, the Centre for Disease Control (CDC) maintains a list of defining symptoms and many medical centres offer CFS clinics, while in the UK the Department of Health officially recognizes it as a 'debilitating and distressing condition'.

CAUSES

No single identifiable cause appears to be at work. Many sufferers insist that there is a physiological reason for their condition and resist any suggestion of a psychological element, but it seems increasingly likely that both mind and body are involved. Medical experts now believe CFS may be a complex interaction between trigger factors such as stress, viral infection, psychological factors, brain chemistry and social attitudes. A number of viruses have been put forward as possible triggers: Epstein–Barr (associated with glandular fever), Coxsackie (associated with chicken pox), a connection with the polio virus, enteroviruses in the bowels and elusive retroviruses are favourite contenders as high levels of antibodies are sometimes found in CFS sufferers. Numerous lines of research have been pursued, but so far nothing concrete has come of them. According to one theory, such viruses may alter the immune system making the body more susceptible to stress, hormonal imbalances, genetic influences, vaccinations, chemicals, bacteria and other toxins, and it's true that researchers have found abnormalities in the immune system and especially the muscle cells of some patients. Treatment for a form of low blood pressure has also proved helpful for a number of people with CFS symptoms.

On the other hand it may be that stress initially reduces resistance to a viral infection. Doctors refer to a particular CFS personality profile—perfectionist, conscientious people who feel obliged to take on too much, come under a lot of stress, find it hard to relax and are inclined to get depressed and introverted. A disproportionate number of patients are young professional women and the majority are clinically depressed.

CONVENTIONAL TREATMENT

Before diagnosing CFS it is important to rule out any treatable or serious diseases that cause similar symptoms, such as glandular fever, clinical depression (up to 75% of CFS patients are clinically depressed—whether as a cause or consequence of their fatigue), anaemia,

hormonal disorders or cancer. Defining factors include physical and mental fatigue that reduces daily activity by at least 50%, illness lasting more than 6 months and associated symptoms in the muscles, nerves and cardiovascular systems, despite all the usual medical examinations and investigations appearing normal. There is no conventional treatment as such, although doctors are now becoming more accepting and supportive. Rest, a balanced diet, vitamin supplements, counselling and antidepressants are usually suggested and the results are promising though slow. Some form of gentle but gradually increasing exercise is recommended, as avoiding all activity possibly causes the problems to get worse as levels of fitness and morale inevitably decline. Furthermore, disuse of muscles is bound to mean that eventually any movement provokes muscle aches and pains.

SELF-HELP AND PREVENTION

If you are under pressure of work, learn to pace yourself, allowing time to relax during the day. Look at your lifestyle for ways to ease stress and delegate commitments (see Stress management self-help sheet). Don't try to battle on if you are ill but get plenty of rest if you catch a viral infection such as a heavy cold or flu. These minor illnesses may be nature's way of saying 'slow down for a few days'. So listen. After you have taken time out, gentle exercise—walking, swimming or stretching—stimulates the release of endorphins, the body's natural pain killers, improves blood flow, increases production of killer T-cells in the immune system and prevents muscles from wasting. Good health requires that we let ourselves be a little ill from time to time.

COMPLEMENTARY THERAPIES

Fatigue involves the whole person; your lifestyle, diet, past emotional history, relationships and attitudes are all factors that may be particularly relevant in CFS. Most practitioners admit that CFS is a difficult disease to treat bearing in mind that any improvement could take months and there is too little evidence to decide which is the best complementary 'cure' for CFS.

Diet and nutrition

Sometimes a nutritional deficiency (e.g. of iron or magnesium) makes fatigue worse.

Food intolerances are all factors that may be particularly relevant in CFS. Most practitioners that certain foods make you feel worse (see Exclusion rotation diet self-help sheet)

A hypoglycaemic tendency is possible if the exhaustion is worse or there is increased irritability after a missed meal or 3 hours after eating.

A diet for low blood sugar involves high-protein, low-sugar, frequent snacks. Try an 'anti-candida' diet (if history suggests onset after large amounts of antibiotics (see questionnaire and self-help sheet).

Bodywork and exercise

Overbreathing produces a number of symptoms including tiredness, cramps, lack of concentration and anxiety. Do you tend to breathe with your upper chest? Do you get breathless under pressure? Consider hyperventilation (see Breathing self-help sheet).

Is there an obvious element of physical tension (posture, body language, clenching teeth, rapid heart, etc.)? Consider relaxation methods (see self-help sheet). Constant muscle tension uses up energy, so it actually makes you tired. If you find it difficult to relax, massage may help kickstart the process so that relaxation self-help gets easier.

Abdominal Muscle Toning

Self-Help Sheet

ABDOMINAL TONING

These exercises are designed to help strengthen the abdominal muscles if they are weak, as well as stretching the lower back. This helps tone up the abdominal muscles by taking away back tension, which actually weakens the belly muscles.

THE EXERCISES

1. For low back tightness and abdominal weakness

- Lie on your back on a carpeted floor, with a pillow under your head.
- Bend one knee and hip and hold the knee with both hands.
- Inhale deeply and as you exhale draw that knee to the shoulder on the same side, as far is comfortably possible.
- Repeat this two more times.
- Rest that leg on the floor, perform the same sequence with the other leg and replace this on the floor.
- Now bend both legs at both the knee and hip and clasp one knee with each hand.
- Hold the knees comfortably (shoulder width) apart and draw the knees towards your shoulders—not your chest.
- When you have reached a point where a slight stretch is felt in the low back, inhale deeply and hold the position for 10 seconds, before slowly releasing the breath and as you do so easing the knees a little closer towards your shoulders.
- Repeat the inhalation and held-breath sequence followed by the easing of the knees closer to the shoulders a further four times (five times altogether).
- After the fifth stretch to the shoulders stay in the final position for about half a minute while breathing deeply and slowly.

This exercise effectively stretches many of the lower and middle muscles of the back and this helps to tone the abdominal muscles which the back muscle tightness may have weakened.

2. For low back and pelvic muscles

- Lie on the floor on your back with a pillow under your head.
- Keep your low back flat to the floor throughout the exercise.

- As you exhale draw your right hip upwards—as though you are 'shrugging it' while at the same time stretching your left leg (push the heel away not the pointed toe) away from you, trying to make it longer.
- Hold this for a few seconds before inhaling again and relaxing both efforts.
- Repeat in the same way on the other side, drawing the left hip up and pushing the right leg away.
- Repeat the sequence five times altogether.

This exercise stretches and tones the muscles just above the pelvis and is very useful following a period of inactivity due to back problems.

3. For abdominal muscles and pelvis

- Lie on your back on a carpeted floor, no pillow, knees bent, arms folded over abdomen, at the same time inhaling and holding your breath.
- Pull your abdomen in ('as though you are trying to staple your navel to your spine').
- Tilt the pelvis forwards by flattening your back to the floor.
- Squeeze your buttocks tightly together and at the same time lift your hips towards the ceiling.
- Hold this combined contraction for a slow count of five before exhaling and relaxing on to the floor for a further cycle of breathing.
- Repeat 5–10 times.

4. To tone abdominal muscles

- Lie on the floor with your knees bent and arms folded across your chest.
- Push your low back towards the floor and tighten your buttock muscles, and as you inhale raise your head and neck and if possible your shoulders from the floor—even if it is only a small amount.
- Hold this for 5 seconds and as you exhale relax all tight muscles and lie on the floor for a full cycle of relaxed breathing before repeating.
- Do this up to ten times to strengthen the abdominal muscles.
- When you can do this easily add a variation in which as you lift yourself from the floor you ease your right elbow towards your left knee—hold as above and then relax.
- The next lift should take the left elbow towards the right knee.

This strengthens the oblique abdominal muscles. Do up to 10 cycles of this exercise daily.

HOW LONG WILL IT BE BEFORE I SEE IMPROVEMENT?

As long as you exercise regularly you should see some improvement in your general fitness within a couple of months.

Aerobic/
Cardiovascular
Exercise

Self-Help Sheet

AEROBIC EXERCISE

- Involves an active exercise of your choice.
- Takes 20 minutes three times a week.
- Does not require any special equipment.
- Is good for your heart.
- Is good for reducing feelings of stress.
- Can be as easy as taking a 20-minute walk.

WHAT IS AEROBIC EXERCISE?

The term 'aerobic exercise' applies to any active exercise which makes your heart beat faster and so gives your heart the kind of boost it needs to work at its best. You do not have to be superfit to start this kind of exercising and it does not mean having to go to a special kind of 'aerobics class' at a gym or buying fancy sports clothes.

WHY SHOULD I DO IT?

Exercise causes the release in the body of natural substances which have a direct antistress effect. So it is useful in helping us to handle stress more effectively and as well as being good for the long-term health of your heart and circulation. Research suggests that precisely the same calming effects which are achieved by meditation could be acquired by regular swimming, jogging, walking or yoga. However, there are some people who prefer meditation and others who find exercise a better option. Regular exercise builds up your heart and lung capacity to exert yourself. At the same time, the body burns away the waste products built up by stress and inactivity. Aerobic exercise can lower blood pressure, burn off fat, raise your metabolic rate and make you feel powerful.

WHAT IF I HAVEN'T EXERCISED REGULARLY FOR A LONG TIME?

If you have any doubts at all about what might be the most sensible way of starting to take exercise please see your doctor. As a general rule it is best to build up the length of your exercise. You may want to start with walking, increasing how much you do each time. Or you may start with walking and when you feel more confident start to go swimming, or some other activity.

WHICH TYPE OF EXERCISE COULD I CONSIDER?

The exercise chosen should be active. This can mean working out at a gym, or participation in organized sport, or just as usefully could involve skipping at home, learning a dance routine, for example, salsa, folk, ballroom, jazzercise, etc., or going cycling, swimming or walking.

HOW CAN I TELL IF I AM DOING 'AEROBIC' ACTIVITY?

The most important thing is not so much the type of exercise you choose but how regularly you do it. The ideal is 20 minutes of vigorous exercise three times a week. If you can possibly fit it into your life try not to have a break of more than 2 days between each session because each session boosts your metabolism for about 48 hours. Before you start any activity, however, you will need to work out the pulse rate that is safe for you to have when you exercise. There is a formula which you can use to discover what your pulse rate should be to obtain benefit safely and, most importantly, what you must not exceed to stay safe when exercising.

FINDING YOUR SAFETY PULSE RATES FOR AEROBIC ACTIVITY

Everyone, at whatever level of fitness, can do aerobic exercise. But to be safe and effective you should work out your safe pulse rates.

You will first need to work out your resting pulse rate.

Substitute *your* pulse rate and *your* age for the numbers used in the example given below.

- Take your pulse in the morning before doing anything active for a few days and find the average. (In the example given here we will say that it is 72.)
- Add this number to your age. (If you are now 36, we have 72 + 36 = 108.)
- Subtract this number from 220 (220 − 108 = 112).
- Calculate 60% (divide by 10 and multiply by 6) of 112.
- Calculate 80% (divide by 10 and multiply by 8) of this number 112:
  60% of 112 = 67
  80% of 112 = 90.
- Now add your morning pulse to these two numbers (72 was our example):
  67 + 72 = 139
  90 + 72 = 162.

These last two numbers will give you the lowest pulse rate and the highest pulse rate that you can have to exercise safely and still get the benefits of aerobic exercise. The 36 year old in our example needs to exercise at a level which gets the pulse rate up to at least 139 but not over 162 to achieve the benefits of aerobic exercise. You will need to exercise above the lowest level (139 beats in our example) for the 20 minutes of your exercise. Do not at any time exceed the upper level (162 in our example).

- Try it out! Stop regularly to check your pulse (either by means of a special pulse monitor from any sports store) or by learning to take your pulse for 10 seconds and multiply by six.
- The key numbers (139 and 162 in our example) will change as you get fitter and older, because the numbers will change. So recalculate every year.

Please fill in the blank spaces below to calculate your key numbers

- My resting pulse is ......
- My pulse...... + my age...... = ...
- This number ...... taken away from 220 = ...
- 60% of this last number is ......
- 80% of this last number is ......
- Add your resting pulse rate to the 60% number......

This is the rate of pulse you need to achieve to exercise aerobically.

- Add your resting pulse rate to the 80% number......

This is the rate of pulse you must not exceed when exercising.

HOW WILL I KNOW IF I AM DOING MY EXERCISE CORRECTLY?

As long as you calculate the range of safety according to the guidance then whether you walk, jog, swim or dance you will be exercising safely. You can use your numbers to keep a check on your progress. As you get fitter your pulse rate will probably change, and as you get older you will need to recalculate the figures.

© Harcourt Publishers Ltd 2002 Peters D, Chaitow L, Harris G, Morrison S Integrating Complementary Therapies in Primary Care: A Practical Guide for Health Professionals

Antiarousal Breathing

Self-Help Sheet

ANTIAROUSAL BREATHING

- Is easy to learn.
- Is under your control.
- Fits in with your daily life.
- Needs no equipment and costs nothing.
- Takes a few minutes to do.

WHAT IS ANTIAROUSAL BREATHING?

Antiarousal breathing is a very simple technique designed to help calm you down when you are feeling anxious or stressed. It does not take long to learn but it does require you to practise it regularly to get the most benefit.

ABOUT THE EXERCISE
Counting as you breathe

It is important during this exercise that you count how long it takes you to breathe in and breathe out. An easy way of counting 1 second at a time is to say (silently) 'one hundred, two hundred, three hundred, etc.' Each count lasts about 1 second. You are aiming (after some weeks of daily practice) to achieve:

- an inhalation phase which lasts for 2–3 seconds
- an exhalation phase lasts from 6 to 7 seconds—without any strain.

Most importantly the exhalation should be slow and continuous. The exercise does not work if you breathe the air out in 2 seconds and then wait until the count reaches 6, 7 or 8 before inhaling again.

THE TECHNIQUE OF ANTIAROUSAL BREATHING

1. Place yourself in a comfortable (ideally sitting/reclining) position. First breathe out very slowly and *fully* through your partially open mouth, lips just barely separated. You can imagine that a candle flame is about 6 inches/15 cm from your mouth and you breathe out without blowing the candle out. As you exhale count silently to yourself to establish the length of the outbreath.
2. Having exhaled fully, without causing any sense of strain to yourself in any way, allow the inhalation which follows to be full, free and uncontrolled. Once again count to yourself to establish how long your inbreath lasts.
3. Without pausing to hold the breath, exhale *fully* through the mouth, blowing the air in a thin stream as if you were whistling (again you should count to yourself at the same speed).
4. Continue to repeat the inhalation and the exhalation for not less than 30 cycles of in and out.

DIAPHRAGMATIC BREATHING

The diaphragm is a dome-shaped muscle which separates our chest and abdominal cavities. When we breathe in (inspiration) the diaphragm contracts, flattens and descends, sucking air into the lungs. As the diaphragm descends it pushes the abdominal contents down, which forces the abdominal wall out.

When we breathe out (expiration), the diaphragm relaxes, air is forced out of the lungs and the abdominal wall flattens.

Diaphragmatic breathing is in itself relaxing compared with the 'emergency mode'—breathing with the upper chest. It is also the most efficient and relaxed way of getting enough air.

DIAPHRAGMATIC BREATHING TRAINING

1. Find a quiet room where you will be undisturbed for about 10–15 minutes. Lie down on the bed or floor. Undo any tight clothing and remove your shoes. Spend a few moments settling yourself down.
2. Close your eyes, spread your feet 12–18 inches (30–45 cm) apart, and check that your head, neck and spine are in a straight line. Focus your attention on your breathing. Do not try and change your breathing for the moment. Become aware of how fast or slow you are breathing, and whether you are breathing with your chest or diaphragm. Notice whether there are any gaps or pauses between your inhalation or exhalation.
3. Now, put one hand on your upper chest, and one hand on your abdomen just below your rib cage. Relax the shoulders and hands. As you exhale gently, press the lower hand to flatten your abdomen. As you inhale, allow the abdomen to rise, and as you exhale, allow the abdomen to flatten. There should be little or no movement in the chest.
4. Allow yourself a little time to get into a regular rhythm. It may help to imagine that as you are breathing in you draw half a circle with your breath around your body, and as you breathe out, you complete the other half of the circle. Allow your breath to become smooth, easy and regular.
5. Now, let your exhalation slow down then be conscious of a comfortable pause before allowing your inhalation to follow smoothly and easily. If any distractions, thoughts or worries come into your mind allow them to come, then allow them to go again and bring your attention back to your breathing.
6. When you are ready to end this exercise, take a few deeper breaths in. Bring some awareness of movement back into your fingers and toes. Open your eyes slowly, and turn over on to one side before gently sitting up.

WHEN SHOULD I PRACTISE THE EXERCISES?

You can practise these exercises briefly on waking and before bedtime. They are invisible so no one will notice if you also do them before meals everyday. The effect will increase with practice.

HOW QUICKLY WILL I SEE RESULTS?

By the time you have completed 15 or so cycles any sense of anxiety you previously felt should be much reduced. Also if pain is a problem this should also have lessened.

USING THESE TECHNIQUES AS 'FIRST AID'

Apart from regular daily practice, it is useful to repeat either exercise for a few minutes (about five cycles of inhalation/exhalation takes a minute) every hour if you are anxious or whenever 'stress' seems to be building up.

Back & Joint Pain Exercises

Self-Help Sheet

BACK AND JOINT PAIN EXERCISES

General spinal stretching

This series of exercises allows multiple releases of tight structures. Perform each exercise as many times as your practitioner suggests.

1. Lie on your back with a pillow under your head/neck, knees bent, feet flat on the floor and your arms out to the sides, palms facing upwards. Allow both knees to fall to the right, while keeping the soles of your feet, shoulders and low back on the floor. (This is to prevent you twisting too much.) Breathe deeply and slowly three times, then take a deep breath and hold it for 10–15 seconds. As you let the breath go allow your knees to ease further toward the floor for 10–15 seconds. Keeping your low back in contact with the floor, bring your knees back to the midline. Repeat on the left side.

2. Lying as shown, keep your outstretched legs together and take them to the right side, as far as possible from the midline, and rest them there. Then take a deep breath and hold it for 10–15 seconds. Keeping your knees to ease slowly to the right as far as is comfortable. Maintain this C-shaped posture while taking three very slow, deep breaths. Hold this position for 10–15 seconds, exhale, and try to take your legs and upper body slightly further to the side. Hold this breath for 10–15 seconds. (Variation: Extend your left arm above your head to obtain even more stretch on the left side.) Come slowly back to the midline and reverse directions to stretch to your right side.

3. Lie on one side with a pillow under your head and your knees bent. Keeping your legs together, curl up so that your back is rounded and your nose is as close to your knees as possible. Make sure the pillow supports your head at all times. Take three slow, deep breaths, then take a deep breath and hold for 10–15 seconds. On exhalation, try to curl a little further.

4. Return to a straight position and, keeping your legs together, extend them backwards behind your midline as far as is comfortable. At the same time take your head and shoulders backward. Make sure that the pillow supports your head at all times. Take three slow, deep breaths; then take a deep breath and hold it for 10–15 seconds. On exhalation try to stretch a little further, and stay in this position for 10–15 seconds.

General self-mobilization of the torso

The following exercises are a modification of those presented by Chester Kirk DO in 1977 in the Journal of the American Osteopathic Association. All should be done in a relaxed manner, with a gentle degree of effort.

1. Sitting in a straight chair, rest the palms of your hands on your thighs, with your fingers facing inward. Allow the weight of your upper body to be supported by your arms, letting your elbows bend outwards as your head and chest come forward, until a slight stretch is felt in your lower back. Hold for 3–5 sec-

onds, breathing normally, then bring your upper body back to the starting position. Repeat this . . . times.

2. Sit on the floor on your right buttock with your right arm and hand extended to take some of your weight. Sit with your knees bent and your feet and legs to the left. Relax your left arm and your legs. By pushing off your right hand (or fist), take your left arm and torso into an upright position until a slight sense of strain or stretch is felt in your low back and left hip or knee. Push rhythmically thus at a rate of two per second, always keeping your right arm straight, until you have done ten. Rest and repeat . . . times. Reverse directions to do the left side.

3. Lie on your back with your arms outstretched, your knees bent and your feet flat on the floor. Cross your left leg over your right and allow the weight of your left leg to take it down toward the floor, which will bring your right knee toward the floor too. Lift your left foot from the floor 3–6 inches (7–15 cm) and gently pulse toward the floor . . . times. If any pain is felt, stop immediately. A gentle stretch should be felt on your left torso/low back as the rhythmic movement is performed. Reverse the direction to do your right side.

4. Lie on your back with your knees and your hands locked behind your neck. Bring your elbows together and raise your head about 2 inches (5 cm). Slowly and rhythmically twist your trunk in opposite directions so that one elbow strikes the floor, then the other. Keep your head and neck relaxed. Repeat this so that this happens . . . times on each side.

5. On your hands and knees with your thighs and arms perpendicular to the floor and fingers pointing towards each other, first inhale, then exhale and take your chin as close to your hands as possible, keeping your head as upright as the position allows. Slowly roll an invisible pea with your chin toward your knees with your chin. Inhale and lift your head and shoulders, then exhale and take your chin toward your knees, slowly pushing the imaginary pea with your chin towards your hands. Remember to exhale as you take your head toward the floor and exhale as you lift your head from the floor. Return to starting position on an inhale. Repeat . . . times.

6. Sit with your left leg crossed over your right and your right hand on the floor between crossed knees. Place your left hand behind your body on the floor 6–8 inches behind your buttocks, fingers pointed backwards. Twist your trunk and shoulders as far as possible to the left without pain, and then follow with your head looking over your left shoulder. Stay in this position while taking five slow breaths. Then try to twist all elements a little further to the left. Reverse the directions to twist to the right. Repeat . . . times.

© Harcourt Publishers Ltd 2002 Peters D, Chaitow L, Harris G, Morrison S Integrating Complementary Therapies in Primary Care: A Practical Guide for Health Professionals

Exercise three—repeat twice daily following flexion and extension exercises.

Rotation exercises—whole body

Please remember:

• *It is most important that when performing these exercises no force is used; just take yourself to what is best described as an 'easy barrier'—and never 'as far as you can force yourself'.*

• *The gains that are achieved by slowly pushing the barrier back, as you become more supple, are achievable over a period of weeks or even months, not days, and at first you should anticipate that you will feel a little stiff and achy in newly stretched muscles the day after first performing them. This will soon pass and does not require treatment of any sort.*

• Sit on a carpeted floor with legs oustretched.

• Cross your left leg over your right leg at the knees.

• Bring your right arm across your body and place your right hand between your crossed knees, so locking the knees in position.

• Your left hand should be taken behind your trunk and placed on the floor about 12–15 cm behind your buttocks with your fingers pointing backwards. This twists your upper body to the left.

• Now turn your shoulders as far to the left as is comfortable, without pain. Then turn your head to look over your left shoulder, as far as possible, again make sure that no pain is being produced, just stretch.

• Stay in this position for five full, slow, breaths, after which, as you breathe out, turn your shoulders and your head a little further to the left, to their new 'restriction barriers'.

• Stay in this final position for a further five full, slow, breaths before gently unwinding yourself and repeating the whole exercise to the right, reversing all elements of the instructions (i.e. cross your right leg over your left, place your left hand between your knees, turn to the right, etc.).

Exercise four—ideally repeat twice daily following the flexion and extension exercises and the previous rotation exercise.

• Lie face upwards on a carpeted floor with a small pillow or book under your head.

• Flex your knees so that your feet, which should be together, are flat on the floor.

• Keep your shoulders in contact with the floor during the exercise. This is helped by having your arms out to the side slightly, palms upwards.

• Carefully allow your knees to fall to the right as far as possible without pain—keeping your shoulders and your lower back in contact with the floor. Your should feel a tolerable twisting sensation, but not a pain, in the muscles of the lower and middle parts of the back.

• Hold this position while you breathe deeply and slowly for about 30 seconds, as the weight of your legs 'drags' on the rest of your body, which is stationary so stretching a number of back muscles.

• On an exhalation slowly bring your knees back to the midline and then repeat the process in exactly the same manner, to the left side.

• Repeat the exercise to both right and left one more time, on each side, before straightening out and resting of a few seconds.

Back Prevention/ Maintenance

Self-Help Sheet

EXERCISES FOR THE GOOD HEALTH OF YOUR BACK

- Easy to learn.
- Takes up to 30 minutes a day.
- Long-term benefit.
- No equipment needed.
- Under your control.
- No side-effects.
- No cost.

BACK PAIN

Back problems are very common and potentially debilitating. The spine can flex (bend forwards), extend (bend backwards), sidebend to each side as well as rotating (twisting) but only when it is healthy and supple. The exercises in this leaflet are designed to help your back maintain suppleness.

For best results the four exercises need to be done in sequence every day.

WHY EXERCISE?

As we age and especially as we adapt to the multiple mechanical stresses and injuries caused by everyday living, such as repeatedly carrying heavy loads, poor posture, difficult working positions, the muscles which support and move the spine, and the joints themselves, can lose their ability to perform all movements efficiently. The exercises described here can help maintain flexibility.

IS IT SAFE?

Yes but it is most important to remember:

- If any of the exercises described hurt while performing them, or leave you with pain after their use, stop doing them. Either they are unsuitable for your particular condition or you are performing them too energetically or excessively.
- These exercises are 'prevention' exercises, meant to be performed in a sequence so that all the natural movements of the spine can benefit, and are *not* designed for treatment of back problems. Exercises for improving back problems are described in other leaflets. You practitioner will give you these if they are appropriate for your condition.

HOW LONG WILL I HAVE TO DO THESE EXERCISES FOR?

As these exercises are designed to prevent back problems if you have a history of back pain and are getting benefit from these exercises you may want to incorporate them into your daily routine so that they become a regular habit.

WHAT CAN I DO TO HELP MYSELF DO THE EXERCISES REGULARLY?

Even though you may be getting benefit from the exercises there will be some days that you miss doing them. This is normal.

Changing daily habits takes some effort especially when the benefits you get from the exercises are long term and can't immediately be seen. If you are having difficulty keeping up the exercises please ask for our leaflet 'Making changes'.

HOW DO I KNOW IF I AM DOING THE EXERCISES CORRECTLY?

As the exercises are described only by a written explanation you may not be quite sure if you are doing them correctly. You may want to check with your practitioner if you have any doubts.

© Harcourt Publishers Ltd 2002 Peters D, Chaitow L, Harris G, Morrison S Integrating Complementary Therapies in Primary Care: A Practical Guide for Health Professionals

THE EXERCISES

Exercise one—this flexion exercise should be performed twice daily but not after a meal

Sequence A

- Sit on the floor with both legs straight out in front of you, toes pointing towards the ceiling.
- Bend forwards as far as is comfortable and grasp one leg with each hand.
- Hold this position for about 30 seconds—approximately four slow deep-breathing cycles.

You should be aware of a stretch on the back of the legs and the back. Be sure to let your head hang down. You should feel no actual pain.

- As you release the fourth breath ease yourself a little further down the legs and grasp again.
- Stay here for a further half minute or so before slowly returning to an upright position.

Sequence B

- Bend one leg and place the foot against the inside of the other knee, the bent knee as close to the floor as possible.
- Stretch forwards down the straight leg and grasp it with both hands. Hold for 30 seconds as before and then, on an exhalation stretch further down the leg and hold for a further 30 seconds.
- Slowly return to an upright position and alter the legs so that the straight one is now bent and the bent one straight.
- Perform the same sequence as described above.
- Repeat sequence A.

Exercise two—repeat twice daily after flexion exercise

Please remember excessive backwards bending of the spine is not desirable. All exercises are designed to be performed very gently, without any force or discomfort at all. If any pain is felt then stop doing the exercise.

Whole body

- Lie on your side (either side will do) on a carpeted floor with a small cushion to support your head and neck. Your legs should be together, one on the other.
- Bend your knees as far as comfortably possible—bringing your heels towards your back-side. Now with your thighs together and in this knees bent position move your thighs backwards as far as you can, without producing pain, so that your back is slightly arched. Your upper arm should rest along your side.
- Now take your head and shoulders backwards to increase the backward bending of your spine—again this should be done slowly and without pain—although you should be aware of a stretching sensation in front of your body and some 'crowding' in the middle of the back.
- Hold this position for approximately three to four full breaths, and then hold your breath for about 15 seconds.
- As you release this try to ease first your legs and then your upper body into a little more backwards bending.
- Hold this final position for about half a minute, breathing slowly and deeply all the while.
- Bring yourself back to a straight side-lying position before turning or to your back and resting before moving into a seated position for the rotation exercise.

Breathing Exercises

Self-Help Sheet

WHY ARE THERE EXERCISES ON BREATHING?

Most of us don't think about how we breathe unless we have a chest infection or a condition like hay fever. The way we breathe, however, can profoundly affect how we are feeling emotionally as well as having an impact on the condition of our bodies. So it is very important for long-term health maintenance.

Ideally our breathing should be relaxed and regular, but a lot of people breathe in an erratic shallow way using only the upper part of the chest. However, with some practice, deeper and more regular breathing can be achieved. There is strong evidence that the breathing exercises described can reduce stress levels.

BREATHING EXERCISES

The following exercises are:

- easy to learn
- cost nothing and do not require any special equipment
- take only a short time to complete
- are designed to fit in with daily living.

Ideally the first two exercises are performed in the morning and evening.

Exercise 1

- Stand upright.
- Take a deep breath through your nose and bend slowly to the right, running your right hand down the outside of the leg and raising the left arm above your head, so that the body stretches to the right.
- As the movement is continued more breath should be slowly drawn in.
- Now bend slowly to the left and allow the left hand to go down the left leg and right arm to come over the head, to take your body over to the left.
- During this movement breathe out slowly through the mouth.
- Continue in this fashion, breathing in as you bend to the right and out as you bend to the left ten times.
- The sequence of breathing should then be changed, breathing in as you bend to the left, and out when bending to the right.
- Do this ten times as well.

This will take about 6–8 minutes depending on how long each breath lasts.

Exercise 2

- Stand erect with your thumbs near your spine at the level of your waist; fingers should point towards the front of your body.
- Close your mouth and take in air, in small amounts, as if sniffing a flower.
- Continue to fill the lungs until no more can be taken.
- While you are breathing in, bend gradually backwards without straining yourself.

- When you feel you have breathed in fully breathe out slowly through your mouth, at the same time bending slowly forwards without strain.
- Do this 10–15 times at least once a day.

Exercise 3 Walking and breathing exercise

- As you walk breathe in through your nose as you take three or four steps, to fill your lungs comfortably.
- The number of steps you take as you inhale will vary with the speed of walking and your general condition. Above all it must be a comfortable, unstrained pattern.
- Hold the breath for one or two steps and then exhale, still through the nose, as you take two or three steps.
- This pattern of counting and breathing as you walk, should be carried out for only a minute or two at a time during the walk (that is around ten cycles of inhalation/exhalation) or until it stops feeling easy to maintain the rhythm.
- Repeat this several times during a half hour walk.
- As your fitness increases, and your lung capacity improves, so you will be able to do more and more of this type of controlled breathing during exercise.

HOW LONG WILL IT BE BEFORE I SEE ANY CHANGES?

The key to success is doing the exercises as regularly as possible for at least a month. You should feel some benefit within this time perhaps feeling less stressed could result, but also other things such as better sleep or better mood.

WHAT CAN I DO IF I FORGET TO DO THE EXERCISES?

Most of us live life with our own habits and routines and making changes takes not only time but commitment. Changing habits takes time and it is normal to be a bit irregular at the beginning. If you find, however, that you are regularly not doing these exercises even though you want to please ask us for our leaflet called 'Making changes', which might help you.

HOW LONG WILL I HAVE TO DO THESE EXERCISES?

The best possible outcome would be that you make the exercises so much part of your routine that you do them automatically or at least when you feel you need to. New breathing patterns will emerge with practice that will help you maintain your sense of well-being and fitness.

HOW CAN I TELL IF I AM DOING IT CORRECTLY?

If you have any doubts about how you are doing your exercises please ask your practitioner who will be glad to help and instruct you. Remember, please only do the exercises within a range of movement and at a rate that you feel comfortable with.

Please note: Anyone with a diagnosis of asthma may need personal instruction in doing these exercises before starting to use them.

Special instructions:

4. Spinal massage

Trigger points and other tender areas along the spine may be treated using two tennis balls stuffed into a sock. The balls are placed on either side of the spine as shown. One may either gently move up and down, or hold the pressure for as long as is tolerable. The shoulder and gluteal areas may also be massaged in this manner, care being taken to avoid bruising, especially in the gluteal region.

Chronic Neck Pain Exercises

Self-Help Sheet

CHRONIC NECK PAIN EXERCISES

Muscle energy technique: exercises for general mobility

Do each exercise slowly and without force using only 20% of your strength at any time or less if indicated. With each contraction take a deep breath and hold this for 7 seconds while you push against your own hand(s). No movement should take place. Let go the breath and effort slowly; at the same time, relax for a second or two and then gently stretch the muscle that has just been contracting—without force.

Caution Holding the head and neck in a backwards position can sometimes cause stress on the blood vessels which carry circulation to the head. Exercises that employ a backward tilt should only carried out following instruction by a licensed health care professional. If you experience light-headedness, dizziness or nausea when carrying out such procedures, stop immediately and rest.

1. Try to tilt your head to the right but stop this with your right hand resting against the right side of your face/head. Now gently bend your neck to the left to stretch the muscles you have just contracted. Repeat . . . times. Reverse directions for your left side.

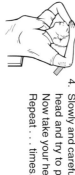

2. Bend your neck forward slightly. Put your hands on your forehead and push against your hands. Now stretch the muscles in the front of your neck by taking your head and back to an easy barrier. Please see caution note above. Repeat . . . times.

3. Bend your neck forward, chin near your chest and place your hands at the back of your head. Push backwards. Now stretch the muscles in the back of your neck by taking your chin further towards your chest without pain. Repeat . . . times.

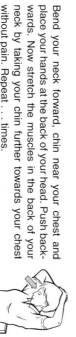

4. Slowly and carefully look up at the ceiling. Place your hands on your forehead and try to push your head upright. Now take your head further back without pain. Please see caution above. Repeat . . . times.

5. Sit upright and pull your chin backwards as though going through the back of your neck. Place your hand on your chin and restrain your effort to return to its normal position. Use only 10% of your strength. Now pull your chin further back to stretch the muscles at the back of your neck. Repeat . . . times.

6. Place your left hand on your left cheek and restrain a turning of your head to the left. Stretch by turning to the right. Repeat . . . times. Reverse directions for a right stretch.

Note Instead of a steady pressure, a pulsing pressure may be used. This is a very light push with no wobble or bounce and just the barest activation of the muscles. This method was first described by T.J. Ruddy, DO. Try to produce 20 pulsations—tiny pushes against resistance—in a 10 second period and then gently stretch the area. Repeat several times if needed.

Self-mobilization techniques

Care should be used in these exercises not to involve force. The essence of self-treatment methods is that they should be safe and gentle. Pain indicates a clear message to stop. Exercises should be repeated every other day, or at least several times per week.

1. Cervicothoracic junction

Stretch your arms sideways with your fingers widely spread and rotate your arms at the shoulder in opposite directions. Arms should be straight. Turn your head toward the side with your thumb down. Hold for 3–5 seconds, then rotate your arms in opposite directions and turn your head to the other side (on which thumb is now down). Synchronize the movement of your head and arms with a deep breath in, blowing out as position is held, then breathing in as you turn your head. Repeat . . . times.

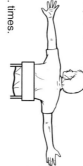

2. Lower cervical/upper thoracic spine

Lie face down with elbows together resting just forward of a line running from shoulder to shoulder. With your head hanging, breathe in and raise your head an inch or so, holding your breath for 7–10 seconds. Breathe out and allow your head to hang freely for 10 seconds. Repeat . . . times.

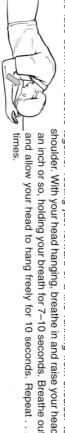

3. Upper trapezius

Lie on a bed or the floor with pillows as shown, left hand holding the side of the bed or tucked under the left buttock, while your right hand reaches across the top of your head and pulls it painlessly as far to the right as possible. Turn your eyes to the left as you hold a deep breath for 7 seconds. On breathing out take your eyes to the right and pull you head further to the right. Relax and repeat . . . times. Reverse directions for the right upper trapezius.

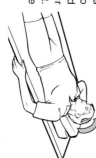

© Harcourt Publishers Ltd 2002 Peters D, Chaitow L, Harris G, Morrison S Integrating Complementary Therapies in Primary Care: A Practical Guide for Health Professionals

Exercises for Relaxing Muscles

Self-Help Sheet

AN EXERCISE FOR WHEN YOUR MUSCLES FEEL STIFF AND PAINFUL

Muscle stiffness is a very common symptom. The exercise described in this leaflet has been designed for you to do if you have a stiff neck but the same method can be used to relax tight muscles anywhere in the body.

ABOUT THE TECHNIQUE

- It is very easy and takes just 5 minutes to learn.
- It takes only a couple of minutes to do.
- It is within your control and is safe.
- You can tell if you are doing it right.
- You can experience immediate relief.
- It can be done anytime you feel you need to do it.
- You do not have to be super fit.
- It does not require any special clothing.

The technique is called 'muscle energy technique' or MET for short. When you are doing this exercise your muscles are meant to get tighter (for a short while) but without moving. So it won't be like doing a workout but remember you still need to be careful.

HOW DO I BENEFIT?

You can ideally do MET before any gentle stretching exercises as it will assist you to perform exercises more easily.

HOW DOES THIS EXERCISE WORK?

It may seem strange to tighten muscles which are already stiff but if you can gently contract muscles then they will relax more afterwards, allowing you more flexibility and less pain. By making the resisted movements with both your right and left hands on each side you are helping all the muscles that need relaxing.

MET NECK RELAXATION EXERCISE

Sit close to a table with your elbows on the table and rest your hands on each side of your face. Your hands remain in this position for the whole of this exercise.

1. Turn your head as far as you can to the right letting your hands move with your face until you reach the point just before your neck begins to feel painful.

2. Now as you try to turn your head back again to the left use your left hand to gently stop the movement. Turn your head slowly using about a quarter of your strength and resist the movement with your left hand.

3. Hold this push, with no movement taking place, for about 7–10 seconds and then slowly stop trying to turn your head to the left.

Now turn your head to the right again, the original direction, as far as is comfortable. You should find that you can turn a good deal further than the first time you tried.

4. With your head turned comfortably to the right you can now use your right hand to resist you turning your head even further to the right. Again turn your head slowly and with a quarter of your strength use your right hand to stop the movement. Hold this movement for 7–10 seconds.

You should now be able to turn your head to the right a bit further than the first two attempts.

You can now repeat the exercise on the left.

Low Back Rehabilitation

Self-Help Sheet

CHAIR EXERCISES FOR BACK PAIN

- Helps to reduce pain.
- Easy to learn.
- Takes up to 30 minutes to do.
- Only equipment required is a chair.
- Under your control.
- Causes no discomfort.

WHY DO THE EXERCISES?

Back pain can be very exhausting. Doctors' advice used to be that you should rest your back when it is painful. Research has shown, however, that gentle exercise is better. The exercises in this leaflet are designed for when you have back pain or if you have had it recently. It is important to do them regularly to get the most benefit, even if it is only for a short time. They will help you get your back into better shape especially when it feels stiff and stuck.

PLEASE REMEMBER

A painful back is very sensitive. These exercises should be used only if they produce no pain or if they offer appreciable relief. If you are feeling very tired wait until you feel a bit more lively to do them. The only equipment you need is a chair.

FOR HOW LONG WILL I NEED TO DO THESE EXERCISES?

These exercises are designed to be performed when you are experiencing pain and stiffness. We have some other exercises you can try which help maintain the suppleness of your back once it feels better. Practitioners will give you these if they think they will suit you.

HOW WILL I KNOW IF I AM DOING THEM RIGHT?

If your back feels better and you are not experiencing pain then you will be performing the exercises OK. Just take it easy. If you have any doubts please discuss them with your practitioner.

THE CHAIR EXERCISES

1. Chair exercise to improve spinal flexion

- Sit in a straight chair so that your feet are about 20 centimetres apart. The palms of your hands should rest on your knees so that the fingers are facing each other.
- Lean forward so that the weight of your upper body is supported by the arms and allow the elbows to bend outwards as your head and chest come forwards—make sure that your head is hanging freely forwards.
- Hold the position where you feel the first signs of a stretch in your lower back and breathe in and out slowly and deeply two or three times.
- On an exhalation ease yourself further forwards until you feel a slightly increased, but not painful, stretch in the back and repeat the breathing.

2. Chair exercise for spinal mobility

- Sit in an upright chair, feet about 20 centimetres apart.
- Twist slightly to the right and bend forwards as far as comfortably possible so that your left arm hangs between your legs.
- Make sure your neck is free so that your head hangs down.
- You should feel stretching between the shoulders and in the low back.
- Stay in this position for about 30 seconds (four slow deep breaths).
- On an exhalation ease your left hand towards your right foot a little more and stay in this position for a further 30 seconds.
- On an exhalation stop the left hand stretch and now ease your right hand towards the floor just to the right of your right foot, and hold this position for another 30 seconds.
- Slowly sit up again and turn a little to your left, bend forwards so that this time your right arm hangs between your legs. Make sure your neck is free so that your head hangs down. Once again you should feel stretching between the shoulders and in the low back.
- Stay in this position for about 30 seconds and on an exhalation ease your right hand towards your left foot and stay in this position for another 30 seconds.
- On another exhalation stop this stretch with your right hand and begin to stretch your left hand to the floor just to the left of your left foot and hold this position for another 30 seconds.
- Sit up slowly and rest for a minute or so before resuming normal activities or doing the next exercise.

3. Chair exercise to encourage spinal mobility in all directions

- Sit in an upright chair and lean sideways so that your right hand grasps the back right leg of the chair.
- On an exhalation slowly slide your hand down the leg as far as is comfortable, and hold this position, partly supporting yourself with your hand-hold.
- Stay in this position for two or three breaths before sitting up on an exhalation.
- Now ease yourself forwards and grasp the front right chair leg with your right hand, and repeat the exercise as described above.
- Follow this by holding on to the left front leg and finally the left back leg with your left hand and repeating all the elements as described.
- Make two or three 'circuits' of the chair in this way to slowly increase your range of movement.

- After a few breaths ease further forwards, repeat the breathing—and keep repeating the pattern until you cannot go further without feeling discomfort.
- When and if you can fully bend in this position you should adjust the exercise so that, sitting as described above, you are leaning forwards, your head between your legs, with the backs of your hands resting on the floor.
- All other aspects of the exercise are the same with you easing forwards and down, bit by bit, staying in each new position for three to four breaths, before allowing a little more movement to take place.
- Never let the amount of stretch be painful.

4. Disturbances—it is important to find a quiet place to meditate. Try to minimize disturbances—it will help you keep your attention on the exercise.

5. Emotions—sometimes upsetting thoughts or feelings may surface. Don't dwell on them—simply let them go, and let your attention return gently to the exercise.

6. Support—try to enlist the support of your family, friends and coworkers. Tell them that meditation is going to help you feel and cope better. Ask them to help you get the periods of quiet that will be needed.

Meditation

Self-Help Sheet

WHY MEDITATE?

Meditation when practised regularly will result in a relaxation response which can counteract some of the stresses of everyday living.

Meditation allows us to achieve a sense of mastery over our attention. For many people, distressing thoughts, feelings and worries about the past or future are a major source of unhappiness. The practice of meditation allows us to help free the mind from these disturbing and distressing thoughts. It has proved very effective in controlling and reducing stress and tension, as well as in treating medical conditions, e.g. high blood pressure.

WHAT IS MEDITATION?

Meditation has been known in various forms and in many cultures for thousands of years. Although there has been a very strong tradition of meditative practices in Western religions, people generally associate it with Eastern religions, probably because the recent revival of interest in meditation has been largely encouraged by teachers from the East where meditation has always been more extensively practised.

Sometimes people misunderstand what meditation is.

MEDITATION IS NOT

- a religion—you will not lose your religion, nor does it matter whether you are devout or atheistic
- just resting or sleeping, it is the practice of active attention
- a hypnotic trance.

The effects of meditation have been well researched. The many changes that occur in the body, e.g. lowering of blood pressure, a fall in stress chemicals in the bloodstream, a deep quietening of breathing processes and an increase in regularity and coherence of brain activity, are now well recognized by scientists. All this has been amply demonstrated and so have the psychological benefits of meditation: a decrease in anxiety, an enhanced sense of being in control of life, less depression and more sense of meaningfulness in life.

Far from undermining a person's religious feelings, people report that their spiritual life is made more valuable and their worship or prayer fuller through the practice of meditation.

What is more, the belief that meditation makes people unworldly has been repeatedly disproved. Meditating business executives, designers and artists generally find they are more productive, applying themselves more efficiently and fruitfully to their work.

Meditating brings into your life regular periods of rest during which the mind is relaxed and calm, and the body is free from tension. In its simplest form meditation requires some focus to which your attention is continually drawn back. This could be a repetitive prayer, a word, a sound, or a beautiful object like a flower or a work of art.

MEDITATION AND STRESS MANAGEMENT

It seems there is nothing new about stress. The following words were written by a Chinese physician 4600 years ago!

The present world is a difficult one.

Grief, calamity, and evil cause inner bitterness . . .

there is disobedience and rebellion . . . .

Evil influences strike from early morning until late at night . . .

they injure the mind and reduce its intelligence and they also injure the muscles and the flesh.

A simple meditation technique

This method of meditation has been refined and simplified and philosophical and religious connotations have been removed.

In order to achieve the relaxation response by meditation it is necessary to have four basic components:

1. A quiet environment with calmness and as few distractions as possible.
2. A mental device to prevent the mind wandering. This should be a constant stimulus such as a word or phrase repeated silently or aloud or even fixed gazing at an object. In the method outlined, the word 'one' is used but any suitable word or phrase that suits you could be substituted.
3. A passive attitude: distracting thoughts will occur. It is important not to worry about these but to redirect the attention to the repetition or the gazing. Do not worry how well you are performing the technique but try and adopt a 'let it happen' attitude. The passive attitude is perhaps the most important element in achieving the relaxation response.
4. A comfortable position is important so that there is no unnecessary muscle tension. If you lie down there will be a tendency to fall asleep. So sit upright and well supported.

1. Sit quietly in a comfortable position.
2. Close your eyes.
3. Deeply relax all muscles, beginning at the feet and progressing slowly up the legs, trunk and arms to the face. Keep them relaxed by gently repeating the process.
4. Breathe through your nose. Become aware of your breathing. Then as you breathe out slowly say the word 'one' silently to yourself. Each time you breathe out say the word 'one'. Breathe easily and naturally.
5. Continue for a few minutes. You can gradually build up to 10–20 minutes. You may open your eyes to check the time. Do not use an alarm. When you finish, sit quietly for several minutes, at first with eyes closed then opened.
6. Practise once or twice daily but not within 2 hours after any meal. Do not worry about whether you succeed in achieving a deep level of relaxation. Maintain a passive attitude and permit relaxation to occur at its own pace. When distracting thoughts occur, don't push them away, but don't dwell on them either. Simply allow your 'inner focus' to return by once more repeating 'one'.

[Adapted from 'The relaxation response' by H. Benson]

SOME COMMON DIFFICULTIES WHEN STARTING TO MEDITATE

1. Attentiveness—it is very common for the mind to wander away from your focus to other thoughts, feelings and minor disturbances. This is perfectly normal. When you notice that you have wandered in this manner, simply let go of the distractions, and return your attention to your word and your breathing.
2. Do not try to push the thoughts and feelings away; let them come and let them go—be patient with yourself. Remember the process of meditation is easy so don't push the river; it flows by itself.
3. Bodily distractions—it is common to become more aware of itches and other minor body distractions or discomforts. Try to return your attention to the exercise by letting go of the distraction. If you get an ache in some part of your body, try to imagine breathing out through that area of pain.

© Harcourt Publishers Ltd 2002 Peters D, Chaitow L, Harris G, Morrison S Integrating Complementary Therapies in Primary Care: A Practical Guide for Health Professionals

Positional Release for Pain Relief

Self-Help Sheet

WHAT IS POSITIONAL RELEASE?

Positional release refers to a technique that helps you when you have pain in tight muscles. When we feel pain the area affected will usually have some degree of local muscle tension, even spasm, and there is probably a degree of local cramp and poor circulation. Massage and stretching methods can often assist in helping these situations, even if only temporarily, but massage may not always be available and if the pain problem is severe then stretching may be too uncomfortable. Positional release technique (PRT) is designed to help ease tense, tight muscles and improve local circulation.

WHY SHOULD I PRACTISE POSITIONAL RELEASE?

Osteopaths find that almost all painful conditions happen in areas which have been in some way strained or stressed, either suddenly in an accident or gradually over time because of poor habits of use, posture, etc. When these 'strains', whether acute or long term, develop some tissues are stretched and others are shortened. It is not surprising that such a pattern causes pain. Tissues will have lost their normal elasticity, at least in part, in the shortened structures. It is not uncommon for new strains of the back (or elsewhere) to occur where tissues are already chronically under ongoing stress. What has been found in PRT is that if the tissues which are short are gently eased to a position in which they are made even shorter, a degree of comfort or 'ease' is achieved which can remove pain from the area.

THE EXERCISES

What do I need to know before I start?

How can I tell which direction is needed to move tissues which are very painful and tense?

There are some very simple rules and we can apply these to ourselves in a simple experiment.

THE PRT EXPERIMENT

1. Sit in a chair and press into your neck just behind your jaw, directly below your ear lobe. Most of us have painful muscles here. Press just hard enough to hurt a little, and grade this pain for your self as a '10' (where 0 is no pain at all).

2. While still pressing the point bend your neck forwards—very slowly—so that your chin moves towards your chest. Keep deciding what the 'score' is in the painful point.

3. As soon as you feel it ease a little start turning your head a little towards the side of the pain, until the pain drops some more.

By 'fine tuning' your head position, a little turning, or sidebending, or bending forwards you should be able to get the score close to '0'.

When you find that position you have taken the pain point to its position of 'ease' and if you were to stay in that position (you don't have to keep pressing the point) for about half a minute, when you *slowly* return to sitting up straight the painful area should be less sensitive, less tense, and therefore the area will have been flushed with fresh oxygenated blood.

If this were a real painful area—and not an 'experimental' one—the pain would ease over the next day or so.

You can do this to any pain point anywhere on the body. It may not cure the problem (sometimes it will) but it will usually take the edge off the pain.

HOW DO I PERFORM PRT SAFELY?

If you follow these instructions carefully, creating no new pain when finding your positions of ease, and do not press too hard, you cannot harm yourself and might release tense, tight and painful muscles.

1. Locate a painful point and press just hard enough to score '10'. If the point is on the front of the body bend forwards to ease it, and the further it is from the midline of your body the more you should ease yourself *towards* that side.

2. If the point is on the back of the body ease slightly backwards until the 'score' drops a little, and then turn *away* from the side of the pain and then 'fine tune' to achieve ease.

3. Hold the 'position of ease' for not less than 30 seconds and very slowly return to the neutral starting position.

Make sure that no pain is being produced elsewhere when you are fine tuning to find the position of ease.

FOR HOW LONG SHOULD I PRACTISE?

Do not treat more than five pain points on any one day as your body will need to adapt to these self-treatments.

HOW LONG WILL IT BE BEFORE I SEE ANY IMPROVEMENT?

Expect improvement in function—ease of movement—fairly soon (minutes) after such self-treatment, but reduction in pain may take a day or so and you may actually feel a little stiff or achy in the previously painful area the next day—this will soon pass.

WHAT CAN I DO IF I FIND IT DIFFICULT TO KEEP UP THIS PRACTICE?

Most of us have patterns and routines in our daily life and changing them to incorporate new ones can sometimes be difficult. Some inconsistency is normal but if you are finding making these changes particularly difficult you may want to have a look at our leaflet called 'Making changes'.

Progressive Muscular Relaxation

Self-Help Sheet

WHAT IS PROGRESSIVE MUSCULAR RELAXATION?

Progressive muscular relaxation (PMR) is a technique you can learn to relax muscles that are tight and tense which can cause you pain and contribute to feeling stressed.

- Easy to learn
- Takes 20 minutes to do
- Best performed daily
- Does not require any special equipment or clothing
- Under your own control
- Anyone can do it.

WHY IS IT A GOOD IDEA?

When we are anxious muscles become tense, and often uncomfortable, and certainly waste a lot of energy. It is not possible for a muscle to be both relaxed and tense at the same time, and so learning to release tension in muscles is a major step towards coping with stress. We all realize that when we respond to a stressful situation, or to inner worries, our muscles tense. Over time this can become chronic and habitual so that after a while we are not even aware of the tension, and cannot easily 'let go' and release it.

If you are very tense and you are asked to 'relax' you will probably tighten your muscles even more—mainly because you have forgotten what 'relaxation' feels like. It is as though your body has forgotten what to do to achieve release of tension in your own muscles.

Relaxation has to be relearned. PMR is one way to achieve this. It uses a series of muscle contractions to exaggerate the tension in particular areas. As they are released you learn to become aware of the difference between 'tension' and 'release' of the particular muscle group.

HOW DO I DO PROGRESSIVE MUSCULAR RELAXATION?

Preparation

Wear loose clothing. Lie on a carpet or rug. Make sure there are no draughts, and that you are unlikely to be disturbed for about 20 minutes.

- Lie comfortably so that you arms and legs are comfortably outstretched. Use a small pillow under your neck and your knees if you want to.
- Tense the fist of your right hand and hold this in a tight squeeze for about 10 seconds.
- Release this clenched fist and stay in this released state for about half a minute; try to notice the sense of release you feel there.
- Repeat this once more for half a minute, tensing and relaxing your hand and notice the sense of ease.
- Do the same to your left hand twice.
- Now do the same with your right foot. Draw your toes upwards towards the knee, tightening the muscles and holding for 10 seconds.
- Release and relax for half a minute and then repeat at least once more before going to the other foot.
- Perform this same sequence in at least five other sites such as:

back of lower legs—by pointing toes instead of drawing them up
upper leg—by pulling your kneecaps towards the hip
buttocks—by squeezing them together

chest/shoulders—by holding an inhaled breath and at the same time drawing your shoulder blades together
abdominal area—by pulling in or pushing out strongly
arms and shoulders—by shrugging your shoulders strongly
neck area—by drawing it into the shoulders or pushing it against the floor
face—by tightening and contracting the muscles around the eyes and mouth in particular, or by frowning strongly.

After each brief spell of tightening notice the difference when you let go.

WHEN AND HOW MUCH SHOULD I PRACTISE?

For the best results you will want to do these exercises on a daily basis. Twice a day is ideal if you can manage it, but not just after you have eaten.

HOW LONG DOES THIS RELAXATION TAKE?

After a week or so you can start to combine muscle groups, so that the entire hand/arm on both sides can be tensed and then relaxed together, followed by the face and neck, then the chest, shoulders and back and finally the legs and feet. After another week or two the tension part of the exercise can be dropped as you get more used to the feeling of relaxation. You can simply lie down and focus on the different regions and note whether they are tense or not, and get them to relax. Altogether you will need 20 minutes per session.

HOW LONG WILL IT BE BEFORE I SEE ANY IMPROVEMENT?

The process of holding tightness, followed by release, will in time give you an awareness of what tension feels like. You will regain the feeling of what it is like when your muscles are relaxed and be able to tell more easily when you are tense. This allows you to recognize muscle tension as it builds and begin to stop it before it becomes set in. Results come quickly if the exercise is performed regularly!

WHAT ELSE CAN I DO?

As well as learning to relax in this way you can learn to use breathing techniques (see Breathing self-help leaflets). After you have learned to relax in these ways you may want to try to meditate (see Meditation self-help leaflet).

HOW WILL I KNOW IF I AM DOING PMR CORRECTLY?

You will know after a short while if you are doing this technique correctly because your muscles will be less tense and you will be able to tell when they begin to tighten if you are feeling stressed. If you have any doubts please see your practitioner.

HOW LONG WILL I HAVE TO DO THIS?

If you have been experiencing stress over a long period and this technique works for you you may want to make PMR part of your daily routine, especially as the technique needs to be done regularly to experience the benefits. You can also do these exercises in times of greater stress.

© Harcourt Publishers Ltd 2002 Peters D, Chaitow L, Harris G, Morrison S Integrating Complementary Therapies in Primary Care: A Practical Guide for Health Professionals

ful use of the relaxation response by learning how to break into the vicious cycle of stress responses. By learning to switch on the relaxation response the stressed state can—up to a point—be avoided or improved. Internal factors—conflicts, anxieties, attitudes and beliefs—can be helped by counselling or psychotherapy. Time management might be needed to deal with work issues. Other kinds of lifestyle changes—nutrition, exercise—would be part of the package too. It would be wrong to think that relaxation techniques are the answer to everything.

NATURAL REMEDIES

Aromatherapy   Practitioners recommend essential oils of lavender, valerian, lemon balm (melissa), frankincense, bergamot, clary sage, marjoram, neroli and chamomile—inhale, add to the bath or massage in a carrier oil.

Nutritional therapy   Some practitioners say supplements of magnesium and calcium help relieve stress symptoms. Vitamin B supplements including B3 and B6 are traditional tonics.

Herbal medicine   Relaxant herbs include chamomile, kava kava, limeflower, hops, lavender. Chinese angelica is preferable to ginseng as a restorative tonic herb for women.

WHAT IF I FEEL TOO EXHAUSTED TO COPE?

Tiredness can be a feature of the stressed state, because dealing with change—especially if it is unfamiliar or continually demanding—does use up energy. So when life feels stressful the 'energy supply' available may need to be increased by getting the right sort of support, rest and insight into the stressors you are having to deal with; whether they are internal or external stressors.

WHAT DO I DO NEXT?

Talk to your practitioner. Don't try to go it alone! It's their job to help you if they can. There is information and support available. If it seems right for you then read the relaxation technique leaflet. Tapes can be useful too and your practitioner will recommend something.

Stress Management

Self-Help Sheet

PRESSURE, STRESS AND THE STRESS RESPONSE

It is important to understand what is meant by 'stress'. It means anything that puts a strain on your mind or body to adapt. That might be the physical effort of a run, or the mental strain and apprehension of an exam. Anything that puts a demand on the mind or body is strictly speaking 'a stressor'.

- *External stressors*—are stressors in the external environment: noise, air pollution, adverse lighting, difficult relationships, adverse work conditions, major life changes, etc.
- *Internal stressors*—are stressors which come from inside. They include poor diet, a lack of consistency and rhythm in personal or work life, unresolved conflicts, painful memories, pain, powerful but unexpressed feelings, unrealistic goals, negative expectations and pessimism, a tendency to be perfectionist, or an inability to recognize warning signs of tension and tiredness.

THE STRESS RESPONSE

Big stressors—or the accumulation of smaller ones—will provoke an alarm reaction, called the 'stress response'. This usually happens when there is an emergency. We all know how it feels to face one. Picture in your mind's eye a shocking or sudden event—for instance suddenly having to brake to avoid a collision or having to jump back on to the kerb to avoid a speeding car. Perhaps even the thought was enough to speed up your heart and cause some tense feelings. So you can see that a mental picture alone can be enough to trigger the stress response. It is a natural 'need for sudden action' mode, an instinctual preparation for an emergency. But it can also be triggered by any stressor which we feel to be an emergency. In fact whether a threat is actual or imagined the stress response is exactly the same: your heart speeds up, muscles tense, breathing quickens, blood pressure rises, body and mind go on guard and the body's energies are temporarily diverted from maintenance activities (like digestion—hence the 'butterflies in the tummy' feeling) and into survival mode.

EMERGENCY AND AFTER

The stress response is an instinctive survival reaction developed for aggression or escape. Our ancestors used this emergency nervous energy to face sabre-toothed tigers. They literally had to fight or run, after which they would lie down exhausted to rest. With the pressure off, physical and mental energy could be restored and this involved another set of natural responses which switch in to help build us up again. This relaxation response sustains wellbeing by reversing all those flight and fight emergency reactions. It is exactly the opposite of that tension and overalertness we need when we have to 'pull out the stops' in the face of a sudden threat to short term survival.

BUT I FEEL STRESSED ALL THE TIME!

When a lot of stressors are active at once or follow each other in succession and overlap, then the stress response, which should be short lived, starts to linger and may be repeatedly boosted as new stressors accumulate. This can create a vicious cycle—with body and mind always on the alert. Some experts call this the stressed state and this is what people generally mean when they complain about 'being stressed'. Useful though the emergency response can be when dangers are real, if body and mind are constantly behaving as if there is physical danger near then exhaustion and jitters from tense muscles, overactive circulation and senses are the likely result. And when these constant low-level reactions to stress begin to cause discomfort, sleeplessness, irritability and poor concentration a vicious circle starts up as we begin to get tense about our own symptoms of tension!

STRESS REDUCTION

One way to manage this would be by changing the number of external stressors—by cutting down the demands, taking more breaks, getting time off or having a holiday, reviewing priorities so as to match goals to resources. It is well worth examining the pressures you have come to take for granted as inevitable, and to change what you can. But it may not realistically be possible to reduce demands. And if the stressors are internal a better option might be to get help and talk through your predicaments and inner conflicts. Counselling can help here. Nowadays, of course, the 'dangers' we feel we face are more to do with job, relationships, family, traffic, noise, overcrowding...in fact just plain everyday twenty-first century life. And from which—unlike the sabre-tooth tiger—there is no running away! But instincts are instincts so, as pressure builds up, mind and body may begin to switch on the same old primitive preparations for flight or fight.

STRESS ADDICTION

So mostly our 'tigers' don't actually chase us, even though our body–mind may react as if the traffic jam or the missed appointment is a physical threat. To a certain extent the stress response can work in our favour if it gives us the edge to meet a deadline or perform under pressure. The 'adrenaline rush' that stimulates our performance can be useful, giving us that added burst of extra energy in an emergency or letting us give that bit extra even though we are exhausted. It is something we all need from time to time for a short term boost. Some people actually get to depend on a continual adrenaline fix to keep going, and always seem to manage to maintain pressure on themselves and those around them by setting unrealistic targets and turning everything into a competition. This can work for years, until the wear and tear starts to take its toll in the form of high blood pressure, heart and circulation problems.

WHO IS IN CONTROL?

Perhaps you feel that mental and emotional strain are an unavoidable feature of the jungle your life seems to have become, and you know that are suffering because of this tension. It could be that your body–mind has forgotten that stress responses are supposed to be followed in a natural order of things—by a relaxation response. In the hectic time we live in we need to respect this natural fact of life, and relearn how the relaxation response works so as to build it into everyday life. Then strain and tension can be counterbalanced by the reviving and sustaining influence of deep relaxation.

WHY LEARN A RELAXATION TECHNIQUE?

It is important to rediscover the ability to calm the body and mind and know how to tap into processes which quieten the hurry, tension and overarousal which modern day stressors easily provoke in us. When you know how, you can actually learn to let muscles relax, heart and breath calm down and thoughts still themselves as body and mind become quieter.

STRESS MANAGEMENT

It would be wrong to think that relaxation techniques are the answer to everything. Stress management is a combination of stress reduction, insight into your internal stressors and skil-

Balanced Diet [non-vegetarian]

Self-Help Sheet

A BALANCED DIET

So much is written about food, what you should or shouldn't eat, that it's sometimes hard to know where to start. Whether you want to change your diet to make it healthier or to lose weight, this leaflet contains ideas for meals which will provide you with everything you need from your food as well as cutting out a lot of what you don't want, usually too many refined sugars and fats. The following are ideas from which to choose breakfast and two main meals which together will provide you with all the nutritional content to maintain good health.

COULD CHANGING MY DIET BE EXPENSIVE?

Generally speaking eating healthily is no more expensive than when we treat ourselves to popular prepared and snack foods. There may be some additional expense at the beginning when you buy the first stocks of foods that might be new to you. Some of the foods mentioned below may indeed be completely new to you and are explained in our leaflet called 'Unfamiliar food'.

YOUR HOUSEHOLD AND CHANGING WHAT YOU EAT

It may be relatively easy to change what you eat but what about family and friends you may cook and eat with?

- Do you want to invite them to change what they eat?
- Do you cook for children or care for a relative who may not want or be able to make changes?

Please consider how the changes you may want to make may affect those around you and how you would like them to be involved.

WHAT CAN I DO IF I FIND I CAN'T STICK TO THE CHANGES I WANT TO MAKE?

For most people changing long-standing patterns takes effort and it is normal to go back to eating favourite foods or taking an extra helping occasionally. However, if you are finding any changes you want to make too difficult please discuss this with your practitioner and ask for our leaflet called 'Making changes'.

SOME 'GOLDEN RULES' FOR HEALTHY EATING

- Eat slowly, and chew well.
- Ensure that you drink at least 1.5 litres of water every day.
- Try to limit caffeine-rich beverages (tea, coffee, chocolate) and keep sugary foods to a minimum.
- Keep alcohol to safe limits—speak to your doctor about what is safe for you. General recommendations are: a maximum of 14 units of alcohol for women per week and 21 units for men (1 unit = either a small glass of wine or 1 single shot of any spirit or half a pint of beer or lager not including strong pilsner larger).

If you would like more information on how to cut down on your alcohol consumption please ask for our leaflet called 'Safer drinking'.

A BALANCED DIET
Breakfast choices

- Oatmeal porridge (made with water)—add cinnamon and/or freshly ground or whole cashew or almond nuts.
- Natural live yoghurt (low fat) to which add one or two tablespoons of cold-pressed flaxseed oil, which should be blended well with it, and add fruit (berries, raisins, apples, pears, grapes).
- Toasted seed mixture (sunflower, pumpkin, etc.) with yoghurt.
- Wholewheat or rice or oat pancakes.
- Two eggs—any style except fried, e.g. scrambled with mushrooms and tomatoes.
- Wholewheat or millet or rice flakes or fresh muesli mixture and live yoghurt.
- Fruit with particular emphasis on enzyme-rich ones such as avocado, papaya, mango, kiwi or pineapple.
- Baked apple or lightly stewed pears plus fresh nuts and seeds.
- Cooked brown rice, moistened with olive or flaxseed oil, to which add fish (canned tuna or salmon, for example) or kedgeree (traditional Scottish rice and fish dish).
- Ryvita, rice cakes, bread or toast with humus or sugarless jam.

Main meal choices

- Homemade soup.
- Mixed salad and/or vegetables and/or rice (or toasted rice cakes) or yeast-less bread or toast.
- Fish (two to three times weekly) and green salad and/or cooked vegetables and/or rice.
- Poultry (two or three times weekly) or meat (one or two times weekly) and green salad and/or cooked vegetables and/or rice.
- Tofu and green salad and/or vegetables (regular cooking or stir fried) and/or rice.
- Vegetarian stew (vegetables and tofu).
- Eggs and green salad and/or vegetables and/or rice.
- Dips with rice cakes or bread/toast or salad sticks (celery, carrot, cucumber, radish, etc.).
- Rice or millet or regular wholewheat pasta (spaghetti, etc.) and homemade tomato-based sauce.
- Healthier desserts—fruit or those with low sugar.

© Harcourt Publishers Ltd 2002 Peters D, Chaitow L, Harris G, Morrison S Integrating Complementary Therapies in Primary Care: A Practical Guide for Health Professionals

Dairy-free Diet

Self-Help Sheet

WHY A DAIRY-FREE DIET?

Dairy products, especially hard cheeses, contain high levels of saturated fats, which are not good for us and can contribute, amongst other things, to the development of heart disease. Most of us could benefit from cutting down on dairy products or cutting them out of our diet altogether. If your practitioner has suggested this here is a list of food and drink which you can eat and drink instead of milk, cheese, yoghurt, etc.

ALTERNATIVES TO DAIRY PRODUCTS

Instead of dairy products, the following may be substituted.

Instead of milk:

- rice milk
- soya milk
- nut milk—almond milk, cashew milk
- oat milk—but not if on a grain-free diet.

Instead of ice cream:

- fresh fruit sorbets
- frozen or fresh fruit smoothies
- juice popsicles
- fruit ice cubes
- frozen rice desserts (rice milk)
- frozen tofu desserts.

Instead of cheese:

- tofu
- ground sunflower seeds.

COST

Some of these foods, especially the substitutes for milk, will cost you a little more.

CHANGING EATING HABITS

Changing habits, especially those to do with diet, takes time and not a little effort. If you find that this diet helps you but are having some problems sticking to it then please discuss this with your practitioner. We also have a leaflet called 'Making changes' which may help you identify why you are having difficulty and may also help you to solve the problem.

HOW LONG WILL I NEED TO CHANGE MY DIET FOR?

If your practitioner has suggested this diet please give yourself a chance by following it for at least a couple of months so that you will be able, together with your practitioner, to assess your improvement. If you feel a lot better then it means dairy products are a problem for you. So you may not want to reintroduce dairy products to your diet. It may be possible to reintroduce the food to your diet after a period of at least six months absence and this should be done with care. Ideally plan this together with your practitioner.

COOKING AND EATING WITH OTHERS AND EATING OUT?

Changing your eating habits may affect family and friends with whom you cook and eat. Please talk to them about any changes that have been suggested to you by your practitioner which may affect them to see how they feel.

Note If you are putting a child on a dairy-free diet you should ask to see a dietician or nutrition counsellor to make sure the diet is balanced.

Exclusion Rotation Diet

Self-Help Sheet

Scoring your symptoms

- Symptoms such as feelings of unusual fatigue, or irritability, or difficulty in concentrating, or muscular pains or actual breathing difficulties, should be listed and given a daily 'score' out of (say) 10, where 0 = 'no problems' and 10 = 'the worst it has ever been'. Like this:

Irritability

0	1	2	3	4	5	6	7	8	9	10

- Be sure to score each symptom each day to see how it varies, and to link this to when suspect foods are eaten (sometimes reaction to foods takes up to 12 hours to be noticed).
- If such a score sheet is kept and a note is made of suspect foods, a link may be uncovered.
- By comparing the two lists (suspect foods and symptoms) it is often possible to note a pattern connecting particular foods and symptoms at which time the exclusion pattern described above can be started.

FOR HOW LONG WILL I NEED TO CONTINUE WITH THIS WAY OF EATING?

This depends to some extent with how many foods are on your list and how quickly you have been able to identify the offending food. If you started by excluding bread and all your symptoms cleared up you will have needed to follow the 'exclusion practice' for only 3–4 weeks. If, however, bread was not the problem and you need to try other foods you will need to continue excluding foods for some time.

WHAT CAN I DO IF I FIND THAT I CAN'T STICK TO THIS PROCEDURE?

It is normal when making changes to lapse from time to time especially when this may involve a period of not eating foods we particularly like and rely on. If you are finding this particularly difficult we have a leaflet called 'Making changes' which may help you.

COOKING AND EATING WITH OTHERS

If you are going to exclude foods from your diet for a period of time this may affect other people that you eat and cook with. Please discuss any proposed changes with them before you start the exclusion rotation diet.

THE OLIGOANTIGENIC DIET

Another way of 'unmasking' allergy-provoking foods is the oligoantigenic diet developed at Great Ormond Street Hospital for Sick Children. We have a separate leaflet on this that you can ask your practitioner for if you have not already got it.

DO YOU HAVE AN UNHEALTHY REACTION TO FOODS THAT YOU COMMONLY EAT?

If your practitioner has given you this leaflet it may be that you have an 'allergic' reaction to food or drink that commonly occurs in your diet. This means that each time you eat this food or take a drink of a particular type you do not feel at your best. Perhaps you feel tired or your joints ache or you come out in a rash. The identification of foods to which we are allergic or intolerant can be difficult but not impossible. In some cases it is obvious, and we may need to undertake a bit of detective work in order to identify culprits.

THE EXCLUSION DIET

Exclusion describes this diet perfectly as each food you commonly eat is systematically left out of your diet in turn in order to find out which one does not agree with you. It may be you are allergic to more than one.

WHERE DO I START?

It will be helpful for you to know in detail what you commonly eat, including things that you crave. Take some time to answer the following questions making notes as you go.

1. List any foods or drinks that you know disagree with you, or which produce allergic reactions (skin blotches, palpitations, feelings of exhaustion, agitation, or other symptoms).
2. List any food or beverage that you eat or drink at least once a day.
3. List any foods or drink that if you were unable to obtain, would make you feel really deprived.
4. List any foods or drink that you sometimes have a definite craving for.
5. What sort of food or drink is it that you use for snacks? List these.
6. Are there foods which you have begun to eat (or drink) more of recently?

Read the following list of foods and underline twice any that you eat at least every day, and underline once those that you eat three or more times a week:

- bread (and other wheat products)
- milk
- fish
- preserved meat
- rice
- corn or its products
- beetsugar
- soy products

- alcoholic drinks
- other citrus fruits
- potato
- breakfast food
- cheese
- pork
- margarine
- tea
- beef
- cake

- cane sugar and its products
- tomato
- sausages
- coffee
- peanuts
- beetroot
- yoghurt
- chicken
- biscuits

- pasta
- soft drinks
- artificial sweeteners
- lamb
- chocolate
- eggs
- oranges

WHICH FOODS SHOULD I EXCLUDE FIRST?

Look at the list of foods you have made in your notes from questions 1–6 and at the foods you have underlined and this will give you a place to start.

1. Decide which foods on your list are the ones you eat most often.
2. Pick one and leave it out of your diet for at least 3 weeks.

WHAT COULD HAPPEN?

If bread (grains) is your problem:

- You may not feel any benefit from this exclusion for at least a week (caused by withdrawal symptoms) worse for that first week.
- If after a week your symptoms (fatigue, palpitations, skin reactions, breathing difficulty, muscle or joint ache, feelings of agitation, etc.) are lessening and you are feeling better you should maintain the exclusion for several weeks, before reintroducing bread to your diet.
- You can then reintroduce bread to 'challenge' your body—to see whether your symptoms return.
- If your symptoms do return after eating bread again you will know that your body is better, for the time being at least, without eating bread.
- Remove this from your diet (in this case grains, or wheat if that is the only grain you tested) for at least 6 months before testing it again.
- By then you may have become desensitized to it and be able to tolerate it again.

If bread (grains) is not your problem:

- If bread (grains) is not your problem, when you don't eat it for 3 weeks your symptoms will have remained largely the same.
- You can now go on and exclude the next food on your list that you eat the most of to see if this is the problem—this includes 'food mixtures' or 'food families'. Sugar, for example, occurs in many foods and 'citrus' would cover oranges, lemons, grapefruits, limes, etc. You may want to go on to exclude dairy produce, or fish, or citrus, or soy products, etc. for the next 3-week period.

This method is often effective.

- Dairy products, for example, are among the commonest allergens in asthma and hay fever problems.
- A range of gluten-free and dairy-free foods are now available from health stores, which makes such elimination far easier.

ROTATION DIET

There are other ways of reducing the stress of irritant foods, and one of these involves the use of a rotation diet, in which foods from any particular family of suspect foods (already identified) are eaten only once in 5 days or so.

KEEPING A DIARY

This system has been found to be most effective if a detailed 'food and symptom diary' is kept, in which all changes from your normal state of health are noted down as well as all foods eaten.

Let's take an example

For example, let's say that bread is on your list. See what happens when you don't eat anything that includes wheat and also other grains (barley, rye, oats and millet) for at least 3 weeks.

Three-Week Oligoantigenic Diet

Self-Help Sheet

WHAT IS THE OLIGOANTIGENIC DIET?

The oligoantigenic diet was developed at Great Ormond Street Hospital for Sick Children, London and at Addenbrookes Hospital, Cambridge, as a means of identifying foods which might be causing or aggravating the conditions of young patients.

HOW DOES IT WORK?

By avoiding foods which may be provoking symptoms for not less than 5 days all traces of any of the food will have cleared the system and any symptoms caused by these should have vanished.

Symptoms which remain are either caused by something else altogether (infection for example, or hormonal imbalance or emotions) or by other foods or substances. Foods are reintroduced into your diet in a carefully controlled sequence (the 'challenge').

If symptoms reappear they are probably due to a reaction to particular foods which are then eliminated from the diet for at least 6 months.

WHICH FOODS ARE THE MOST LIKELY TO BE CAUSING MY PROBLEMS?

There is some evidence to support the idea that those foods which have become a major part of the human diet since Stone Age times, mainly grains (particularly wheat) of all sorts and dairy produce, are the most likely to provoke reactions. All modern processed foods involving any chemicals, colourings, flavourings, etc. are also suspect.

HOW DO I DO THE OLIGOANTIGENIC DIET?

- The oligoantigenic diet is usually followed for 3 weeks while a careful check is kept on symptoms (pain, stiffness, mobility, etc.).
- If they improve or vanish then one or more of the foods being avoided may be to blame.
- The identification of the food(s) you need to avoid depends upon the symptom(s) returning with the reintroduction (challenge) of the food.

The eating pattern listed below is a modified version of the hospital diet. Use it to evaluate the effect of following a pattern of eating in which the foods listed below are excluded for 3 weeks. You may want to keep a diary to help you do this. It is a tough diet.

Fish
Allowed: white fish, oily fish.
Forbidden: all smoked fish.

Vegetables
None is forbidden but people with bowel problems are asked to avoid beans, lentils, Brussels sprouts and cabbage.

Fruit
Allowed: bananas, passion fruit, peeled pears, pomegranates, paw-paw, mango.
Forbidden: all other fruit.

Cereals
Allowed: rice, sago, millet, buckwheat, quinoa.
Forbidden: wheat, oats, rye, barley, corn.

Oils
Allowed: sunflower, safflower, linseed, olive.
Forbidden: corn, soya, 'vegetable', nut (especially groundnut).

Dairy
Allowed: none.
Forbidden: cow's milk and all its products including yoghurt, butter, most margarine, all goat, sheep and soy milk products; eggs.

Drinks
Allowed: herbal teas such as camomile and peppermint and bottled spring water.
Forbidden: tea, coffee, fruit squashes, citrus drinks, apple juice, alcohol, tap water, carbonated drinks.

Miscellaneous
Allowed: sea salt.
Forbidden: all yeast products, chocolate, preservatives, all food additives, herbs, spices, honey, sugar of any sort.

WHAT DO I DO NEXT?

- If benefits are felt after this exclusion of a range of foods that you would normally eat you can gradually reintroduce one food at a time.
- Leave at least 4 days between each reintroduction. This will allow you to identify those foods which are causing you trouble and should be left out of your diet altogether. If symptoms return do not eat that particular food.
- If a reaction does occur (symptoms returning having eased or vanished during the 3-week exclusion trial) the offending food is eliminated for at least 6 months.
- You should not try to reintroduce another food into your diet for a 5-day period to be able to clear your body of all traces of the offending food you have been able to identify.
- Testing (challenge) can start again, one food at a time, after this 5-day 'free' period. Reintroduce anything which was eliminated by the oligoantigenic diet.

Cautionary note When a food to which you react strongly and which you have been consuming regularly is stopped, you may experience 'withdrawal' symptoms for a week or so, including flu-like symptoms and marked mood swings, anxiety, restlessness, etc. This will pass after a few days. So during the 3-week elimination period at the start of the oligoantigenic diet you may notice some of these symptoms. This can be a strong indication that whatever you have eliminated from your diet is contributing to your problem and may be producing many of your symptoms.

FOR HOW LONG WILL I NEED TO CONTINUE WITH THIS DIET?

After the initial 3-week period of elimination you will need to continue to reintroduce the foods that were left out until you can identify those that were causing your problems.

COOKING AND EATING WITH OTHERS

Eliminating foods from your diet will affect family and friends you eat and cook with. Please discuss your proposed changes with them before you make them.

Wheat-free Diet

Self-Help Sheet

WHY A WHEAT-FREE DIET?

If you have been experiencing ill health, especially with unconnected symptoms like tiredness, aching joints or loose stools, you may have a problem with gluten, a protein found in wheat, oats, rye and barley. Your practitioner may have suggested that you follow a 'wheat-free' diet to improve your general health.

SO WHAT CAN I EAT IF ANYTHING THAT CONTAINS FLOUR IS EXCLUDED FROM MY DIET?

Some of the foods that you may want to try will probably be unfamiliar to you. Please ask for our list which describes these foods if your practitioner has not already given this to you.

Fortunately there are largely gluten-free grains or grain-like foods available including: amaranth, buckwheat, rice, maize, millet, quinoa and spelt (a genetic relative of wheat with less gluten).

There are also a few gluten-free pastas on the market made from corn, quinoa, rice, soy and buckwheat and flours made from brown rice, maize and buckwheat are readily available.

COST

Following a wheat-free diet is generally no more expensive than eating products including wheat but you may have to spend more at the beginning as you replace popular foods that contain gluten with those that are gluten free.

FOOD LABELLING

It is sometimes obvious that foods contain wheat—bread and pastries, for example. However, there are many foods containing flour that you would not expect. For example, wheat products can also be included in soups as a thickening agent and can even be found in some toothpastes.

Please read all food labels carefully and remember common food like pasta is made from wheat.

A SAMPLE MENU

We have prepared a sample menu which is wheat free and provides you with all the nutrients you require to maintain your health.

Breakfast

- Cooked 'safe' grains (quinoa, millet, cornmeal porridge) with maple syrup, fruit or nuts.
- Corn or rice-based cereal moistened with rice milk or soy milk.
- Rice cakes with fruit and nut butter.
- Eggs and potatoes.
- Tofu scramble, rice or tofu and vegetables.
- Wheat-free muffins or pancakes (buckwheat, rice flour or cornmeal).
- Dried or stewed fruits, nuts.
- Beverages: herbal tea, milk, soy milk, diluted fruit juices.

Lunch

- Fresh vegetable salad: lettuce, radicchio, spinach, kale, chicory, chard, mustard greens, nasturtium leaves, borage leaves, carrots, mushrooms, tomatoes, cucumber, cabbage, radishes, beetroot, etc.
- With (choose one from): fish (salmon, tuna, etc.), poultry, tofu, nut butter, eggs, lentils, beans.
- And (choose one from): potato, rice, gluten-free bread, rice cakes or crackers. Other suggestions include: soups (bean, vegetable rice, fish, vegetable, green pea, etc.); gluten-free pasta (buckwheat, soya, quinoa, corn).

Dinner

- Choose one from: fish, poultry, lamb, beef, tofu, tempeh, nut butter, eggs, lentils, beans and rice.
- Choose one from: millet, rice, oats, aubergine, sweet potato, yam, peas, potato, squash (acorn, hubbard, butternut).
- And as many of the following vegetables as appetite dictates: artichoke, asparagus, beets, broccoli, brussels sprouts, carrots, chard, cabbage, celery, etc. or salad as listed in lunch.

Other suggestions include: soups (bean/vegetable/rice/miso/green pea); gluten-free pasta (buckwheat, soya, quinoa, corn).

Snacks

- Fresh seeds (sunflower, pumpkin).
- Fresh nuts (almonds, walnuts, hazels, etc.).
- Fresh fruit.
- Rice cakes and tahini or humus.

CHANGING EATING HABITS

Changing habits, especially those to do with diet, takes time and not a little effort. If you find that this diet helps you but are having some problems sticking to it then please discuss this with your practitioner.

We also have a leaflet called 'Making changes' which may help you identify why you are having difficulty and may also help you to solve the problem.

HOW LONG WILL I NEED TO CHANGE MY DIET FOR?

If your practitioner has suggested this diet please give yourself a chance by following it for at least a couple of months so that you will be able, together with your practitioner, to assess your improvement. If you feel a lot better then it means gluten is a problem for you. So you may not want to reintroduce wheat to your diet. It may be possible to reintroduce the food to your diet after a period of at least 6 months' absence and this should be done with care. Ideally plan this together with your practitioner.

COOKING AND EATING WITH OTHERS AND EATING OUT

Changing your eating habits may affect family and friends with whom you cook and eat. Please talk to them about any changes that have been suggested to you by your practitioner which may affect them to see how they feel.

© Harcourt Publishers Ltd 2002 Peters D, Chaitow L, Harris G, Morrison S Integrating Complementary Therapies in Primary Care: A Practical Guide for Health Professionals

Vegetarian Diet

Self-Help Sheet

VEGETARIAN DIET

If you are thinking of changing your diet to exclude meat and fish you may want some information on balanced eating. If you are already vegetarian you may want to check that your diet is providing everything necessary to maintain good health.

We have prepared a sample diet which provides all the complex carbohydrates, adequate protein, and has a very low fat intake. Anyone wishing to add more dairy proteins to this diet should consider virtually fat-free forms of yoghurt or cheese or cottage cheese.

Some of the foods mentioned may be new to you. Please ask for our leaflet 'Unfamiliar foods', which tells you all about them.

SUMMER	WINTER
Breakfast	
Watermelon or melon	1 cup oatmeal or whole grain cereal seeds
nuts	& soy milk
or	or
2 servings fruit with 1 cup yoghurt	Muesli with grated apple & raisins & soy milk
or	or
Cereal with fruit (&/or nuts)	Brown toast with 1 egg, 1 tablespoon
& plantmilk	flaxseed oil
10:00 a.m. snack	
1–2 servings fruit & seeds	1 baked apple
or	or
fresh fruit or vegetable drink	warm tomato juice with rye
	crispbread & tahini
Lunch	
Cool soup: cucumber or	Warm soup: miso, bean or
gazpacho; vegetable salad with	vegetable; fresh salad or
olive oil; cottage cheese tofu	steamed vegetables dressed
pate, bean spread, or hummus;	with olive oil and lemon juice;
2/3 cups corn, rice, potato	1 cup wholegrain/rice
&/or	&/or
2 slices wholegrain bread	2 slices wholegrain bread, baked beans, tofu
4:00 p.m. snack	
Herb tea with wholegrain cookie	Almonds or other nuts
or	or
Frozen banana or grapes	Herb tea & dried fruits soaked in water:
	dates, figs, raisins
Dinner	
2 types steamed vegetables;	Baked tofu or 1/2 cup lentil,
wholegrain pasta with sauce	pea or bean soup, baked potato;
or cold potato, grain or bean	squash or 1 cup grain (rice,
salad; raw vegetable salad	buckwheat, millet); steamed
with 2 tsp. oil	vegetables or raw vegetable salad with olive
	oil/lemon juice dressing.
Evening snack	
1 serving fruit and nuts	Herbal tea and wholegrain cookie
or	or
Fruit sorbet	Mashed butternut squash, spices
or	or
Frozen soy yoghurt	Rice cake with fruit spread

8

Blank forms and evaluation documentation

INTRODUCTION

The forms in this chapter have contributed to the way in which staff at the Marylebone Health Centre collect and structure data. They also help to shape the team and its ability to keep track of complicated information efficiently. They are included as an example and a possible guide to developing your own approach.

Therapy choice questionnaire

The evidence base for CTs is patchy at best, nor are there comparative studies to help us decide which therapy might be preferable. For instance, RCTs suggest several quite different CTs might be effective treatment for rheumatoid arthritis so how is a patient (or a doctor) to make an informed choice?

One approach aims to take into account the evidence as expressed in Table 2.2 but recognizing its incompleteness and therefore the important part played by patient preference, health beliefs and locus of health control when making therapy choices. The questionnaire in this chapter is a decision making tool we have been developing at Marylebone Health Centre which incorporates these elements.

Mymop

Our group has chosen the MYMOP method for tracking outcomes expressed in the patient's own words. The MYMOP is a user friendly and practical tool but one which requires consistency and determination to build into everyday practice. We have incorporated it into an electronic clinical record which makes reporting easier, but for those who do not use computers there is the choice of plotting scores and comments graphically on paper or of using the summary record presented here.

GP TO IN-HOUSE CT REFERRAL FORM

Date:.. Referring GP:...

If referring to a specific clinician - enter name: ....

Therapy requested (*tick* ☑ *one*)

Massage ☐   Osteopathy ☐   Homeopathy ☐   Naturopathy ☐   Acupuncture ☐

Data Entry Use
Referral ID:................
Name:................
DoB:................
Daytime tel:................

PROBLEM DETAILS *tick* ☐ *relevant box/es*

Musculoskeletal pain:		*Allergies & intolerance:*		*Stress-related problems:*	
Head, neck & back	☐	Asthma	☐	Migraine	☐
Osteo-arthritis	☐	IBS	☐	Non-specific GIT	☐
Rheumatoid-arthritis	☐	Rhinitis & hay fever	☐	Anxiety	☐
Myo-fascial pain	☐			Tension	☐

Women's health:		*Complex chronic illness:*	
PMS	☐	Persistent pain	☐
Dysmenorrhoea	☐	Fatigue syndromes	☐
Peri-menopausal	☐		

Duration of problem	
1–2 Wks	☐
2–4 Wks	☐
1–3 Wks	☐
3–12 Wks	☐
over 1 Yr	☐
not known	☐

Further clarification for presenting problem, including site (e.g. knee)

....

....

....

....

....

....

AIM OF REFERRAL: Advise GP ☐   Advise Patient ☐   Diagnosis ☐   GP Complex case ☐   Patient Support ☐   Treatment ☐

NOS-specify:...

ALTERNATE MANAGEMENT:

Please tick relevant box &
where necessary qualify

☐ Would refer to speciality:...

☐ Would prescribe:...

☐ GP follow-up   ☐   Would refer to in-house counsellor

BACKGROUND INFORMATION, COMMENTS, RED FLAGS, ANYTHING RELEVANT, etc.

....

....

....

....

....

....

....

....

....

....

....

CP NOTES

Date: ....   CP: ....

       Symptoms: ....

          Worries: ....

      Evaluation: ....

      Treatment: ....

       Outcome: ....

Date: ....   CP: ....

       Symptoms: ....

          Worries: ....

      Evaluation: ....

      Treatment: ....

       Outcome: ....

Date: ....   CP: ....

       Symptoms: ....

          Worries: ....

      Evaluation: ....

      Treatment: ....

       Outcome: ....

Date: ....   CP: ....

       Symptoms: ....

          Worries: ....

      Evaluation: ....

      Treatment: ....

       Outcome: ....

SUMMARY REPORT

Date: ....

            Diagnosis/findings ....

....

      Additional information ....

....

                 Treatment ....

....

      Impression of outcome ....

....

Suggestions about further treatment ....

....

THERAPY CHOICE QUESTIONNAIRE

ID No.

We want to find out why people choose certain therapies. The questionnaire we are asking every new patient to fill in will take you 10 minutes at the most to complete. It helps us assess your ideas and attitudes about health. There are no right or wrong answers and the results are completely anonymous. If you don't want to fill it in simply let the receptionist know.

WHICH THERAPY HAVE YOU CHOSEN?

1	Homeopathy	
2	Acupuncture	
3	Herbal medicine	
4	McTimoney chiropractic	
5	Bodywork (massage)	
6	Nutritional therapy	
7	Chinese herbal medicine	
8	Osteopathy / craniosacral therapy	

QUESTIONNAIRE Please circle the boxes where you agree with the statements.

SECTION 1

- *If you had to choose <u>only seven</u> of the following, which would you consider most essential to your health?*

	A	B
Well-balanced diet and healthy eating habits.	Yes	
Plenty of exercise and fresh air.	Yes	
The ability to deal with stress.		Yes
Relaxation techniques and time for myself.		Yes
Material security.	Yes	
Spiritual development.		Yes
Family and friends.		Yes
The flow of healing energy through me.		Yes
Elimination of toxins and waste products.	Yes	
A body structure that functions precisely and efficiently.	Yes	

SECTION 2

● *What controls your health?*

	A	B
If I become ill, I have the power to make myself well again.	Yes	
Often I feel that, no matter what I do, if I am going to get sick I will get sick.		Yes
A good practitioner can help me avoid health problems.	Yes	
It seems that my health is greatly influenced by accidental happenings or events.		Yes
I am directly responsible for my own health.	Yes	
I can only maintain health by consulting a health professional.		Yes
My physical well-being depends on how well I take care of myself.	Yes	
When I feel ill, I know it is because I have not been taking care of myself properly.	Yes	
I can pretty much stay healthy by taking good care of myself.	Yes	
Even when I take care of myself, it's easy to get sick.		Yes
When I'm sick, I have to let nature and time heal my body.		Yes
Health depends mostly on genes, family traits and inherited constitution.		Yes

SECTION 3

● *Please circle where you agree with the following statements.*

	A	B	C
I am happy to be touched and massaged.	Yes		
I don't mind taking medicines and can usually remember to take them regularly.		Yes	
I am comfortable exploring my feelings with another person.			Yes
I like the idea that I can use my mind to influence my health.			Yes
I would be prepared to change my diet radically if required.		Yes	
I can tolerate having needles stuck in me.	Yes		
Taking remedies helps me feel I'm getting better.		Yes	
I am comfortable talking about personal issues.			Yes
I don't mind being unclothed in the presence of a practitioner.	Yes		
I want to be able to talk freely and privately about the things that bother me.			Yes
I am comfortable with a practitioner manipulating my body.	Yes		
I feel my body has to be clean inside to work well.		Yes	

HOW MUCH DO YOU KNOW ABOUT THE TREATMENT?

I think I know more than most people about the treatment I have chosen.	
I know about as much as the average person about the treatment I have chosen.	
I know very little about the treatment I have chosen.	
I have had this kind of treatment before.	
I heard about this treatment from (please tick the appropriate box):	
a newspaper or magazine	
TV	
radio	
a friend or relative	
I heard about some research that said the treatment would help my condition.	

• *(Optional question) Are you doing anything else to improve your condition?*

. . . .

. . . .

. . . .

. . . .

• *(Optional question) Why do you feel you chose this therapy?*

. . . .

. . . .

. . . .

. . . .

• *(Optional question) Is there anything else we should have asked you about?*

. . . .

. . . .

. . . .

. . . .

Thank you very much indeed for doing this questionnaire. Please hand it in at reception.

ANALYSING YOUR RESULTS

Use the results of the three sections to determine which approach is most likely to suit you. You may find that more than one approach appeals.

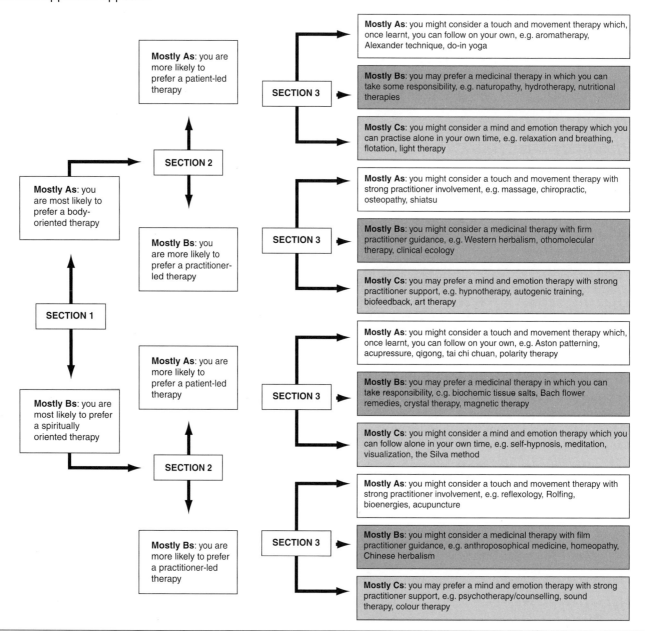

OTHER IMPORTANT FACTORS

You should expect to be able to make informed choices about therapies, but the amount of objective information available is still small. Be an informed 'consumer', aware that stories in the media can make vague statements about unspecified conditions, and that claims for fantastic results and super-human well-being may not be founded on accurate studies.

Nor is it true that all complementary therapies are safe and harmless.

The instincts you have about a therapy or a practitioner are important, as belief and trust play a significant role in healing. Make sure that your practitioner is reputable and well trained.

Consider also the following points:

- Is scientific evidence of a therapy's efficacy important to you? (see Table 2.2)
- Are you influenced by the personal recommendation of a friend?
- Is your doctor's opinion of a therapy's efficacy important?
- Is a particular therapy suitable for any specific health problem you have?

MYMOP GUIDES AND FORMS

Patients spend time filling in the first MYMOP at their first consultation. At each subsequent consultation a MYMOP follow-up form is completed. MYMOP was developed by Dr Charlotte Paterson as a tool for GP consultations and it continues to be adapted by her and is now used by many complementary practitioners as well as GPs. For updated versions of MYMOP, email c.paterson@dial.pipex.com.

USING MYMOP—THE PRACTITIONER GUIDE*

INTRODUCING MYMOP/FIRST CONSULTATION

It is worth spending time introducing MYMOP into the consultation, emphasizing the following. How it is introduced sets the tone for its use over the entire course of treatment. Emphasize:
1) Its value to both patient and practitioner.
2) Its usefulness to the practice and by extension other patients.

WITH THE FORM

1) Patients can pick what is important to them to measure.
2) Don't have to use a medical term.
3) Point out that they will normally be asked to fill the form out before the session but it can be used within the consultation for discussion and you would welcome that if they wanted to.

---

* Reproduced with permission of Dr Charlotte Patterson, Warwick House Medical Centre, Taunton, UK

4) Does not take more than a couple of minutes to fill out once they get used to it.
5) Don't have to fill out everything (if only one problem, etc.).
6) Will get to keep a record of progress if wanted.
7) Patient fills out first form—emphasize there is no right and wrong; it is not a test. Does patient need any assistance to help decide on the problems?
8) Does patient have any questions/comments (check understanding)?

SECOND SESSION

Give patient form at start or, if possible, before the start of the session. If patient does not come weekly then remind patient that the form relates to the last consultation.

In consultation find out what patient thinks about form. Is any more explanation necessary? It may be necessary to say in sessions 1–3 that some people find it difficult to fill out and that you know the form is not perfect but by the end of treatment the results of using the forms do reflect what is going on and therefore may be of value to patient, but are definitely of value to the practice.

THIRD TO FIFTH SESSION

MYMOP graphs produced ideally between 3–5 sessions to give to patients.
a) So they can see the results.
b) Check validity of their experience against graph.
c) Shows that we value their input.
d) Also remind patients they can change the problem if they want.

LAST SESSION OR END OF BOOKLET

Give patient booklet. Thank patient again for participation. Ongoing evaluation?

About MYMOP

We would appreciate your help with some medical research. We are trying to find out how best to use the complementary therapy service. MYMOP stands for 'Measure Yourself Medical Outcome Profile' and it is a new way of measuring how and in what way your treatment is helping you. The MYMOP form asks you to pick two symptoms or problems that are most bothering you and helps you to measure the changes in them.

The first time you fill in MYMOP your practitioner will explain it to you and help you. The booklet will be kept in your confidential file until your next visit. Your practitioner will ask you to fill in a MYMOP page at each visit, which takes only a few minutes. This will generally be done before your consultation begins.

ARE MY DETAILS KEPT PRIVATE?

Yes. The MYMOP forms will only be seen by the person treating you, the project coordinator and the research assistant. Any reports written about the research will not include information where individuals can be identified. That is, your name and other personal details will not be included.

Please tell us if you do not want to do this. There is no problem if you wish to say no. Saying 'no' will in no way affect the treatment you receive either now or in the future.

If you agree to participate and then change your mind you can withdraw from the research project and again this will not affect the treatment you receive.

If you have any questions your practitioner will be glad to answer them. Alternatively you can see the project coordinator who is in the health centre every..

Name...

I agree to take part in the research project on the use of complementary medicine.

Signed..

I do not wish to take part in the research project in complementary medicine

Signed..

Date...

MYMOP:
Measure Yourself
Medical Outcome Profile

HOW TO FILL IN THE MYMOP FORMS

This booklet contains six MYMOP forms. The first time you fill one in your practitioner will assist you. If you want further help at any time, please ask.

Filling in the MYMOP forms helps you discuss whether your health is getting better with the treatment you are receiving.

The first thing your practitioner will help you do is choose the symptom that you have come for help for which bothers you the most. This is called **symptom one** and will be written in your own words below. Then you can choose a second symptom which you think is part of the same problem. This is called **symptom two**.

Very often illness prevents us from doing things we need or like to do. Can you think of anything? If you can this is written next to **activity I cannot do**

Symptom one..

Symptom two..

Activity I cannot do...

These will be the things that you measure every week with this booklet. Each time you fill in a MYMOP form you should copy them from here on to the form. Please don't change these. If your symptoms change there is room on the form to add another one called **symptom three**.

FILLING IN THE FORM

Each form has a carbon copy attached and you have a piece of card to put under the form when you fill it in. This means you place the card under the first pink sheet when filling in the first form and when you come back again for treatment under the first yellow sheet. The top copy is left in the booklet which will be kept with your notes. The carbon copy is sent to the researcher.

Once you have chosen your symptoms you can score how good or bad they are by choosing a number from 0 to 6. Also score your general feeling of well-being: how are you feeling in yourself? Then complete the rest of the questions.

You will be asked to fill in a new form each time you come for treatment with your homeopath/acupuncturist /osteopath/naturopath/massage therapist. This will usually be just before you see your practitioner.

With some therapies you may see your practitioner every week, with others it may be less often. The form asks you how severe your problem has been over the last week but we would like you to fill it in to indicate how severe your problem has been since **the last time** you were treated—not just over the last week, as the booklet indicates.

Thank you for filling in this booklet. If at any time you would like any help filling in the booklet, have any other questions, or would like more information about the research project, please ask your practitioner.

FIRST MYMOP

Name and address...

d.o.b..................................... Date................................... Practitioner seen ....

Choose one or two symptoms that bother you the most. Write them on the dotted lines.

Now consider how bad each symptom has been, over the last week, and score it by circling your chosen number.

SYMPTOM 1:......................   **0**   **1**   **2**   **3**   **4**   **5**   **6**

....   As good as   As bad as
....   it could be   it could be

SYMPTOM 2:......................   **0**   **1**   **2**   **3**   **4**   **5**   **6**

....   As good as   As bad as
....   it could be   it could be

Now choose one activity of daily living that your problem prevents you from doing.

Score how bad it has been in the last week.

ACTIVITY: I cannot: **0**   **1**   **2**   **3**   **4**   **5**   **6**

....   As good as   As bad as
....   it could be   it could be

Lastly, how would you rate your general feeling of well-being during the last week?

                                   0   **1**   **2**   **3**   **4**   **5**   **6**

                                   As good as   As bad as
                                   it could be   it could be

How long have you had your Symptom 1, either all the time or on and off?

1–2 weeks ☐   2–4 weeks ☐   4–12 weeks ☐

3 months–1 year ☐   Over 1 year ☐

Have you had any previous help or treatment for this problem? If so, who from?..............................

....

....

MYMOP. Follow-up

Name ....   Date...

Please circle the number to show how severe your problem has been IN THE LAST WEEK.

This should be YOUR opinion, no-one else's!

SYMPTOM 1:.........................   **0   1   2   3   4   5   6**

....   As good as   As bad as
....   it could be   it could be

SYMPTOM 2:.........................   **0   1   2   3   4   5   6**

....   As good as   As bad as
....   it could be   it could be

ACTIVITY: *I cannot:* **0   1   2   3   4   5   6**

....   As good as   As bad as
....   it could be   it could be

WELL-BEING : how   **0   1   2   3   4   5   6**
would you rate your
general feeling of   As good as   As bad as
well-being?   it could be   it could be

If an important new symptom has appeared you may describe it and mark how bad it is below.

Otherwise do not use this line

SYMPTOM 3:.........................   **0   1   2   3   4   5   6**

....   As good as   As bad as
....   it could be   it could be

The treatment / help I am having for this problem is: (please include anyone, or anything, that you have
used to try and help this problem since you last filled in a MYMOP form)

....

....

© Harcourt Publishers Ltd 2002 Peters D, Chaitow L, Harris G, Morrison S Integrating Complementary Therapies in Primary Care: A Practical Guide for Health Professionals

MYMOP. Follow-up

Name .... Date ....

Please circle the number to show how severe your problem has been IN THE LAST WEEK.

This should be YOUR opinion, no-one else's!

SYMPTOM 1: **0**   **1**   **2**   **3**   **4**   **5**   **6**

.... As good as   As bad as
.... it could be   it could be

SYMPTOM 2: **0**   **1**   **2**   **3**   **4**   **5**   **6**

.... As good as   As bad as
.... it could be   it could be

ACTIVITY: *I cannot:* **0**   **1**   **2**   **3**   **4**   **5**   **6**

.... As good as   As bad as
.... it could be   it could be

WELL-BEING : how   **0**   **1**   **2**   **3**   **4**   **5**   **6**
would you rate your
general feeling of   As good as   As bad as
well-being   it could be   it could be

If an important new symptom has appeared you may describe it and mark how bad it is below.

Otherwise do not use this line

SYMPTOM 3: **0**   **1**   **2**   **3**   **4**   **5**   **6**

.... As good as   As bad as
.... it could be   it could be

The treatment / help I am having for this problem is: (please include anyone, or anything, that you have used to try and help this problem since you last filled in a MYMOP form)

....

....

MYMOP. Follow-up

Name .... Date ....

Please circle the number to show how severe your problem has been IN THE LAST WEEK.

This should be YOUR opinion, no-one else's!

SYMPTOM 1:...............................   **0**   **1**   **2**   **3**   **4**   **5**   **6**

.... As good as   As bad as
.... it could be   it could be

SYMPTOM 2:...............................   **0**   **1**   **2**   **3**   **4**   **5**   **6**

.... As good as   As bad as
.... it could be   it could be

ACTIVITY: *I cannot:* **0**   **1**   **2**   **3**   **4**   **5**   **6**

.... As good as   As bad as
.... it could be   it could be

WELL-BEING : how   **0**   **1**   **2**   **3**   **4**   **5**   **6**
would you rate your
general feeling of   As good as   As bad as
well-being   it could be   it could be

If an important new symptom has appeared you may describe it and mark how bad it is below.

Otherwise do not use this line

SYMPTOM 3:...............................   **0**   **1**   **2**   **3**   **4**   **5**   **6**

.... As good as   As bad as
.... it could be   it could be

The treatment / help I am having for this problem is: (please include anyone, or anything, that you have used to try and help this problem since you last filled in a MYMOP form)

....

....

MYMOP. Follow-up

Name .... Date ....

Please circle the number to show how severe your problem has been IN THE LAST WEEK.

This should be YOUR opinion, no-one else's!

SYMPTOM 1:...............................   **0**   **1**   **2**   **3**   **4**   **5**   **6**

....   As good as   As bad as

....   it could be   it could be

SYMPTOM 2:...............................   **0**   **1**   **2**   **3**   **4**   **5**   **6**

....   As good as   As bad as

....   it could be   it could be

ACTIVITY: *I cannot:* **0**   **1**   **2**   **3**   **4**   **5**   **6**

....   As good as   As bad as

....   it could be   it could be

WELL-BEING : how   **0**   **1**   **2**   **3**   **4**   **5**   **6**

would you rate your

general feeling of   As good as   As bad as

well-being   it could be   it could be

If an important new symptom has appeared you may describe it and mark how bad it is below.

Otherwise do not use this line

SYMPTOM 3:...............................   **0**   **1**   **2**   **3**   **4**   **5**   **6**

....   As good as   As bad as

....   it could be   it could be

The treatment / help I am having for this problem is: (please include anyone, or anything, that you have used to try and help this problem since you last filled in a MYMOP form)

....

....

MYMOP. Follow-up

Name _____   Date_____

Please circle the number to show how severe your problem has been IN THE LAST WEEK.

This should be YOUR opinion, no-one else's!

SYMPTOM 1:_____   **0   1   2   3   4   5   6**

_____
As good as   As bad as
it could be   it could be

_____

SYMPTOM 2:_____   **0   1   2   3   4   5   6**

_____
As good as   As bad as
it could be   it could be

_____

ACTIVITY: *I cannot:* _____   **0   1   2   3   4   5   6**

_____
As good as   As bad as
it could be   it could be

_____

WELL-BEING : how   **0   1   2   3   4   5   6**
would you rate your
general feeling of   As good as   As bad as
well-being   it could be   it could be

If an important new symptom has appeared you may describe it and mark how bad it is below.

Otherwise do not use this line

SYMPTOM 3:_____   **0   1   2   3   4   5   6**

_____
As good as   As bad as
it could be   it could be

_____

The treatment / help I am having for this problem is: (please include anyone, or anything, that you have used to try and help this problem since you last filled in a MYMOP form)

_____

_____

NEW MYMOP TRACKING FORM

Patient name:		Therapist:
Date of birth:		Practice no:

Date:	**Score 0–6**	**Patient's own words**
MYMOP 1:		What is the main symptom of your problem?
MYMOP 2:		Is there any other symptom you hope will improve?
Activity:		Is there anything your problem stops you from doing?
Well-being		And how are you in yourself?

Date:	**Score 0–6**	**Practitioner comment**
MYMOP 1:		
MYMOP 2:		
MYMOP 3:		
Function:		
Well-being:		

Date:	**Score 0–6**	**Practitioner comment**
MYMOP 1:		
MYMOP 2:		
MYMOP 3:		
Function:		
Well-being:		

Date:	**Score 0–6**	**Practitioner comment**
MYMOP 1:		
MYMOP 2:		
MYMOP 3:		

Function:		
Well-being:		
Date:	**Score 0–6**	**Practitioner comment**
MYMOP 1:		
MYMOP 2:		
MYMOP 3:		
Function:		
Well-being:		
Date:	**Score 0–6**	**Practitioner comment**
MYMOP 1:		
MYMOP 2:		
MYMOP 3:		
Function:		
Well-being:		
Discharge summary	**Score 0–6**	**Comment**
MYMOP 1 change		
MYMOP 2 change		
MYMOP 3		
Activity change		
Well-being change		
GHHOS score		
Main treatment		
Main self-care advice		
Future management suggestion to GP		

Please fill in each time you see the patient.

MYMOP CHART

Symptom 1 .... chart colour =

Symptom 2 .... chart colour =

Activity restricted: I cannot .... chart colour =

Well-being   chart colour =

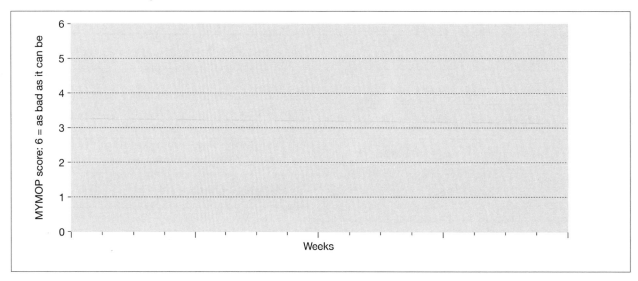

Figure 8.4 MYMOP graph.

THE SMITH PROJECT CP GUIDE TO CLINICAL DATA ENTRY (FILEMAKER PRO 4.1) (EXAMPLE)

PART ONE: GETTING INTO THE PROGRAM

1. Turn the computer on by pressing the Start key, which is the top right-hand key on the keyboard marked with a small triangle.
2. The computer will now check its systems and become usable when the small clock icon turns into an arrow.
3. Once the computer has become useable use the keypad to move the arrow and click twice on the 'hard disk' icon, which is in the top right hand corner of the screen
4. If you have successfully opened the hard disk, rows of files will now be showing on the screen. Using the keypad to move the arrow, click twice on the Filemaker Pro 4.1.
5. If you have successfully opened Filemaker there will be another group of files on the screen. Go to MHC system with the arrow and click twice to open.
6. You should now be in the MHC system.

ENTERING THE DATA

*What to do with a **new** patient*

7. You will need to enter information on two pages for each patient on the first visit. Click with the arrow on Patcase FP3 (see printed sheet attached) to enter data from the yellow form.

Patcase FP3—to be filled out on patient's first visit

8. **You must create a new page for each patient**.

To create a new page press the 'apple' symbol and N simultaneously.

The patient code number, which is crucial to making the whole system work, is the patient number on the front of the patient file.

Enter this first. The date will automatically appear in the date field when you ask for a new page. Please also enter this as part of the patient code.

Entering the patient number and date prevents the episodes of treatment with different practitioners from getting mixed up.

e.g

Patient referral number 54389

Date of treatment   110199

Patient referral code becomes 54389.110199

9. Use the Tab key to move between fields.

10. The therapy field, GP and condition all have drop-down menus. These will only work, however, if you click on them once. More than that and the menu does not work.
11. Select from the drop-down menu by clicking once on the desired statement.
12. When entering the MYMOP problems these are the ones that *you*, the CP, discuss with the patient.
13. When you have finished entering data on Patcase FP3 take the arrow to close and click. This will take you back to the home page.

This form needs to be filled out with the patient in the room. The minimum you must fill in is the patient number and the MYMOP problems. The rest can be filled out after the session. You can't fill in the treatment sheet until the MYMOP problems are entered on this page.

ENTERING DATA ON THE TREATMENT PAGE

Each time a patient attends for treatment you need to enter data on the Treatment page.

14. Click on Treatment to open.
15. Use tab key to move around the page. To create a new record use the keypad to direct the cursor to Mode, which is on the bar at the top of the page. Click twice on Mode and scroll down to New record on the menu that appears. Clicking on this opens a new record that has only the date entered.
16. Type in the patient reference number on this page first.
17. Complete this page and close.

REPORT PAGES

Reports can be produced automatically by this database. Closing a page will automatically bring you back to the home page, from where you can click to the reports menu.

Referrals page

18. Click on this page to find out about a patient's previous referral history with CT treatment (will only show up from the start of this database being in operation). Enter the patient number and name.

View treatments

19. Click on here to review a patient's progress. Enter the patient number and the data will change automatically to show you a review of treatment including MYMOP results. You may need to go to this page to remind you and the patient of the patient scores on the MYMOP form.

SEEING A PATIENT FOR FOLLOW-UP

Follow steps 1–6 to get into the program.

20. Click on to TREATMENT FP3 to go straight to a treatment sheet. Fill it in according to the directions above 14–17.

21. If you need to see the patient, click MYMOP results close, which takes you to the home page, and click on View treatments.

22. Closing this program will bring you back to the home page; click on treatment to continue filling in the data from today's treatment.

MOVING BETWEEN PAGES

How to find data already entered on a patient is most important for this system to work effectively.

There are two ways of doing this.

Go to the treatment page on the program Treatment FP3.

1. Go to Browse at the bottom of the page. Click on to the drop-down menu and click on Find.

2. Go to the treatment page and create a new page.
3. Type in patient code (patient number plus date of first treatment).
4. Click on the find button on the left-hand side of the screen.

This will bring up the patient's notes on to the screen.

or

1. Click on the icon next to the Browse button (right-hand side).
2. This will bring on to the screen an icon that looks like an open book in the top left-hand corner.
3. You can scroll through all of your patient files by clicking on either of the 'pages'.
4. The record number underneath the book will change as you scroll. You can then note the record number for future use.

This example is available, updated, on screen. The application is available from Hal Andrews at andrewh@wmin.ac.uk

(Figures 8.1–8.3 show examples of screens from the Filemaker program.)

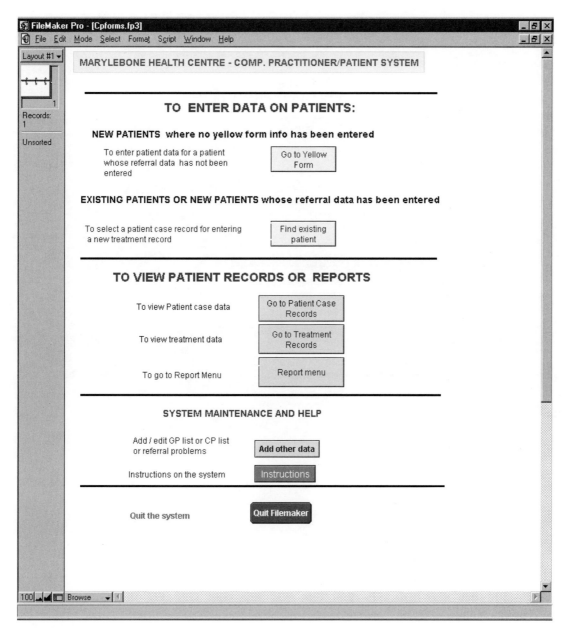

Figure 8.1   System menu screen.

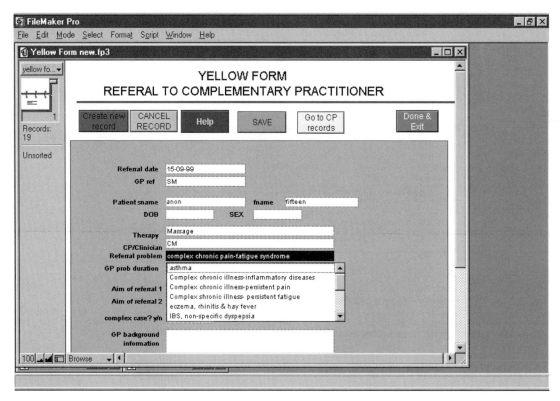

Figure 8.2 Referral screen.

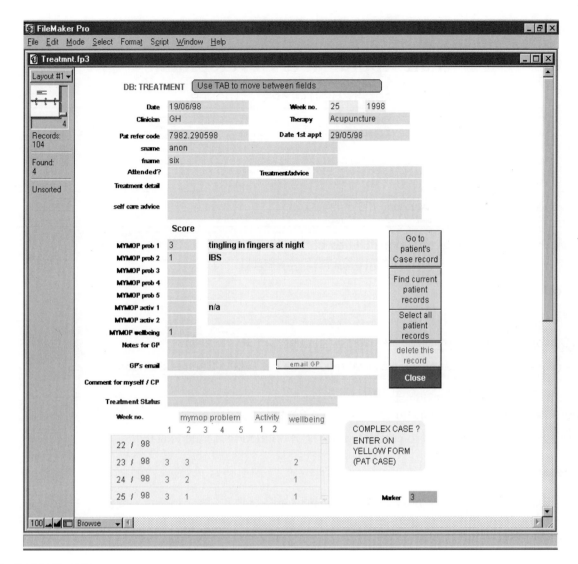

Figure 8.3 Treatment screen.

STAFF APPRAISAL AND DEVELOPMENT FORM

Staff Appraisal & Development

Name	
Post	
Date of Appointment	
Review Period	Annually (30 mins)

1. List the main duties and responsibilities of the post

Clinical

- Treat patients referred by GPs.
- Conform with treatment guidelines agreed through CP/GP meetings.
- Accurately record treatments in clinical records as per Health Centres Standard.
  - Using CP summary boxes at each consultation.
  - Completing discharge summary box, when treatment series ends.
  - Instructing each patient to complete a MYMOP form for every consultation.

Professional

- To take part in continuing professional education, relevant to your clinical practice.

Organizational

- To attend the regular clinical and process meetings as well as occasional Staff Development sessions organized.
- To encourage those patients who can afford to contribute to the patient donation account, which supports Complementary Therapy services.
- To work with the Practitioner Team for the further development of clinical services.

Research

- To ensure that your clinical work is subject to continuing medical audit, by taking part in our programme of service evaluation.

Performance measures to be developed collaboratively and agreed by each practitioner to form basis of objectives for next review period.

Staff Appraisal & Development

2. List any objectives with your appraiser for the review period just ending. Include any performance indicators where agreed.

This section relates to section 1; how does each of the items in section 1 work in relation to the way you work and your professional development in the coming year?

3. Comment on your own performance in relation to your main work responsibilities and the objectives specified in sections 1 and 2. Identify the areas where you have and have not achieved the agreed objectives.

You may wish to consider: your most important achievements; the parts of your work that you enjoy most/least; which particular skills and abilities make a significant contribution to your work; your relationship with other members of staff.

Staff Appraisal & Development

3 (continued)

4. **Comment on any organizational factors which have affected your work and any suggestions for improvement.**

e.g. Resources, Premises, Communication

Staff Appraisal & Development

5. Give an indication of how you plan to develop your work over the next 2 years. Include time-scales, resource requirements and any obstacles to their achievement.

6. Thinking of your present post, please indicate those areas where, in your view, you could benefit from additional training or staff development, more experience or further guidance. Please give reasons.

Signature	Date
Appraisee: Appraiser:	

Appendices

Summary and recommendations of a report by the House of Lords Select Committee on complementary and alternative medicine, November 2000*

SUMMARY OF DELIVERY SECTION

- Current patterns of access
- Methods of delivery
- Primary care organizations
- Criteria for NHS provision
- Recommendations

METHODS OF DELIVERY

- Mainly private sector
- Mainly without GP referral
- Patchy NHS access (1995 . . . '40% of GPs . . . ')

Private sector access (Thomas 2000. >90%)

- Fees for services: single-handed independents and 'specialist centres'
- ± GP referral
- ± PMI re-imbursement
- Via beauty and fitness industries
- OTC self-medication

NHS access

- Via GP/primary care team member
- During hospital care
- Potentially via community health initiatives[a] ([a] 9.7 DoH 'CT welcome to bid into e.g. Healthy Living Centres, Healthy Workplace, Healthy Schools?')

Two models discussed in detail

Marylebone Health Centre
NHS general practice
Primary care team:
- homeopathy
- osteopathy
- naturopathy
- acupuncture
- massage

---

* Reproduced with permission of the HMSO.

Southampton Centre for the Study of CM
Private sector but also contracted to HAs
Team approach:
- homeopathy
- osteopathy
- nutritional and environmental medicine
- acupuncture
- massage.

Important similarities in approach:

- appropriate lines of communication for referral and feedback
- audit and evaluation.

Similar range of conditions:

- stated range of conditions
- often complex and chronic
- need for an evidence base
- GPs say patients have benefited
- 'integrated projects provide evidence'.

PRIMARY CARE ORGANIZATIONS

Concern expressed over:

- attrition of CT services
- PCGs reversing trend for innovation.

Primary care culture favours CM (M Dixon):

- Primary care and CM (from their own perspectives) 'holistic'
- committed to idea of self-care
- therapeutic relationship stronger in primary care.

Currently limited secondary care application of CM:

- manipulative therapies in orthopaedics and physical medicine
- acupuncture and relaxation therapies via pain clinics
- acupuncture and aromatherapy in midwifery and cancer care
- homeopathy and a range of CTs via homeopathic hospitals.

RECOMMENDATIONS

The report acknowledges and accepts the need to provide CAM in the NHS:

- CPs should aim to work more closely with patients' GPs
- encourage patients to discuss their CT with their GP
- encourage open-minded exchange of information

- NHS CT provision to continue via healthcare professional referral (primary, secondary and tertiary care)
- only properly regulated CAM therapies to be accessed in NHS.

INTEGRATION: WAYS FORWARD?

The report implies a need to demonstrate that CAM can meet the same high standards that should apply across all forms of health care, e.g.:

Threats:

- so far PCO consensus has been difficult to achieve
- many GPs see CAM as 'low priority' in medium–long term
- attrition of established CAM services?
- secondary and tertiary care will be difficult to influence.

Opportunities:

- innovation vs equity: the need for pilot units and projects
- Chairs and Chief Executives of PCOs are key agents of change
- identify existing and planned PCO CT initiatives
- local needs and development of HlmPs and 'care pathways'
- use frameworks for quality improvement (practice development planning, personal learning plans, clinical governance)
- > patient involvement as PCGs become PCTs
- map initiatives and best practice in PCOs delivering CAM
- evaluate key units
- build a network to share good practice and approaches for clinical governance
- develop large collective data sets
- collaborate with key CAM professional bodies in e.g. CPD, and research and development pilot projects
- support GP education programmes and practice development planning
- develop CAM pathways and guidelines (e.g. via NHS Direct)
- reliable information service (info on CAM relevance, accessing regulated CPs, therapies, evidence . . .)
- develop more equitable access outside NHS?
- develop learning packs to support integrative projects
- networks for clinical governance of CAM in the NHS
- approaches to evidence-based commissioning and evidence-based practice, practice development and personal learning
- promote a national system for integration outcomes evaluation
- care pathway development for national priority conditions where conventional treatments unsatisfactory, costly (e.g. pain, cancer, moderate mental health problems)
- support targeted community health initiatives, e.g. Healthy Living Centres.

Useful addresses

General

British Complementary Medicine Association (BCMA)
249 Fosse Road South, Leicester LE3 1AE
tel: 0116 282 5511

Centre for the Study of Complementary Medicine
51 Bedford Place, Southampton
tel: 01703 334752

Council for Complementary and Alternative Medicine (CCAM)
63 Jeddo Road, London W12 6HQ
tel: 020 8735 0632

Natural Medicine Society
Regency House, 97–107 Hagely Road, Edgbaston, Birmingham B16

Research Council for Complementary Medicine
email: info@rccm.org.uk / website: http://www.rccm.org.uk

Training
(Degree level)
University of Westminster School of Integrated Health
115 New Cavendish St, London W1M 8JS
tel: 020 7911 5883
email: cav-admissions@wmin.ac.uk / website: www.wmin.ac.uk

(see also under individual therapies)

Overseas
Canadian Holistic Medical Association
491 Eglington Avenue West, Apt 407, Toronto, Ontario M5N 1A8, Canada
tel: (1) 416 485 3071

Acupuncture

Acupuncture Association of Chartered Physiotherapists
Chartered Society of Physiotherapists, 14 Bedford Row, London WC1R 4ED
tel: 020 7242 1941

British Acupuncture Council
Park House, 206–208 Latimer Road, London W10 6RE
tel: 020 8964 0222/fax: 020 8964 0333
email:info@acupuncture.org.uk/website: www.acupuncture.org.uk

(For doctors only)
British Medical Acupuncture Society
Newton House, Whitley, Warrington WA4 4JA
tel: 01925 730727/fax: 01925 730492
email: bmasadmin@aol.com/website: www.medical-acupuncture.co.uk

Training
(Degree level)
University of Middlesex
White Hart Lane, London N17 8HR
website: www.mdx.ac.uk
(Degree level)
London School of Acupuncture and Traditional Chinese Medicine

University of Westminster School of Integrated Health
115 New Cavendish St, London W1M 8JS
tel: 020 7911 5883
email: cav-admissions@wmin.ac.uk/website: www.wmin.ac.uk

British Academy of Western Acupuncture
12 Poulton Green Close, Spital, Wirral L63 9FS
tel: 0151 3439168

College of Integrated Chinese Medicine
19 Castle St, Reading, Berks RG1 7SB
tel: 0118 950 8880/fax:0118 950 8890
email:admin@cicm.org.uk/website: www.cicm.org.uk

London College of Traditional Acupuncture and Oriental Medicine
HR House, 447 High Road, London N12 0AZ
Tel: 020 8371 0820/fax: 020 8371 0830
email: college@lcta.com / website: www.lca.com

Northern College of Acupuncture
124 Acomb Rd, York YO2 4EY
tel: 01904 784828

Overseas
American Association of Acupuncture and Oriental Medicine
433 Front St, Catasauqua, PA 18032, USA

Herbalism

National Institute of Medical Herbalists (NIMH)
56 Longbrook Street, Exeter EX4 6AH
tel: 01392 426022/fax: 01392 498963
email: nimh@ukexeter.freeserve.co.uk
website: www.btinternet.com/~nimh/

Register of Chinese Herbal Medicine
PO Box 400, Wembley, Middlesex HA9 9NZ
tel: 020 7470 8740
website: www.rchm.co.uk

European Herbal Practitioners Association
Midsummer Cottage Clinic, Nether Westcote, Chipping Norton OX7 6SD
tel: 01993 830419/fax: 01993 830957
website: www.users.globalnet.co.uk/~epha/

Training
(Degree level)
University of Middlesex
White Hart Lane, London N17 8HR
website: www.mdx.ac.uk

(Degree level)
University of Westminster School of Integrated Health
115 New Cavendish St, London W1M 8JS
tel: 020 7911 5883
email: cav-admissions@wmin.ac.uk/website:www.wmin.ac.uk

College of Practitioners of Phytotherapy
Bucksteep Manor, Bodle Street Green,
Hailsham, East Sussex
tel: 01323 833812

(Chinese herbalism)
(Degree level)
University of Middlesex
White Hart Lane, London N17 8HR
website: www.mdx.ac.uk

College of Integrated Chinese Medicine
19 Castle St, Reading, Berks RG1 7SB
tel: 0118 950 8880/fax: 0118 950 8890
email: admin@cicm.org.uk / website: www.cicm.org.uk

London College of Traditional Acupuncture and Oriental Medicine
HR House, 447 High Road, London N12 04Z
Tel: 020 8371 0820/fax: 020 8371 0830
email: college@lcta.com/website: www.lca.com

London School of Acupuncture and Traditional Chinese Medicine
University of Westminster School of Integrated Health
115 New Cavendish St, London W1M 8JS
tel: 020 7911 5883
email: cav-admissions@wmin.ac.uk /website: www.wmin.ac.uk

Northern College of Acupuncture
124 Acomb Rd, York YO2 4EY
tel: 01904 784828

Overseas
American Herb Association
PO Box 673, Nevada City, NA 95959, USA

North American Herbalists' Guild
PO Box 1683, Sequel, CA 95073, USA

National Herbalists' Association of Australia
Suite 305, BST House, 3 Smail St, Broadway, NSW 2007, Australia
tel: (61) 2 211 6437

Homeopathy

(For medically trained homeopaths)
Faculty of Homoeopathy
15 Clerkenwell Close, London EC1R 0AA
tel: 020 7566 7800/fax: 020 7566 7815
email: info@trusthomeopathy.org

UK Homœopathic Medical Association (UKHMA)
6 Livingstone Road, Gravesend, Kent DA12 5DZ
tel: 01474 560336

(Mainly for non-medically qualified homeopaths)
Society of Homoeopaths
2 Artizan Road, Northampton NN1 4HU
tel: 01604 621400/fax: 01604 622622
email: societyofhomoeopaths@btinternet.com /website:
www.homoeopathy.org.uk

Training
(Degree level)
London College of Classical Homoeopathy
University of Westminster School of Integrated health
115 New Cavendish St, London W1M 8JS
tel: 020 7911 5883
email: cav-admissions@wmin.ac.uk/website: www.wmin.ac.uk

Overseas
US Institute of Homeopathy and College of Homeopathy
520 Washington Boulevard, Suite 423, Marina Del Rey, CA 90292, USA
tel: (1) 310/306 5408

International Foundation for Homeopathy
2366 East Lake Avenue East
Suite 30, Seattle, WA 98102, USA
tel: (1) 206/324 8230

National Center for Homeopathy
801 N. Fairfax St, Suite 306, Alexander, VA 22314, USA
tel: (1) 703/548 7790

Australian Institute of Homeopathy
21 Bulah Heights, Berdwa Heights, NSW 2082, Australia

Osteopathy and chiropractic

General Chiropractic Council
3rd Floor North, 344–354 Gray's Inn Road, London WC1X 8BP
tel: 020 7713 5155 (for queries about regulation 0845 601 1796)/fax:
020 7713 5844/email: enquiries@gcc-uk.freeserve.co.uk

General Osteopathic Council
Osteopathy House, 176 Tower Bridge Road, London SE1 3LU
tel: 020 7357 6655/fax: 020 7357 0011
email: info@osteopathy.org.uk /website: www.osteopathy.org.uk

British Association for Applied Chiropractors
The Old Post Office, Cherry St, Stratton, Audley, nr Bicester, Oxon OX6 9BA
tel: 01869 277111

British Chiropractic Association, Blagrave House, 17 Blagrave St,
Reading RG1 1QB
tel: 0118 950 5950

(Educational organizations for doctors)
British Institute of Musculoskeletal Medicine
27 Green Lane, Northwood, Middlesex HA6 2PX
tel/fax: 01923 220999
email: BIMM@compuserve.com

British Osteopathic Association
Langham House East, Mill St, Luton, Beds LU1 2NA
tel: 01582 488455

Craniosacral Therapy Association of the UK
Monomark House, 27 Old Gloucester St, London WC1N 3XX
tel: 07000 78435

Manipulative Association of Chartered Physiotherapists
c/o Professional Affairs, Chartered Society of Physiotherapists,
14 Bedford Row, London WC1R 4ED
tel: 020 7242 1941/fax: 020 7306 6611

McTimoney Chiropractic Association
21 High St, Eynsham, Oxon OX8 1HE
tel: 01865 880974

Osteopathic Information Service
PO Box 2074, Reading, Berks RG1 4YR
tel: 01734 512051

Society of Orthopaedic Medicine
c/o Amanda Sherwood, administrator.
tel: 01454 610255
website: www.soc-ortho-med.org

Training:
(Degree level)
University of Middlesex
White Hart Lane, London N17 8HR
website: www.mdx.ac.uk

(Degree level)
University of Westminster School of Integrated Health
115 New Cavendish St, London W1M 8JS
tel: 020 7911 5883
email: cav-admissions@wmin.ac.uk/website: www.wmin.ac.uk

Anglo-European College of Chiropractic
13–15 Parkwood Rd, Bournemouth BH5 2DF
tel: 01202 436275

London College of Osteopathic Medicine
8-10 Boston Place, London NW1 6QH
tel: 020 7262 5250/fax: 020 7723 7492

McTimoney Chiropractic School
14 Park End St, Oxford OX1 1HH
tel: 01865 246786

Overseas
American Chiropractic Association
1701 Clarendon Boulevard, Arlington, VA 22209, USA

International Chiropractors' Association
110 N. Glebe Rd, Suite 1000, Arlington, VA 22201, USA

Chiropractors' Association of Australia
PO Box 241, Springwood, NSW 2777, Australia
tel: (61) 47 515644

New Zealand Chiropractors' Association
PO Box 7144, Wellesley St, Auckland, New Zealand
tel: (64) 9 37334343

Exercise systems

British Wheel of Yoga
1 Hamilton Place, Boston Rd, Sleaford, Lincs NG34 7ES
tel: 01529 306851

Tai Chi Union
131 Tunstall Rd, Knypersley, Stoke-on-Trent ST8 7AA

Yoga Biomedical Trust
PO Box 140, Cambridge CB4 3SY

Yoga Therapy Centre
60 Great Ormond St, London WC1N 3HR

Overseas
American Yoga Association
513 South Orange Ave, Sarasota, FL 34236, USA
email: Am Yoga Assn@aol.com

Healing

British Alliance of Healing Associations
15 Lawrence Ave, Mill Hill, London NW7 4NL
tel: 020 8906 8141

Doctor–Healer Network
27 Montefire Court, Stamford Hill, London N16 5TY
tel: 020 8800 3569

Healer Practitioner Association
1A Northcote St, Cardiff CF24 3BH
tel: 029 2049 7837

Training
College of Healing
Croft House, Fromes Hill, Herefordshire HR8 1HP
tel: 01531 640067

Hypnosis and relaxation

British Association of Counselling (BAC)
1 Regent Place, Rugby, Warwickshire CV21 2PJ
tel: 01788 550899/fax: 01788 562189
website: www.counselling.co.uk

British Psychological Society (BPS)
St Andrews House, 48 Princess Road East, Leicester LE1 7DR
tel: 0116 254 9568/fax: 0116 247 0787
website: www.bps.org.uk

British Society of Medical and Clinical Hypnosis (BSMCH)
23 Broadfields Heights, 53/58 Broadfields Ave, Edgware, Middx
HA8 8PF
tel: 020 8905 4342
or 17 Keppel View Rd, Kimberworth S61 2AP
tel: 07000 560309

Central Register of Advanced Hypnotherapists
28 Finsbury Park Rd, London N4 2JX
tel: 020 7226 6963

National Register of Hypnotherapists and Psychotherapists
12 Cross St, Nelson, Lancs BB9 7EN
tel: 01282 716839

UK Confederation of Hypnotherapy Organisations (UKCHO)
Suite 401, 302 Regent St, London W1R 6HH
tel: 0800 952 0560
website: www.ukcho.co.uk

United Kingdom Council of Psychotherapy (UKCP)
167–9 Great Portland Street, London W1N 5FB
tel: 020 7436 3002/fax: 020 7436 3013
website: www.psychotherapy.org.uk

Training
London College of Clinical Hypnosis
229A Sussex Gardens, Lancaster Gate, London W2 2RL
tel: 020 7402 9037/fax: 020 7262 1237
email: lcch@compuserve.com / website: www.lcch.co.uk

Overseas
Society for Clinical and Experimental Hypnosis
University of Colorado Medical Center, Colorado, USA

Massage- and touch-based therapies

Aromatherapy Organizations Council
PO Box 19834, London SE25 6WF
tel: 020 8251 7912/fax: 020 8251 7942
website: www.aromatherapy-uk.org

Association of Reflexologists
27 Old Gloucester St, London WC1N 3XX
tel: 0870 567 3320
email: aor@reflexology.org /website: www.reflexology.org/aor

British Massage Therapy Council
17 Rymers Lane, Oxford OX4 3JU
tel: 01865 774123 (for lists of registered practitioners 020 8992 2554)
website: www.bmtc.co.uk

British Reflexology Association
Monks Orchard, Whitbourne, Worcester WR6 5RB
tel: 01886 821207

Feldenkrais Guild UK
PO Box 370, London N10 3XA

Fellowship of Sports Masseurs and Therapists (FSMT)
BM Soigneur, London WC1N 3XX
tel: 020 8886 3120

International Federation of Reflexologists
76–78 Edridge Rd, Croydon, Surrey CR0 1EF
tel: 020 8667 9458

Irish Reflexologists Institute
3 Blakglen Court, Lambs Cross, Sandyford, Dublin, Ireland

London and Counties Society of Physiologists (LCSP)
LCSP Administrative Office, 330 Lytham Road, Blackpool FY4 1DW
tel: 01253 408443

Massage Therapy Institute GB (MTIGB)
PO Box 2726, London NW2 4NR
tel: 020 8208 1607

Register of Tuina and Thai Massage Practitioners
Bodyharmonics Centre, 54 Flecker's Drive, Hatherley, Cheltenham GL51 5BD
tel: 01242 582168

Scottish Massage Therapists Organisation (SMTO)
70 Lochside Road, Denmore Park, Bridge of Don,
Aberdeen AB23 8QW
tel: 01224 822956

Shiatsu Society
31 Pullman Lane, Godalming, Surrey GU7 1XY
tel: 01734 730836

Society of Teachers of the Alexander Technique
20 London House, 266 Fulham Rd, London SW10 9EL
tel: 020 7352 1556

Trager Association UK, 20 Summerdale Road, Hove, East Sussex BN3 8LG
tel: 01273 411193
website: www.trager.com

Westcountry Massage Association
38 South Street, Exeter, Devon EX1 1ED
tel: 01392 410954

Zero Balancing Association UK
10 Victoria Grove, Bridport, Dorset DT6 3AA
tel: 01398 420007

Training
(Degree level)
University of Westminster School of Integrated Health
115 New Cavendish St, London W1M 8JS
tel: 020 7911 5883
email: cav-admissions@wmin.ac.uk / website: www.wmin.ac.uk

(HND)
University of Middlesex
White Hart Lane, London N17 8HR
website: www.mdx.ac.uk

Acupressure Massage Training School
82 The Spinney, Beaconsfield, Bucks HP9 1SA
tel: 01494 678221/fax: 01494 681284
email: abercromby@btinternet.com
website: www.acupressure-training.co.uk

Alexander Teaching Network
PO Box 53, Kendal, Cumbria LA9 4UP

Bayly School of Reflexology
Monks Orchard, Whitbourne, Worcester WR6 5RB
tel: 01886 821207

(For nurses and midwives)
British School of Reflex Zone Therapy
23 Marsh Hall, Talisman Way, Wembley Park HA9 8JJ
tel: 020 8904 4825

London College of Massage and Shiatsu
21 Portland Place, London W1N 3AF

Massage Training Institute (MTI)
90–92 Islington High Street, London N1 8EG
tel: 020 7226 5313

Northern Institute of Massage
100 Waterloo Rd, Blackpool, Lancs FY4 1AW

Tisserand Institute
65 Church Rd, Hove, East Sussex BN3 2BD
tel: 01273 206640

Overseas
American Alliance of Aromatherapy
PO Box 750428, Petalumo, CA 94975, USA

American Aromatherapy Association
PO Box 3679, South Pasadena, CA 91031, USA

American Massage Therapy Association
820 Davis St, Suite 100, Evanston, IL 60201, USA

International School of Reflexology
PO Box 12642, St Petersburgh, FL 33733, USA

National Association of Holistic Aromatherapy
219 Carl St, San Francisco, CA 94117, USA
tel: (1) 415/564 6785

Naturopathy

General Council and Register of Naturopaths
2 Goswell Road, Street, Somerset BA16 0JG
tel: 01458 840072/fax: 01458 840075
email: admin@naturopathy.org.uk/website: www.naturopathy.org.uk

Training
British College of Naturopathy and Osteopathy
Frazer House, 6 Netherall Gardens, London NW3 5RR
tel: 0207 435 6464

Overseas
American Association of Naturopathic Physicians
PO Box 20386, Seattle, WA 98112, USA
tel: (1) 206 323 7610

Australian Natural Therapists Association
PO Box 308, Melrose Park, South Australia
tel: (61) 8 371 3222

Canadian Naturopathic Association
205, 1234 17th Avenue South West, PO Box 3143, Station C, Calgary, Alberta, Canada
tel: (1) 413 244 4487

Nutritional medicine

British Association of Nutritional Therapists
BCM BANT, London WC1N 3XX
tel: 0870 606 1284

(Membership organization for doctors only)
British Society for Allergy, Environmental and Nutritional Medicine (BSAENM)
For publications: PO Box 28, Totton, Southampton SO40 2ZA
tel: 01703 812124
For inquiries: PO Box 7, Knighton LD7 1WT
tel: 0906 3020010

British Society for Nutritional Medicine
PO Box 3AP, London W1A 3AP

Training
(Degree level)
University of Westminster School of Integrated Health
115 New Cavendish St, London W1M 8JS
tel: 020 7911 5883
email: cav-admissions@wmin.ac.uk / website: www.wmin.ac.uk

Institute for Optimum Nutrition
Blades Court, Deodar Road, Putney,
London SW15 2NU
tel: 020 8877 9993/fax: 020 8877 9980
email: ion@cableinet.co.uk

Plaskett Nutritional Medicine College
Three Quoins House, Trevallett, Launceston, Cornwall PL15 8JS
tel: 01566 86118

Appendix III

Information sources

Integrative teams need evidence! Here are ways of finding the latest research-derived data by using website databases, search engines and journals, as well as journals and books in print.

THE WORLD WIDE WEB

Your browser will find tens of thousands of alternative and complementary therapy listings. We have tried to narrow down the field for you. There is a list of useful websites in Andrew Vickers' article 'Recent advances in CM' on the BMJ site at: http://www.bmj.com/cgi/content/full/321/7262/683

Our favourite search engines and databases

AMED
AMED (British Library) has over 500 journal listings including many CT papers, and includes other subjects such as physio.

CINAHL
CINAHL is broad ranging. Information on the CINAHL database including journal coverage is contained on the website at: http://www.cinahl.com
 From the homepage, click on Products and Services, then the CINAHL database. For a complete list of journals in pdf format, visit their Library and click on Journal List. The Journal Directory has a listing of journals by subject. They currently index 32 journals in the area of complementary/alternative therapies/medicine.

CISCOM
RCCM's CISCOM database of nearly 70 000 published research references in CAM is drawn from many sources including hand searches. CISCOM is being revised, updated and restructured. This process is being carried out in three stages and at the end of February 2001 stage 1 will have been completed and the CISCOM service will again be available to professionals and the public.
 Stage 1: Newly restructured database that will include a thesaurus of keywords to ensure accuracy and consistency in entering and accessing data. Expanded information range to include 'grey' literature and new journals. From the end of February, enquirers will be able to request searches that bring together therapy, condition and associated research.
 Stage 2: CD-ROM version of CISCOM available for PC and Apple platforms with customized browsing, search and print facilities. New information will include type and quality of the research study being reported. Quarterly updates.
 Stage 3: Launch of the CISCOM database on-line, backed up by access to electronic versions of journal articles as these become available.

 A small fee will be charged to cover search costs. External funding is being sought to cover the updating, maintenance and administration of the database. Timing of stages 2 and 3 will depend upon the success of fundraising. Website: http://www.rccm.org.uk

Cochrane resources
The Cochrane Collaboration have begun systematic reviews of CTs for certain health problems, at: http://hiru.mcmaster.ca/cochrane/cochrane/whatcdsr.htm#CAT

Reviews currently include:
Acupuncture for chronic asthma
Acupuncture for smoking cessation
The effectiveness of acupuncture in the treatment of low back pain
Homeopathy for chronic asthma
Homoeopathic Oscillococcinum for preventing and treating influenza and influenza-like syndromes
Alexander technique for chronic asthma
Intercessory prayer for the alleviation of ill health.

The Cochrane Collaboration and the Cochrane Library include most published CAM trials, at: http://www.cochrane.org
The Cochrane Collaboration field on complementary medicine is at: http://www.compmed.ummc.umaryland.edu/compmed/cochrane/cochranefr.htm

MEDLINE
Includes some published research on complementary medicine, and papers from CT journals. You can get online MEDLINE via PubMed (EMBASE and CINAHL both have MEDLINE too) or via EMBASE (Elsevier) at Elsevier.com

NIH
We like the NIH database in Washington DC at: http://www.ncbi.nlm.nih.gov

Also:

Memorial Sloan-Kettering Cancer Center, New York, United States Integrative Medicine Service at:
http://www.mskcc.org/patients_n_public/patient_care_services/outpatient_services_and_facilities/integrative_medicine_service/index.html
National Center for Complementary and Alternative Medicine at: nccam.nih.gov
Your Life – Your Choice (Canadian practitioners' site) at: http://www.life-choices.com

PubMed
PubMed is the National Library of Medicine's search service that provides access to over 11 million citations in MEDLINE, PreMEDLINE, and other related databases, with links to participating online journals, at: http://www.ncbi.nlm.nih.gov

Other databases and search engines
AlphaSearch at: http://www.calvin.edu/Library/ searreso/internet/as
Argus Clearing House at: http://www.clearinghouse.net
Google at: http://www.google.com
MedHunt at: http://www.hon.ch/MedHunt
Medical Matrix (search on 'alternative medicine') at: http://www.medmatrix.org
Medical World Search (a very clever search engine, with multiple search words) at: http://www.mwsearch.com
Northern Light at: www.northernlight.com
SUMSearch (University of Texas search for evidence-based info, it splits results according to the source) at: http://sumsearch.uthscsa.edu
TRIP (an amalgamation of 26 databases of hyperlinks from 'evidence-based' sites around the world) at: http://www.ceres.uwcm.ac.uk

Here are some comments from colleagues in the front line:
'There is only one worth talking about: it is called google.com and has some weird way of telepathically reading your mind. Everyone I have directed to this search engine has raved about it.

WARNING: Google can ruin your life! Having instant access to virtually any information will prevent a curious and undisciplined mind from achieving anything.'

'Another popular search engine is Ovid. Then use PubMed to get papers.'

'The RCCM CISCOM database has been the most effective database in this area for some time; it is not currently available to professionals or the public but will be soon! I also use Medline/AMED via Ovid, which I find easy to use from home via academic library access, but many social science journals are not covered through these, so Psychlit and Psychinfo are also useful. Search engines such as Google are good, but the quality of information is sometimes questionable.'

'The best FREE search facility that I know is the British Library. They have access to all the major indexes, papers back to 1966, simple to use (not like Ovid), and fast.'

Websites on individual CTs

Acupuncture
Acupuncture Association of Chartered Physiotherapists at: http://www.aacp.uk.com
Acupuncture.com (a broad TCM site) at: http://www.acupuncture.com
British Acupuncture Council at: http://www.acupuncture.org.uk/
British Medical Acupuncture Society at: http://www.medical-acupuncture.co.uk
International acupuncture associations at: http://directory.google.com/Top/Health/Alternative/Acupuncture_and_Chinese_Medicine/Professional_Organizations/
A new acupuncture site is at: http://www.acubriefs.com/newsletter.htm.

Subscription to the newsletter is free, but does require that you provide some identifying data: Subscribers are expected to have email software and, preferably, a browser that allows you to view cited links.

Chiropractic
General Chiropractic Council at: http://www.gcc-uk.org
UK chiropractic website at: http://www.chiropractic.org.uk
International chiropractic organizations at: http://directory.google.com/Top/Health/Alternative/Chiropractic/Organizations_and_Associations/
Mantis—the site I would add is at: http://www.healthindex.com Health Index, which is excellent since its recent makeover; this holds the chiropractic database called Mantis. You will have to subscribe though.

Herbal medicine
American Botanical Council at: http://www.herbalgram.org/
BiomedNet—you can check out Medline free and very effectively at Evaluated Medline here at: http://www.bmn.com/
I started as an individual and now have been taken up within our university site licence. You can check if they still take on individuals.
BIOSIS—access to this, the largest biological sciences database, is free if you can get on to Edinburgh University's Edinburgh Data and Information Access at: http://edina.ed.ac.uk/

You can get ready access to this and many other science sites free as an academic by registering with Athens if you have a Domain administrator at your institution; to check that out or even apply to be an administrator yourself go to: http://www.niss.ac.uk/athens/siteadmlst.html
Phytonet at: http://www.exeter.ac.uk/phytonet/

Homeopathy
Faculty of Homeopathy at: http://www.trusthomeopathy.org
Homeopathic Trust at: http://www.trusthomeopathy.org/
National Center for Homeopathy in the US at: http://www.homeopathic.org/
Society of Homeopaths at: http://www.homeopathy-soh.org
Glasgow Homeopathic Hospital HOM_Inform is useful for specific searches—when it works! Last time I tried it the literature search function was not functioning.

Hypnosis
British Society of Medical and Dental Hypnosis at: http://www.bsmdh.org/
US Society for Clinical and Experimental Hypnosis at: http://sunsite.utk.edu/ijceh/scehframe.htm

Massage
American Massage Therapy Association at: http://www.amtamassage.org/
Aromatherapy Organisations Council at: http://www.aromatherapy-uk.org

Nutrition
http://www.nutritionnewsfocus.com/cgi-bin/birdcast.cgi

Osteopathy
General Osteopathic Council at: http://www.osteopathy.org.uk
Osteopathic Information Service available at: http://www.osteopa-thy.org.uk/
US osteopathic medicine at the Student Doctor Network at: http://osteopathic.com/

Other websites and databases

General
Alternative Medicine Foundation at: http://www.amfoundation.org
Alternative Medicine Homepage at: http://www.pitt.edu/-cbw/altm.html
Bandolier (evidence-based medicine monthly reports) site for comp medicine at:
http://www.jr2.ox.ac.uk/Bandolier/booth/booths/altmed.html
BMJ collection of articles on CAM at:
http://www.bmj.com/cgi/collection/complementary_medicine
CAM and cancer at: http://www.cancer.org
Clinical governance at:
http://www.shef.ac.uk/uni/projects/wrp/clingov.html
Columbia University site via NCCAM at:
http://nccam.nih.gov/nccam/fi/
Health A to Z (conventional and complementary medicine site) at: http://www.healthatoz.com
Integrative Medicine Communications aims to help health care practitioners combine the best of complementary and alternative therapies with conventional medicine; for more information about products and services, go to: http://www.onemedicine.com
Jeff Bland's content. His site is on:
http://www.healthcomm.com/hc/bio1.html
Journal of Alternative and Complementary Medicine: Research on Paradigm, Practice and Policy (see Journals below) at:
http://www.liebertpub.com
National Center for Complementary Medicine at:
http://www.nccam.nih.gov/ncam
Lifeonline at: http://lifeonline.guardianunlimited.co.uk/healthandfitness/0,6488,116886,00.html
Medical Matrix at: http://www.medmatrix.org
Omni (a catalogue of sites covering health and medicine) at: http://omni.ac.uk
Quackwatch (information on unusual complementary treatments) at: http://www.quackwatch.com
Research Council for Complementary Medicine at:
http://www.rccm.org.uk
Thriveonline at: http://www.thriveonline.com
Well-aware is a new UK-based site offering an evidence-based site to both complementary and conventional treatments at:
http://well-aware.co.uk

If you want a good central site for references and practices of action research, try **Jack Whitehead's homepage** at:
http://www.bath.ac.uk/~edsajw

It is not specifically about CT but contains a wealth of references to inquiry practices addressing questions such as 'how do I improve my practice?'

Academic
University of Exeter Centre for Complementary Health Studies at: http://www.ex.ac.uk/chs and Department of Complementary Medicine at: http://www.ex.ac.uk/pgms/comphome.htm
University of Maryland Complementary Medicine Program at: http://www.compmed.ummc.umaryland.edu/ and the School of Medicine
University of Middlesex (degree programmes in CTs) at: http://www.mdx.ac.uk
University of Westminster (degree programmes in CTs) at: http://www.westminster.ac.uk
USA Institute for Alternative Futures at: http://www.altfutures.com

PRINTED INFORMATION SOURCES

Books and reports

Mills S, Budd S 2000 Professional organisation of complementary and alternative medicine in the United Kingdom 2000. University of Exeter Centre for Complementary Health Studies, Exeter

Royal London Homeopathic Hospital 1999 The evidence base of complementary medicine. RLHH, London

Zollman C, Vickers A 2000 ABC of complementary medicine. BMJ, London (The contents of this book are also available as articles on the bmj.com website.)

Also, get hold of the magnificent piece of work from the USA Institute for Alternative Futures: The future of complementary and alternative approaches in US Health care, July 1998.

Journals and bulletins

Bandolier (evidence-based medicine monthly reports, free within NHS) at: Pain Research, The Churchill, Headington, Oxford OX3 7LJ; tel: 01865 226132
Complementary Therapies in Medicine (aimed at GPs, nurses, allied health professionals, four issues per year) at:
Journals Subscription Department, Harcourt Publishers Ltd, Foots Cray High St, Sidcup, Kent DA14 5HP; tel: 020 8308 5700
Compmed Bulletin (evidence base of selected clinical topics, bimonthly) at: Church Farm Cottage, Weethley Hamlet, Evesham Rd, Alcester, Warwickshire B49 5NA; tel: 01789 400295
CAM: The Magazine for Practitioners of Complementary and Alternative Medicine Register for free subscription at: http://www.cam-mag.com or contact Target Publishing, PO Box 12932, London N8 8WL
Journal of Alternative and Complementary Medicine: Research on Paradigm, Practice and Policy (reports on CAM treatments, case reports, and current concepts, six issues per year) at:
http://www.liebertpub.com

Index

Note: page numbers in bold refer to figures and tables.

Search engines, internet, 325–326
Self-help advice
    common disorders management, 181–198
    conditions, 219–246
Self-help leaflets, patients' feedback, 153
Self-help sheet, 247–284
    diets, 273–284
    exercises, 247–272
Self-regulation, symptoms as signs of, 28–30
Self-repair, body's capacity, 27
Service adaptation, CTs, 147–177
Service delivery, CTs, 111–145
    examples, integrated delivery, 121–142
    process, 112–121
Service design, CTs, 73–109
    example, 101–106
    key issues, 74–75
    models, integration and delivery, 76–79
    people issues, 79–83
Service development, for GPs, 135–138
Service evaluation, CTs, 111–145
Service innovation, CTs development, 75
Service reflection, CTs, 147–177
Side-effects, CTs, 113
Skills, CTs, 83
Smith project, clinical data entry, 305–309
Somatization, 'complex' cases, 163–164, 168
Somerset Coast Primary Care Group,
    collaborative practice, 78
South Norfolk Primary Care Group,
    collaborative practice, 78
Southampton Centre for the Study of
    Complementary Medicine,
    collaborative practice, 78
Specialists, CPs as, 80
Spondylosis, cervical, patient advice sheet,
    241–242
St Margarets Surgery, Wiltshire, collaborative
    practice, 78
Staff appraisal and development forms,
    310–313
Stereotypes, unresolved issue, 156
Stress
    and digestion, **29**
    patient advice sheet, 231–232
    theory, 32–33

Stress management
    meditation and, 265–266
    self-help sheet, 271–272
Stroke, patient advice sheet, 229–230
Structural factors, common disorders
    management, 181–198
Structures, CTs development, 74
Suitability of CTs, key issue, 16–17
'Supportive' containment, 'complex' cases,
    164
Symptoms, as signs of self-regulation,
    28–30

T

Tai chi
    information for doctors, 92–93
    models and research, 54
Theories of healing, CTs, 26–34
Therapeutic ambition, unresolved issue,
    156–157
Therapies, patient advice sheet, 199–218
Therapy choice questionnaire, 285, 288–291
Thrush, patient advice sheet, 231–232
Tiredness
    management information sheet, 198
    patient advice sheet, 245–246
    research, 47
Toning muscles, self-help sheet, 247–248
Touch-based therapies
    consultations, 95
    contraindications, 113
    information for doctors, 94–96
    models and research, 55–56
    side-effects, 113
    useful addresses, 321–322
Training
    acupuncture, 87
    chiropractic, 92
    exercise systems, 92–93
    healing, 93
    herbal medicine, 89
    homeopathy, 90
    hypnotherapy, 94
    information for doctors, 86–98

    key issue, 18
    massage, 95
    naturopathy, 96–97
    nutritional therapies, 98
    osteopathy, 92
    relaxation therapies, 94
    touch-based therapies, 95
'Transformative' containment, 'complex'
    cases, 165
Transforming approach, CTs service delivery,
    76
Treatment numbers, deciding on, 81–82
Trends, 4
    CTs, 6–7
    international, 7
Trigger point pain, patient advice sheet,
    239–240
Types, CTs, **79**

U

Unmet needs, key issue, 13–14
Unresolved and difficult issues, 156–172
Useful addresses, 319–323

V

Vegetarian diet, self-help sheet, 283–284
Vitalistic explanations, healing, 31–32
Voluntary sector funding, 84

W

Wheat-free diet, self-help sheet, 281–282
World wide web, information source,
    325–327

Y

Yoga
    information for doctors, 92–93
    models and research, 54